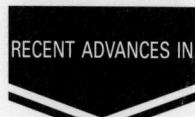
RECENT ADVANCES IN

Critical Care Medicine

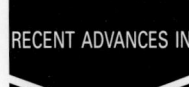

RECENT ADVANCES IN

Critical Care Medicine

Edited by

T. W. Evans BSc MD FRCP PhD
Professor of Intensive Care Medicine,
National Heart and Lung Institute;
Consultant in Intensive Care and Thoracic Medicine,
Royal Brompton Hospital, London, UK

C. J. Hinds FRCP FRCA
Director of Intensive Care,
St Bartholomew's Hospital, London, UK

NUMBER 4

CHURCHILL LIVINGSTONE
NEW YORK EDINBURGH LONDON MADRID MELBOURNE MILAN AND TOKYO

CHURCHILL LIVINGSTONE
Medical Division of Pearson Professional UK Limited

Distributed in the United States of America by
Churchill Livingstone Inc., 650 Avenue of the Americas,
New York, N.Y. 10011, and by associated companies,
branches and representatives throughout the world.

First published 1996

ISBN 0443 047111
ISSN 0309-2305

British Library Cataloguing in Publication Data
A catalogue record for this book is available from the British
Library

Library of Congress Cataloging in Publication Data
is available

Note
Medical knowledge is constantly changing. As new
information becomes available, changes in treatment,
procedures, equipment and the use of drugs become
necessary. The editors, contributors and the publishers
have, as far as it is possible, taken care to ensure that the
information given in this text is accurate and up to date.
However, readers are strongly advised to confirm that the
information, especially with regard to drug usage, complies
with latest legislation and standards of practice.

The
publisher's
policy is to use
paper manufactured
from sustainable forests

Produced by Longman Singapore Publisher Pte Ltd
Printed in Singapore

Contents

Preface

The enormous expansion of medical research worldwide, reflected in the ever increasing number and size of specialist journals, has made it increasingly difficult for busy clinicians to keep abreast of all the relevant developments in their field, especially when important new information may appear in any one of a huge variety of specialist and non-specialist journals. In no field is this more true than critical care medicine. Since the last edition of *Recent Advances in Critical Care Medicine* was published in 1988 there have been many important advances in our understanding of underlying pathophysiological processes, a variety of new therapeutic approaches have been developed, many of the established techniques have been refined and there have been significant improvements in the methods used to evaluate the impact of these strategies on morbidity and mortality. To make judgements about the relative importance of these various scientific and clinical advances, and to commission top quality authors from an international field, was an invidious task. Our eventual selection was necessarily personal but there was a surprisingly large measure of agreement between us as to those topic which most merited inclusion and the choice of contributors.

Firstly, we felt it appropriate to re-evaluate the techniques used to support patients with acute lung injury and to consider not only recent refinements to conventional methods of mechanical ventilatory support but also the role of extra and intra corporeal gas exchange, and administration of inhaled nitric oxide and surfactant supplementation. Furthermore, the increasing appreciation that the acute respiratory distress syndrome may only be the respiratory manifestation of a panendothelial insult lead us to commission articles regarding the important advances which have been made in understanding the factors which can influence the inflammatory response to endotoxin and the effects of the resulting endothelial damage on vascular control mechanisms.

Epidemiological evidence of an increase in the incidence of acute severe asthma suggested to us that a reevaluation of clinical practice in this area, especially in relation to intensive care management was warranted. A chapter dealing with the advances that have markedly reduced the incidence of barotrauma and severe pulmonary damage in ventilated asthmatics is therefore included, along with a thorough review of the management of acute severe asthma in the context of guidelines appearing from both the British and American Thoracic Societies.

Since the last edition of Recent Advances was published one of the most extensively debated and investigated clinical controversies has been disordered oxygen transport, its relationship to outcome from critical illness and the influence of attempts to manipulate oxygen transport on morbidity and mortality. It would therefore have been a glaring omission if we had not included a chapter on this topic.

The prevention and management of acute renal failure in the critically ill is increasingly the domain of intensivists rather than renal physicians and new techniques of ultra and haemofiltration should ensure that this trend continues. We therefore thought it appropriate to include reviews of both the causes and effective management of acute renal insufficiency in the intensive care unit.

Given the rapidly escalating cost of health care, the way in which we evaluate new and potentially expensive therapies is assuming ever greater importance, and is likely to have a considerable impact on the future funding of intensive care. One of the most exciting developments in this field has been the use of severity scoring to assist in the design and interpretation of clinical trials and we are delighted to have been able to include a chapter on this important contribution to clinical research.

Finally, we would like to express our gratitude to all the authors who, despite their heavy clinical and research commitments, have in our view without exception produced outstanding, authorative contributions. We would also like to thank the publishers for their support and forbearance during the production of this publication.

T. W. Evans
C. J. Hinds

Contributors

Karoline F Bruin PhD
Center for Hemostasis, Thrombosis, Atherosclerosis and Inflammation
Research, Academic Medical Center, University of Amsterdam,
Amsterdam, The Netherlands

Fabrice Brunet MD
Service de Reanimation Medicale et de Physiologie, Hôpital Cochin,
Paris, France

N P Curzen
MRC Training Fellow, Honorary Registrar in Critical Care and
Cardiology, National Heart & Lung Institute, Royal Brompton National
Heart & Lung Hospital, London, UK

S P Davies MB MRCP
Consultant Physician & Nephrologist, Renal Unit, Royal Shrewsbury
Hospital NHS Trust, Shrewsbury, UK

A T Dinh-Xuan MD PhD
Service de Reanimation Medicale et de Physiologie, Hôpital Cochin
Paris, France

Tim Evans BSc MD FRCP PhD
Professor of Intensive Care Medicine, Unit of Critical Care, National
Heart & Lung Institute, Royal Brompton National Heart & Lung
Hospital, London, UK

Christopher Fanta MD
Clinical Director, Respiratory Division, Brigham and Women's
Hospital, Boston Massachusetts, USA

Michelle Hayes FRCA
Senior Registrar, Department of Anaesthesia, Royal Surrey County
Hospital, Guildford, UK

Keith Hickling MB ChB BSc FRCA FFICANZCA
Intensive Care Unit, Queen Elizabeth Hospital, Kowloon, Hong Kong

Charles Hinds FRCP FRCA
Director of Intensive Care, St Bartholomew's Hospital, London, UK

W A Knaus MD
Professor of Amesthesiology & Computer Medicine, Director, ICU
Research Unit, George Washington University Medical Center,
Washington DC, USA

James F Lewis MD FRCP(C)
Assistant Professor, Departments of Medicine & Physiology, University
of Western Ontario, The Lawson Research Institute, London, Ontario,
Canada

M J Moan MD
Respiratory Division, Brigham and Women's Hospital, Boston
Massachusetts, USA

P E Stevens BSc MRCP
Consultant Nephrologist and Head of Department of Renal Medicine,
Kent and Canterbury Hospitals NHS Trust, Canterbury, Kent, UK

David Taube
Transplant Unit, St Mary's Hospital, London, UK

David V Tuxen MB BS FRACP DipHBM MD
Director, Intensive Care Unit and Hyperbaric Service, Department of
Respiratory Medicine, Alfred Hospital, Prahran, Victoria, Australia

Sander J H van Deventer MD PhD
Center for Hemostasis, Thrombosis, Atherosclerosis and Inflammation
Research, Academic Medical Center, University of Amsterdam,
Amsterdam, The Netherlands

R A W Veldhuizen PhD
Department of Medicine, University of Western Ontario, The Lawson
Research Institute, London, Ontario, Canada

Marijke von der Möhlen MD
Center for Hemostasis, Thrombosis, Atherosclerosis and Inflammation
Research, Academic Medical Center, University of Amsterdam,
Amsterdam, The Netherlands

David Watson
Consultant and Senior Lecturer in Intensive Care and Anaesthesia,
St Bartholomew's Hospital, London, UK

1. Supporting the injured lung: ECMO, IVOX and inhaled NO

F. Brunet   A.T. Dinh-Xuan

(PC-IRV, permissive hypocapnia, HFJV) as effective as (ECMO, ECCO₂R-LFPPV, IVOX)?

Inhaled NO - beneficial, but risk/benefit ratio?

INTRODUCTION

Since it was first described (Ashbaugh et al 1967), the mortality associated *ARDS* with acute respiratory distress syndrome (ARDS) in adults has remained high (Bone et al 1992). However, patients who survive the acute phase of the syndrome generally resume productive lives with no serious pulmonary limitation (Elliott et al 1981). Specific treatments for ARDS would ideally be directed at limiting the initial abnormal inflammatory responses that characterize the condition. However, contemporary therapy for *support* ARDS is essentially supportive with mechanical ventilation assuming a central role. Conventional modes of ventilatory support aim to normalize *PaO_2, $PaCO_2$* arterial blood gas tensions and employ relatively large tidal volumes *FiO_2 ↑* (Slutsky 1994). The application of positive end-expiratory pressure *$PEEP$!* (PEEP) was advocated early on, to achieve adequate arterial oxygenation at the lowest possible fractional inspired oxygen concentration (FiO_2) in order to avoid oxygen toxicity (Petty & Ashbaugh 1971, Shapiro et al 1983). Such an approach, however, frequently requires high airway pres- *Paw* sures and tidal volumes for effective ventilation which may in turn worsen lung injury (Shapiro et al 1983, Gammon et al 1992). New strategies have therefore been developed with the aim of reducing minute ventilation and *MV ↓ ($PaCO_2$↑)* thereby limiting the exposure of the injured lung to high inflation pressures (Gurewitch et al 1986, Dall'Ava-Santucci et al 1990, Hickling et al 1990). Fundamental to the use of these modes of ventilation (described elsewhere in this book) is the concept of permitting 'abnormal' respiratory function characterized by hypercapnia (Pesenti 1990, Marini and Kelsen 1992). To date, comparative studies demonstrating the superiority of these *? evidence?* new strategies have not been performed and tolerance of permissive hypercapnia is still questionable (Pesenti 1990). Moreover, any decrease in the risk of lung injury achieved using limited pressure and volume modes of ventilation remains hypothetical (Brunet et al 1994). Although ARDS has been previously considered to be a process of diffuse lung injury, analysis of CT scans performed in such patients suggests that this is not so (Gattinoni et al 1988). In patients with severe lung injury, total lung capacity may be reduced to one-third of normal and regional alveolar hyperinflation may occur even when ventilatory pressures and volumes are limited to levels considered safe (Brunet et al 1994). Low tidal volumes and pressures may also fail to achieve adequate arterial oxygenation, necessitating an increase in FiO_2 with the potential risk of oxygen toxicity (Brian & Jenkinson 1988).

Extrapulmonary methods to supplement gas exchange in theory may help to 'rest the lungs', especially in patients with greatly reduced lung capacities (Kolobow et al 1978, Gattinoni et al 1984, 1986). Extrapulmonary gas transfer allows decreased ventilator settings thereby limiting ventilation to the remaining compliant part of the lungs (Gattinoni et al 1984, 1986). Extracorporeal support may also permit a reduction in FiO_2 (Zapol et al 1979).

Notwithstanding the fact that early trials of veno-arterial extracorporeal membrane oxygenation (ECMO) failed to improve survival in adults with ARDS (Zapol et al 1979), the efficacy of veno-venous extracorporeal support is still under investigation. Among such techniques, extracorporeal CO_2 removal combined with low-frequency positive-pressure ventilation (ECCO$_2$R-LFPPV) and veno-venous ECMO are the most commonly used (Gattinoni et al 1984, 1986, Bindsley et al 1987, Chevalier et al 1990, Morris et al 1990, Wetterberg & Steen 1991, Brunet et al 1992, 1993, 1994). Clinical, open studies have reported higher survival rates using these techniques compared to historical controls (Gattinoni et al 1984, 1986). However, even these new approaches have their own drawbacks and considerable resource implications. To overcome these problems a simple extrapulmonary, intracorporeal gas exchanger has been recently introduced to clinical practice (Mortensen 1987, High et al 1992, Conrad et al 1993). This device is inserted into the venae cavae and right atrium and allows a reduction in the requirement for pulmonary gas exchange.

The recent introduction of inhaled nitric oxide (NO) represents a great advance in supporting patients with ARDS. Inhalation of NO in mechanically-ventilated patients with lung injury improves arterial oxygenation and reduces both pulmonary vascular resistance and intrapulmonary shunt (Rossaint et al 1993). However, many questions related to its long-term administration, optimal dose and potential side-effects are still unanswered (Gerlach et al 1993, Monchi et al 1993). Moreover, some patients with ARDS do not respond to NO inhalation (Mira et al 1994) and its effects on survival are unknown.

In this chapter, we will discuss the potential benefits and side-effects of these non-conventional techniques for ventilatory support in ARDS. Specifically, we will address two questions: (1) do these strategies improve arterial oxygenation and do they reduce the risk of pulmonary barotrauma? (2) can their complications be limited? The place of, and indications for each method in the general management of patients with ARDS will also be clarified.

EXTRACORPOREAL LUNG SUPPORT

Methods

All extracorporeal modes of respiratory assistance use artificial membranes to achieve gas exchange, but variations do exist between the different methods. Indeed, the goal of extracorporeal support may vary from achieving total gas exchange to CO_2 removal alone. The type of mechanical ventilation used in conjunction with extracorporeal support can also vary. These differences may be confusing in the analysis of results reported in the literature. We will therefore describe the techniques of veno-arterial and veno-venous ECMO and extracorporeal CO_2 removal with ECCO$_2$R-LFPPV before discussing the results of clinical trials using these approaches. Extralung assistance (ELA) and extracorporeal lung assistance (ECLA) have also been described (Wetterberg & Steen 1991), but are similar to veno-venous ECMO.

Extracorporeal circuit   ① va/vv access ② pump ③ membrane

The circuit requires either veno-arterial (Zapol et al 1979) or veno-venous access (Gattinoni et al 1984, 1986). Vascular access is mostly achieved percutaneously, but cannulae can also be surgically inserted (Zapol et al 1979, Gattinoni 1984, 1986, Brunet et al 1992, 1993). The circuitry comprises silicone or polyurethane tubing, with ports for sampling, monitoring and connection to a hemodialyser, if needed. The blood is usually driven by an occlusive pump, but non-occlusive and centrifugal pumps are also used (Chevalier et al 1990). The artificial membranes employed vary in performance as measured by the amount of gas transferred and their life span. The extracorporeal circuit and the membranes can be either heparin-coated (Bindsley et al 1987) or not (Gattinoni et al 1984, Brunet et al 1992, 1993). Blood flow through the extracorporeal circuit varies from about 20% to 50%, and may even be as high as 90% of the cardiac output in ECCO$_2$R-LFPPV, veno-venous and veno-arterial ECMO respectively.

Flow - 20 - 50% (- 90%) CO

Pulmonary management

Different modes of ventilation can be employed in association with extracorporeal support. In veno-arterial ECMO, conventional ventilation was used in the comparative study reported by Zapol et al (1979). In studies of veno-venous ECMO, the mode of ventilation is not always clearly described, but most used pressure-limited, volume-cycled ventilation. ECCO$_2$R-LFPPV uses an original mode of ventilation first described by Kolobow et al (1978), which is close to pseudo-apnoeic oxygenation and has been termed 'low-frequency positive-pressure ventilation'. Using this approach, respiratory rate averages 4 cycles/min with a tidal volume re-

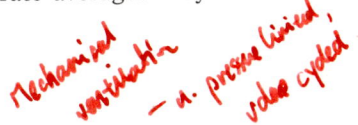

Mechanical ventilation - a. pressure limited, volume cycled

duced to about 5 ml/kg and peak pressure limited to 40 cmH$_2$O. Arterial oxygenation is mainly achieved by a continuous flow of oxygen administered via a small catheter inserted into the trachea just above the carina.

Patient care

During by-pass, the patient is sedated and paralysed, usually with a combination of intravenous pancuronium bromide, benzodiazepines and opiates. To date, extracorporeal support has necessitated continuous anticoagulation obtained by heparin infusion. However, the quantity of heparin required varies with the type of material of the circuit, which can be heparin-coated or not, and the monitoring protocol (Gattinoni et al 1986, Bindsley et al 1987, Brunet et al 1992). Thus, the possibility of heparin-free veno-venous circulation with heparin-bonded material has been reported in pigs (Koul et al 1992), but these results have not been confirmed in clinical practice. Continuous clinical surveillance by a trained team is required during the by-pass period.

The cost

The cost of extracorporeal lung support is seldom reported, but ECCO$_2$R is more expensive than mechanical ventilation (Morris et al 1994) and a medico-economic study in patients with severe ARDS admitted to our ICU has shown that the total cost of extracorporeal support is about 50% higher (personal data).

Clinical results

Despite promising preliminary results, a multicentre comparative trial of veno-arterial ECMO in adults failed to demonstrate its superiority over conventional ventilation (Zapol et al 1979). Mortality rate in the ECMO group was close to that of controls, although ECMO was associated with improved arterial oxygenation in all patients. The severity and frequency of complications seen in the ECMO group may explain this apparent discrepancy. As the arterial access employed was judged responsible for the severity of bleeding and infections in this study, in adults only veno-venous extracorporeal support has been used since.

Using ECCO$_2$R-LFPPV Gattinoni et al (1984) reported in a preliminary study a 70% survival rate in patients with severe ARDS who met ECMO criteria and had an expected survival rate of about 10%. Using veno-venous extracorporeal support in the same circumstances, subsequent studies have reported a survival rate close to 50%. However, these studies were uncontrolled and it has proved difficult to demonstrate convincingly the superiority of ECCO$_2$R-LFPPV over mechanical ventilation in terms of mortality. Indeed, recent studies have demonstrated comparable survival rates with new modes of mechanical ventilation (Gurewitch et al 1986, Hickling et al 1990, Suchyta et al 1992). Comparative studies are the only appropriate way of establishing the superiority of any given therapy, but they require the enrolment of a large population of patients with precise diagnostic criteria for ARDS, as well as inclusion criteria for the provision and escalation of support in both mechanical ventilation and extracorporeal arms. Until now, only one comparative study has been performed in a relatively small group of patients with ARDS. The results did not show beneficial effects of extracorporeal support over a control group treated with mechanical ventilation allowing 'permissive hypercapnia' (Morris et al 1994). However, the survival rate of about 40% in both groups was higher than that expected using ECMO criteria. In the mechanical ventilation group the use of pressure-limited volume-cycled modes with permissive hypercapnia may explain the observed high survival rate, similar to that reported in other studies (Hickling et al 1990). The authors did not show benefits in terms of arterial oxygenation nor in the reduction of peak pressure in the $ECCO_2R$-LFPPV group as reported in other studies using the same method (Gattinoni et al 1984, 1986, Chevalier et al 1990, Brunet et al 1993). These two factors are known to indicate a poor prognosis (Bone et al 1992, Gammon et al 1992, Suchyta et al 1992) and for example, we observed that in 23 patients with severe ARDS the improvement of oxygenation was significantly higher in survivors than in non-survivors (Brunet et al 1993).

Does extracorporeal lung support improve arterial oxygenation?

During veno-arterial ECMO, the membrane supplies the body's total oxygen requirements, allowing a reduction in ventilatory FiO_2. Even partial veno-arterial by-pass can correct hypoxemia and hypercapnia in patients suffering from severe acute respiratory failure (Zapol et al 1979). The effects of veno-venous by-pass on arterial oxygenation are still controversial. Certainly the amount of oxygen provided via the membrane to the mixed venous blood is insufficient to achieve total arterial oxygenation, even though it has been reported that high flows through the extracorporeal circuit and right ventricular insertion of the return cannula might achieve this goal (Wetterberg & Steen 1991). However, all (Gattinoni et al 1984, 1986, Chevalier et al 1990, Brunet et al 1993) but one (Morris et al 1994) clinical study have reported improvements in arterial oxygenation using veno-venous techniques. In 60 consecutive patients treated in our institution, $ECCO_2R$-LFPPV improved arterial oxygenation dramatically in all but two cases, both of whom suffered from severe alveolar haemorrhage with bronchial obstruction. The role of the natural lungs in arterial oxygenation remains important when these veno-venous methods are em-

VV ECMO
$ECCO_2R$-LFPPV $\}$ → PaO_2 ↑

ployed. Thus using $ECCO_2R$-LFPPV, the continuous flow of oxygen administered via an intratracheal catheter is the principal method of oxygenation (Kolobow et al 1978, Gattinoni et al 1986). Oxygen diffusion, which is necessary for this pseudo-apnoeic mode of ventilation requires good airway patency and compensation for any large pleural leaks (Brunet et al 1993). The continuous flow of oxygen administered via the intratracheal catheter increases alveolar oxygen concentration and facilitates better distribution of oxygen to the alveoli by diffusion (Brunet et al 1993) and cardiac motion (Venegas et al 1991). The observed improvement in arterial oxygenation probably results from a better regional distribution of ventilation-perfusion ratios achieved by the combination of artificial and natural pulmonary gas exchange. Oxygen supplied extracorporally helps to decrease hypoxic pulmonary vasoconstriction and improve right ventricular function.

Does extracorporeal lung support reduce pulmonary barotrauma?

Reductions in both airway pressures and insufflated volume are commonly reported in patients treated with extracorporeal support (Gattinoni et al 1984, 1986, Chevalier et al 1990). In 23 patients receiving $ECCO_2R$-LFPPV, peak inspiratory pressures, tidal volume and mean airway pressures were significantly less than they had been using mechanical ventilation a few hours before initiating extracorporeal support (Brunet et al 1993). Reductions in both pressures and volumes theoretically decreases the risk of barotrauma as shown by a reduction in hyaline membrane formation with $ECCO_2R$-LFPPV in animal models (Pesenti et al 1982). Borelli et al (1988) reported a reduction in the incidence of histological pulmonary abnormalities and an improved survival rate in sheep treated with $ECCO_2R$-LFPPV as compared to those treated with mechanical ventilation after initial barotraumatic lung injury. However, no clinical trial has demonstrated such a benefit in patients with ARDS, probably because of the difficulty of defining pulmonary barotrauma in clinical practice (usually reported as the incidence of pneumothoraces, pneumomediastinum, subcutaneous emphysema and airway cysts). Moreover, the underlying lung injury may enhance the development of barotrauma, an effect that cannot be separated easily from ventilator-induced pulmonary damage (Hernandez et al 1990). Secondly, barotrauma may be due to high applied volumes rather than high pressures (Dreyfuss et al 1988). The high level of PEEP used in $ECCO_2R$-LFPPV could be the source of such 'volotrauma' by increasing end-expiratory volume above functional respiratory capacity. In a recent study using respiratory inductive plethysmography (Dall'Ava-Santucci et al 1988) we compared the effects of $ECCO_2R$-LFPPV with that of a limited-pressure mode of mechanical ventilation in 11 patients with severe ARDS (Brunet et al

1994). This study showed that $ECCO_2R$-LFPPV improved arterial oxygenation and significantly reduced both peak and mean airway pressures, tidal and total volumes, including end-expiratory volumes, in all but two patients who had marked increases in airway resistance.

Can the complications of ECMO be reduced?

bleeding + complement activation
pulmonary hypoperfusion

The poor results of early trials of veno-arterial ECMO were in part related to the high incidence of complications. Pulmonary hypoperfusion, bleeding and complement activation were associated with diverting the entire blood flow through an external oxygenator. Veno-venous by-pass aimed to limit the frequency and severity of these complications and to avoid exacerbating pulmonary damage by maintaining normal lung perfusion (Gattinoni et al 1984). Patient tolerance of veno-venous extracorporeal circulation is generally good, even when extracorporeal support is maintained over long periods of time (Gattinoni et al 1984, 1986, Chevalier et al 1990, Brunet et al 1993). In particular, hemodynamics usually improve and infectious complications are rare (Gattinoni et al 1980). However, recent animal experiments have also shown that the extracorporeal circulation of blood might provoke abnormal inflammatory responses and thereby worsen lung injury and hemodynamics (Zwischenberger et al 1993). In clinical practice, hemorrhagic complications remain the major cause of morbidity and mortality (Gattinoni et al 1984, Bindsley et al 1987, Morris et al 1990, Brunet et al 1992, 1993). Multiple factors including lung injury, multiple organ failure and sepsis account for the abnormalities in hemostasis. Activation of the coagulation pathway by contact with foreign surfaces is common in patients with ARDS treated with extracorporeal support. In particular, thrombocytopenia, abnormal platelet function, low fibrinogen and/or antithrombin III concentrations, and the presence of fibrin degradation products are constant features, despite close monitoring of coagulation. In our experience, even dramatically reducing the dose of infused heparin compared with preliminary reports failed to eliminate bleeding. The improvement in biocompatibility of the foreign surfaces and the possibility of using heparin-bonded circuits may help to decrease this risk (Bindsley et al 1987, Koul et al 1992).

Can the indications for ECMO be defined clearly?

The place of extracorporeal lung support in the treatment of patients with ARDS is still controversial. One improvement is arterial oxygenation which can be achieved using these techniques and suggests that they should be employed in patients who remain severely hypoxemic after a trial of all modes of mechanical ventilation. In patients 'at risk' of pulmonary barotrauma, reductions in airway pressures and volumes can be

1) Persistent hypoxaemia on 'best mechanical ventilation'
2) Patient at high risk of barotrauma?

achieved and those should reduce the risk of baro- and volotrauma. However, these results were obtained in open clinical trials and must be confirmed by larger controlled studies. In particular, they must be compared to new modes of mechanical ventilation such as PC-IRV, permissive hypoventi-lation and high frequency jet ventilation.

INTRAVASCULAR GAS EXCHANGER

Methods

A number of new devices aimed at achieving intravascular gas exchange are being developed in Japan and the USA, but only one device is currently under clinical investigation—the intravascular oxygenator IVOX®, produced by Cardiopulmonics Inc, Salt Lake City, USA.

IVOX® technique

The IVOX® is a device containing multiple crimped hollow fibres (length 55–65 cm) consisting of an ultra-thin gas-permeable siloxane polymer membrane supported by a skeleton of microporous polypropylene (Fig. 1.1). Insertion of the device is performed only surgically and requires previous training. Briefly, devices of size #7 to #10 are furled to an outer diameter of 1.1–1.5 cm and inserted through a femoral venotomy to lie through both venae cavae and within the right atrium, where they are unfurled to attain a surface area of 0.21–0.52 m^2. The introducer used for IVOX® insertion into the right common femoral vein is in the shape of a hollow, truncated ram's horn. A 10 cm incision is made over the right common femoral vein, the vessel is dissected free and ligatures are placed proximally and distally to control bleeding while the venotomy is made. The patient is given 400 units/kg heparin via a central venous catheter. A guide wire is inserted through the introducer into the venae cavae, over which the IVOX® is passed until the tip of the device is located in the inferior portion of the superior vena cava, as determined by fluoroscopy. Diffusional gas exchange then occurs between 100% O$_2$ flowing under negative pressure (between –300 and –500 mmHg) inside the hollow fibres and blood flowing between the fibre bundle floating in the central venous blood stream, achieving continuous in vivo blood oxygenation and CO$_2$ extraction. Carbon dioxide elimination is constantly monitored by capnometry. The subatmospheric intra-fibre pressure is used to avoid the risk of gas embolism in case of fibre rupture. The device is maintained in place during the acute phase of the disease and gas transfer is interrupted only during a short period of time each day, to evaluate performance of the device. Removal is also performed surgically with surgical repair of the common femoral vein.

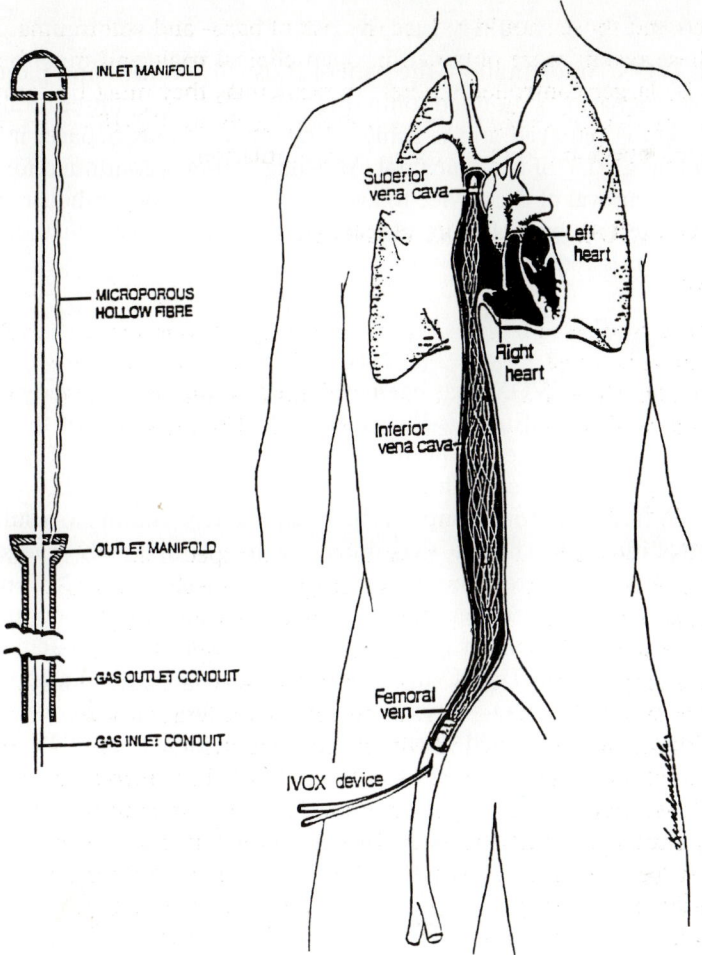

Fig. 1.1 Intravascular oxygenator IVOX® (Cardiopulmonics Inc., Salt Lake City, USA).

Pulmonary management

Different modes of ventilation can be employed in association with IVOX®, but usually pressure-limited volume-cycled ventilation is used. Hypercapnia, which is often associated with these modes of ventilation, can be decreased by CO_2 removal via the IVOX®. In one study, jet ventilation was used with IVOX® (Conrad et al 1993). However, the poor performance of IVOX® does not permit the use of 'low-frequency positive-pressure ventilation' as in ECCO$_2$R-LFPPV.

pressure-limited volume-cycled mechanical ventilation + IVOX (IVCO$_2$R)

but needs high/nasal respiratory frequency

Patient care

During IVOX® implantation, the patient is usually sedated and paralysed. Although heparin is bonded onto the surface of the fibres, full anti-coagulation is required and is achieved by a continuous heparin infusion to maintain a PTT of twice normal. Anticoagulation is continued for seven days after removal of the device to avoid venous thrombo-embolism which can be detected by echo-doppler. Constant clinical surveillance by a trained team is required.

Clinical results

The clinical use of IVOX® has been evaluated in a two-phase study carried out in the USA and Europe. Phase I established the safety of the device and phase II investigated its performance in patients with ARDS who met the appropriate entry criteria (reported in Table 1.1). About 120 patients have been treated in total (unpublished data). The preliminary results are, however, difficult to analyse. Gas transfer achieved by IVOX® ranged between 20 and 30% of total body requirements (High et al 1992, Conrad et al 1993) and was lower than expected on the basis of results obtained in animal models (Mortensen 1987). For example, CO_2 removal achieved in 10 patients treated by IVOX® in our own institution approximated to 20% of CO_2 production. CO_2 removal increased slightly with the size of the device and was unchanged during implantation (Brunet et al 1994). The influence of such a low level of extrapulmonary gas exchange on survival and on the respiratory management of the patients in terms of reduction of pulmonary barotrauma is unclear.

Does IVOX® improve arterial oxygenation?

The effect of IVOX® on oxygenation is poor, when compared to that obtained using extracorporeal support, although precise evaluation of rates of oxygen transfer is difficult. Extrapolating from animal experiments, it seems that the volume of O_2 supplied by IVOX® is low, even using larger devices. High et al (1992) using a more sophisticated method of measurement of oxygen transfer, also found the quantity transferred to be low and questioned its usefulness in the venous circulation. In 10 patients with ARDS treated with IVOX® in our institution, we observed a moderate but

Table 1.1   Phase II IVOX® study entry criteria

Patients entered into phase II study when they met following gas criteria:
$PaO_2 \leq 60$ mmHg with $FiO_2 \geq 0.5$ and PEEP ≥ 10 cmH$_2$O
or when they required following ventilator settings:
PIP ≥ 45 cmH$_2$O or MAP ≥ 30 cmH$_2$O.

not significant increase in PaO_2 (Brunet et al 1994). In the same study, interrupting gas flow through the device was associated with a variable and insignificant decrease in PaO_2/FiO_2. However, the effects of IVOX® may be obscured by spontaneous variations in PaO_2 during these periods, which in turn may induce alterations in regional intrapulmonary shunt by changing the degree of hypoxic vasoconstriction.

Does IVOX® reduce pulmonary barotrauma?

Some clinical studies have reported that IVOX® permitted a reduction in ventilator settings in patients with ARDS. Conrad et al (1993) reported that in 2 patients the use of IVOX® was associated with reductions in ventilatory support, but the final mode of ventilation employed was not described in detail and 1 patient was treated with high-frequency positive-pressure ventilation. High et al (1992) observed that in only 2 of their 5 patients, did IVOX® permit a reduction in ventilatory support. We observed that peak inspiratory pressures could be decreased in our 10 patients treated with 'permissive hypercapnia' and that CO_2 removal by IVOX® allowed $PaCO_2$ and pH to remain stable, despite decreasing minute ventilation. A recent study, using a mathematical model for gas transfer in IVOX® has shown that under conditions of permissive hypercapnia, CO_2 removal can be significantly enhanced above that observed during normocapnia (Bidani et al 1993).

Can the complications of ECMO be reduced using IVOX®?

Tolerance of IVOX® is satisfactory and device implantation and explantation have proved to be simple when the protocol is strictly adhered to. However, some bleeding has been reported during insertion of IVOX® and a reduction in platelet count is frequently observed. None the less, no serious bleeding has been reported. Infection related to the device is infrequent. A decrease in cardiac index may occur after insertion of the device and hypovolaemia due to blood loss during insertion, as well as impaired venous return by the largest devices can occur, although this has not been reported in animal models. Incomplete unfurling of the device after insertion may limit gas transfer and preclude any reduction in ventilator settings. This is quite difficult to detect by fluoroscopy or ultrasound examination and is often only confirmed on removal of the device.

In conclusion, the effects of IVOX® on arterial oxygenation are far less than those of either $ECCO_2R$ or ECMO. CO_2 removal may, however, help to reduce ventilator settings in patients with ARDS. A reduction in the incidence of pulmonary barotrauma and improvements in final outcome using IVOX® needs to be confirmed by a randomized study comparing mechanical ventilation with and without IVOX®.

INHALED NO

The biology of NO

More than a decade ago, the existence of an extremely labile and potent endogenous vasodilator synthesized by the endothelium, termed endothelium-derived relaxing factor (EDRF), was established by Furchgott & Zawadzki (1980). Subsequently, the nature of EDRF remained elusive, until experimental results from several laboratories identified it as NO (Ignarro et al 1987, Palmer et al 1987). The molecular target of NO is the soluble enzyme guanylate cyclase (Moncada et al 1991). Stimulation of the latter by NO increases the level of the second messenger cyclic guanosine monophosphate (cGMP) within vascular smooth muscle, thereby causing vasorelaxation (Murad 1986). The nitrogen atom of NO is derived from the N-guanidino terminal of the amino acid, L-arginine, whereas the oxygen atom is provided by molecular oxygen (O_2) (Moncada et al 1991). NO is synthesized from these two precursors by a newly discovered family of enzymes, the NO synthases (NOS). The complementary DNA for various isoforms of the NOS family has been recently cloned, and its amino acid primary structure sequenced (Förstermann et al 1991). There are two major subgroups of NOS isoforms, the constitutive and the inducible one. Endothelial NOS are predominantly constitutive, and most certainly, play a key role in the modulation of systemic (Moncada & Higgs 1993) and pulmonary (Dinh-Xuan 1992) vascular tone. One of the inducible NOS isoforms probably mediates the cytotoxic activity of activated macrophages against numerous pathogens and intracellular microorganisms (Nathan & Hibbs 1991). Another inducible NOS isoform, which accounts for pathological synthesis of large amounts of NO, is thought to be the major cause of the refractory hypotension seen in human septic shock (Petros et al 1991). The activity of these different NOS isoforms is highly regulated, requiring the presence of specific cofactors, including the calcium/calmodulin complex and reduced nicotinamide adenine dinucleotide phosphate (Moncada et al 1991). The synthesis of NO is stereospecifically inhibited by various L-arginine analogues, which act as competitive inhibitors of both the constitutive and inducible NOS isoforms (Moncada et al 1991).

Physiological role of NO in the human pulmonary circulation

As in other mammalian species, pulmonary endothelium-dependent relaxation mediated by NO is also demonstrable in humans (Dinh-Xuan et al 1990) and in vivo studies suggest that endogenous NO may have physiological importance in the modulation of the human pulmonary circulation (Dinh-Xuan 1992). Indeed, endogenous NO is present in the exhaled air from spontaneously breathing healthy subjects (Gustafsson et al 1991, Garnier et al 1994). Furthermore, significant increases in NO output are observed in conditions which might alter pulmonary and bronchial vasoreactivitiy, such as exertion and hypoxia (Garnier et al 1994). Data from studies using isolated vascular rings or perfused lungs also strongly suggest that endothelium-derived NO probably modulates pulmonary vasoreactivity in normoxia (Dinh-Xuan et al 1991), and during acute alveolar hypoxia (Liu et al 1991). Although some controversies still exist as to its rate of production during chronic hypoxia (Adnot et al 1991, Isaacson et al 1994), endogenous NO probably has a pivotal role in the modulation of pulmonary vascular tone in health and pulmonary vascular disease (Dinh-Xuan 1992, 1993). Indeed, most authors agree that NO is probably the major paracrine mediator and that its rate of synthesis and/or release can rapidly adapt in response to acute increases in pulmonary vascular tone. Hence, a possible physiological role for NO would be to protect the pulmonary vasculature from the disproportionate vasoconstriction that might result from various chemical and physical stimuli (Dinh-Xuan 1992, 1993).

Pulmonary vasodilatation

Inhaled NO

Pulmonary hypertension may complicate various chronic and acute pulmonary disorders, including ARDS. The treatment of pulmonary hypertension, irrespective of its aetiology, has always represented a formidable challenge for physicians, the main difficulties stemming from the fact that no pulmonary vasodilator is devoid of systemic side-effects. The 'ideal' pulmonary vasodilator must therefore be selective, its activity being restricted to the pulmonary circulation. Knowing that NO is rapidly inactivated by haemoglobin (Martin et al 1986), it has been hypothesized that NO, given by inhalation, could act as such a selective pulmonary vasodilator (Higenbottam et al 1988). After entering the airways, inhaled NO primarily reaches the pulmonary vascular smooth muscle through diffusion from alveolar spaces, thereby causing pulmonary vasodilatation. Once it reaches the luminal side of pulmonary endothelial cells, NO is rapidly bound and therefore inactivated, by circulating haemoglobin. Thus, no downstream vasodilatory effect is likely to occur with inhaled NO. However, the recent suggestion that NO could be carried away by serum albumin, which subsequently releases NO downstream, makes systemic hypotension a theoretical possibility (Stamler et al 1992a). However, to the best of our knowledge, no such effect has been reported.

PHT↓

Inhaled NO has been successfully applied in animals to reverse hypoxic (Frostell et al 1991) and thromboxane-induced pulmonary vasoconstriction (Frostell et al 1991). In humans, the short-term inhalation of NO also produces significant and selective pulmonary vasodilatory effects in the newborn with persistent pulmonary hypertension (Kinsella et al 1992,

HPV ↓
T_xPV ↓

1°. 2° PHT↓

Roberts et al 1992), and in adults with pulmonary hypertension, either primary (Pepke-Zaba et al 1991), or secondary to chronic obstructive lung disease (Adnot et al 1993) and ARDS (Rossaint et al 1993, Fierobe et al 1995). Furthermore, when given by inhalation, NO has a unique ability to improve gas exchange and arterial oxygenation (Kinsella et al 1992, Roberts et al 1992, Adnot et al 1993, Rossaint et al 1993). Thus, unlike infused prostacyclin, which dilates pulmonary vessels of ventilated as well as non-ventilated lung units, inhaled NO preferentially induces vasodilatation in the former. As a result, ventilation/perfusion mismatching is reduced, as shown by a decrease in intrapulmonary shunting (Q_S/Q_T); and

V̇/Q̇ improved

Q_S/Q_T ↓

PaO_2/FiO_2 ↑

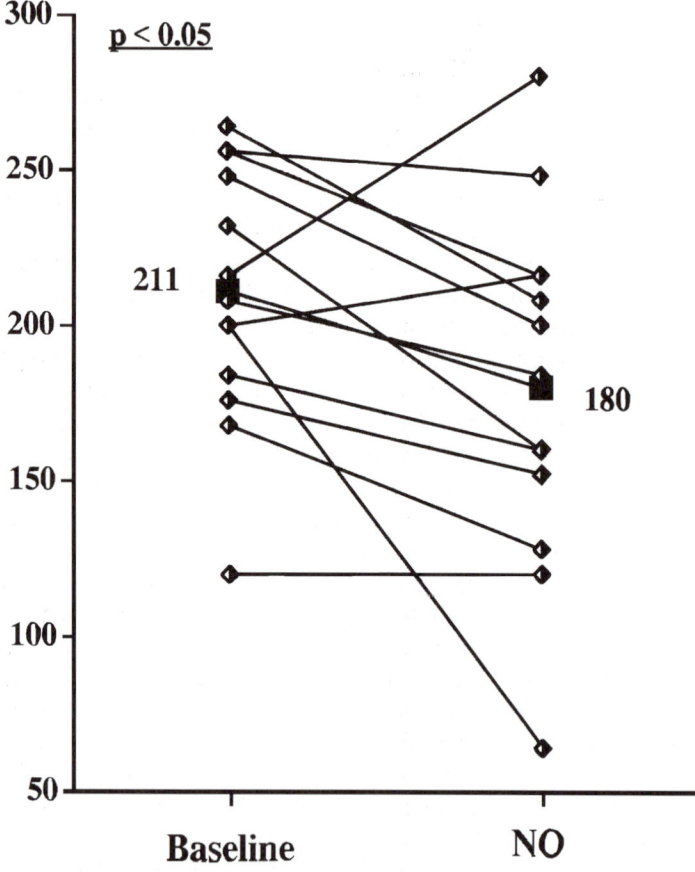

Fig. 1.2   Pulmonary vascular resistance during baseline and NO (5 ppm). Effects of inhaled NO (5 ppm) on vascular resistance (PVR) in all but 3 patients. From Fierobe et al 1995.

[handwritten annotations at top: P_aO_2: PGI_2 aerosol $\equiv$ inhaled NO]
[handwritten: P_aCO_2: inhaled NO > PGI_2 (bronchodilatation)]

gas exchange is improved with an increase in PaO_2/FiO_2 (Rossaint et al 1993). It is possible that the inhaled route of administration as much as NO itself is instrumental in obtaining such beneficial effects on arterial oxygenation, as improvements of similar magnitude are observed in ARDS using aerosolized prostacyclin (Walmrath et al 1993). On the other hand, it is likely that the bronchodilatory effects of NO (Högman et al 1993) may account for the observed decrease in $PaCO_2$ (Fierobe et al 1995) by opening up lung segments which were previously poorly ventilated. An elegant way to improve arterial oxygenation is to combine the use of inhaled NO with infused almitrine (Payen et al 1993), a known pulmonary vasoconstrictor. The resulting constriction induced by almitrine which predominates in the shunting vascular bed will further reduce Q_S/Q_T and improve arterial oxygenation.

The remaining unsolved questions

To date, three main difficulties with the use of inhaled NO in ARDS need to be addressed. First, despite initial optimistic reports (Rossaint et al 1993), it is now apparent that not all patients are likely to benefit from inhaled NO, even with doses higher than 40 ppm (Mira et al 1994). Secondly, weaning patients who are treated with long-term inhaled NO may be fraught with difficulties, as exogenous administration of NO could switch off endogenous production (Bult et al 1991). Finally, potentially harmful effects of this oxygen-derived free radical remain to be defined. Under physiological conditions, there are at least three redox forms of NO which, either by gaining or losing an electron, are converted to nitroxyl anion (NO^-) or nitrosonium (NO^+), respectively (Stamler et al 1992b). A better understanding of the biochemistry of nitrogen oxides (NO_x), which include NO, is mandatory in order to predict, and therefore avoid, the toxicity induced by these molecules. Indeed, experimental data suggest that both endogenous and exogenous NO_x react readily with oxygen, superoxide, water, nucleotides, metalloproteins, thiols, amines and lipids (Stamler et al 1992b). Biochemical end-products of these reactions may account for an array of toxic effects, including impaired mitochondrial respiration, lipid peroxidation, and mutagenesis (Stamler et al 1992b). In the meantime, the most practical way of reducing NO toxicity is to limit the concentration of NO administered to patients. In this regard, a recent study which reports significant beneficial affects of NO on gas exchange with doses ranging from 60 to 230 parts per billion (Gerlach et al 1993), i.e. several hundred times less than doses previously used in ARDS (Rossaint et al 1993), is encouraging.

In conclusion, the use of inhaled NO is undoubtedly a dramatic breakthrough in the management of patients with ARDS; at least in terms of its specific and beneficial effects on pulmonary hemodynamics and gas exchange. However, as with other therapeutic advances, inhaled NO must

[handwritten margin annotations: "variable response"; "NO dependence?"; "toxicity: NO^-, NO^+, NO_x"; "? $\ll 40$ ppm"]

still be evaluated in large, multicentre, controlled trials before we can determine whether the future management of ARDS will include the use of a gas which was not long ago regarded by many physicians as an atmospheric pollutant.

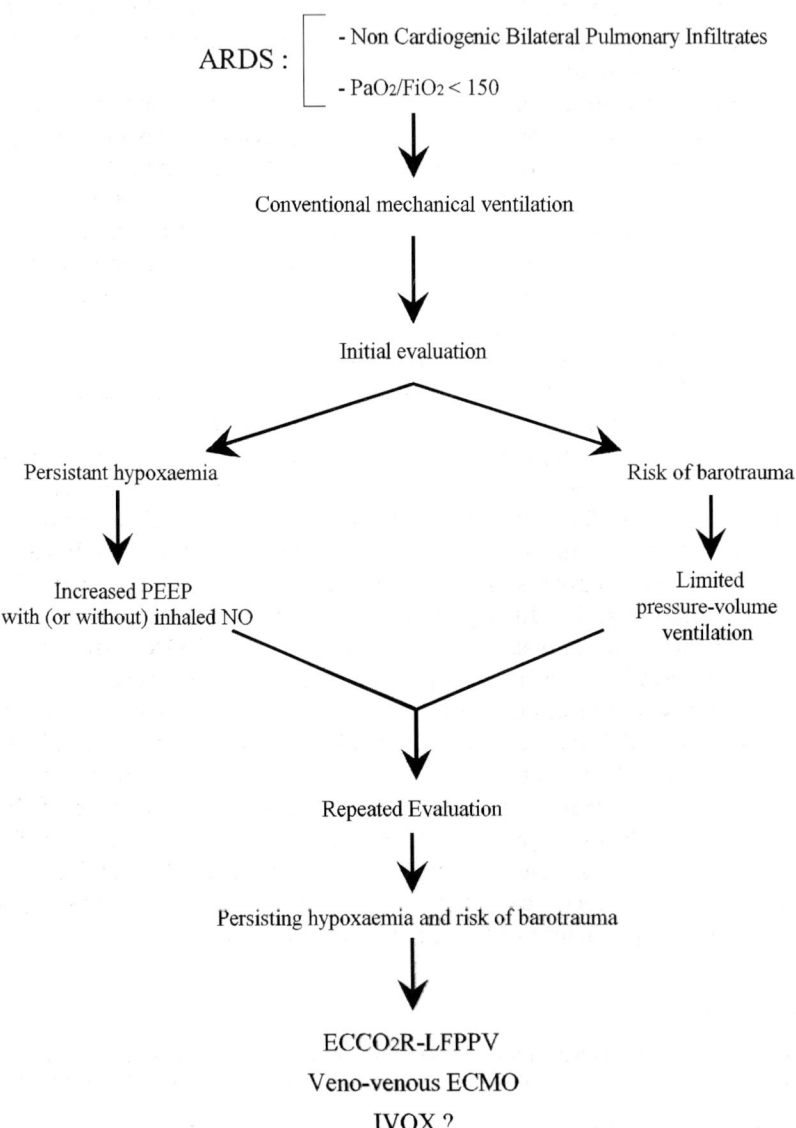

Fig. 1.3   Therapeutic approaches in ARDS.

KEY POINTS FOR CLINICAL PRACTICE: INDICATIONS
FOR ECMO, IVOX® AND INHALED NO IN ARDS (Fig. 1.3)

- Supportive treatment in ARDS must aim to achieve optimal tissue oxygenation while limiting the risk of pulmonary barotrauma. In most patients, conventional mechanical ventilation with PEEP allows adequate oxygenation, but may be deleterious when high airway pressures and volumes are required.
- Pressure- and volume-limited modes may help to mitigate the risk of barotrauma, but can expose the patient to hypercapnia and an increased FiO_2, with the risk of oxygen toxicity. Inhaled NO may help to improve both hemodynamics and arterial oxygenation and may be indicated in patients who remain hypoxaemic. The benefits of NO on oxygenation must be balanced against the potential risks, and NO administration must be included in a general strategy that aims to reduce both oxygen toxicity and pulmonary barotrauma.
- Extrapulmonary gas exchange is indicated (1) in patients in whom different modes of mechanical ventilation have failed to achieve adequate oxygenation (defined as PaO_2/FiO_2 remaining lower than 150) and (2) those who are ventilated with a high risk of baro- and volutrauma. In the absence of defined 'at risk' ventilator settings, the following criteria can be proposed: PIP ≥ 50 cmH$_2$O and tidal volume ≥ 12 ml/kg needed to maintain $PaO_2 \geq 60$ mmHg with pH ≥ 7.2 whatever the level of $PaCO_2$.
- Extracorporeal support is more effective than IVOX®, both in maintaining oxygenation and reducing the risk of barotrauma, but is more invasive and carries an increased risk of severe bleeding. IVOX® can be used to reduce ventilator settings in patients with mild to severe ARDS in whom arterial oxygenation is mainly achieved by mechanical ventilation.
- ECCO$_2$R-LFPPV and veno-venous ECMO are now indicated only in the most severely ill patients with extremely poor lung mechanics in whom other techniques are ineffective. A better understanding of the evolution of ARDS, together with improved definitions of criteria for inclusion and management, as well as a reduction in the incidence of bleeding through technical improvements, may broaden the indications for these highly efficient extracorporeal techniques.

REFERENCES

Adnot S, Raffestin B, Eddhahibi S et al 1991 Loss of endothelium-dependent relaxant activity in the pulmonary circulation of rats exposed to chronic hypoxia. J Clin Invest 87: 155–162

Adnot S, Kouyoumdjian C, Defouilloy C et al 1993 Hemodynamic and gas exchange respones to infusion of acetylcholine and inhalation of nitric oxide in patients with chronic obstructive lung disease and pulmonary hypertension. Am Rev Respir Dis 148: 310–316

Ashbaugh D G, Bigelow D B, Petty T L, Levine B E 1967 Acute respiratory distress in adults. Lancet 2: 319–323

Bidani A, Niranjan S C, Clark J W et al 1993 Model analysis of the effects of permissive hypercapnia on CO_2 removal by IVOX®, an intracorporeal gas exchange device (abstract). Critical Care Medicine 21: S125

Bindsley L, Eklund J, Norlander O et al 1987 Treatment of acute respiratorsy failure by extracorporeal carbon dioxide elimination performed with a surface heparinized artificial lung. Anesthesiology 67: 117–120

Bone R C, Balk R, Slotman G et al 1992 Adult respiratory distress syndrome: sequence and importance of development of multiple organ failure. Chest 101: 320–326

Borelli M, Kolobow T, Spatola R et al 1988 Severe acute respiratory failure managed with continuous positive airway pressure and partial extracorporeal carbon dioxide removal by an artificial membrane lung: a controlled, randomized animal study. Am Rev Respir Dis 138: 1480–1487

Brian C L, Jenkinson S G 1988 Oxygen toxicity. Clin Chest Med 9: 141–152

Brunet F, Mira J P, Belghith M et al 1992 Effects of aprotinin on haemorrhagic complications in ARDS patients during prolonged extracorporeal CO_2 removal. Intensive Care Med 18: 364–367

Brunet F, Belghith M, Mira J P et al 1993 $ECCO_2R$-LFPPV improves arterial oxygenation while reducing risk of pulmonary barotrauma in patients with ARDS. Chest 104: 889–898

Brunet F, Mira J P, Belghith M et al 1994 Extracorporeal CO_2 removal technique improves oxygenation without causing overinflation. Am J Respir Crit Care Med 149: 1557–1562

Bult H, de Meyer G R Y, Jordaens F, Herman A G 1991 Chronic exposure to exogenous nitric oxide may suppress its endogenous release and efficacy. J Cardiovasc Pharmacol 17 (Suppl 3): S79–S82

Chevalier J Y, Durandy Y, Batisse A et al 1990 Preliminary reports: extracorporeal lung support for neonatal acute respiratory failure. Lancet 335: 1364–1366

Conrad S A, Eggerstedt J M, Morris V F, Romero M D 1993 Prolonged intracorporeal support of gas exchange with an intravenacaval oxygenator. Chest 103: 158–161

Dall'Ava-Santucci J, Armaganidis A, Brunet F et al 1988 Causes of error of respiratory pressure volume curves in paralyzed subjects. J Appl Physiol 64: 42–49

Dall'Ava-Santucci J, Armaganidis A, Brunet F et al 1990 Mechanical effects of PEEP in patients with adult respiratory distress syndrome. J Appl Physiol 68: 843–848.

Dinh-Xuan A T 1992 Endothelial modulation of pulmonary vascular tone. Eur Respir J 5: 757–762

Dinh-Xuan A T 1993 Disorders of endothelium-dependent relaxation in pulmonary disease. Circulation 87 (Suppl V): V81–V87

Dinh-Xuan A T, Higenbottam T W, Clelland C A et al 1990 Acetylcholine and adenosine diphosphate cause endothelium-dependent relaxation of isolated human pulmonary arteries. Eur Respir J 3: 633–638

Dinh-Xuan A T, Higenbottam T W, Clelland C A et al 1991 Impairment of endothelium-dependent pulmonary-artery relaxation in chronic obstructive lung disease. N Engl J Med 324: 1539–1547

Dreyfuss D, Soler P, Basset G, Saumon G 1988 High inflation pressure pulmonary edema: respective effects of high airway pressure, high tidal volume and positive end-expiratory pressure. Am Rev Respir Dis 137: 1159–1164

Elliott C, Morris A H, Cengiz M 1981 Pulmonary function and exercise gas exchange in survivors of adult respiratory distress syndrome. Am Rev Respir Dis 123: 492–495

Fierobe L, Monchi M, Belghith M et al 1995 Inhaled NO and right ventricular function in patients with ARDS (abstract). Am J Respir Crit Care Med 151: 1414–1419

Förstermann U, Schmidt H H H W, Pollock J S et al 1991 Isoforms of nitric oxide synthase: characterization and purification from different cell types. Biochem Pharmacol 10: 1849–1857

Frostell C G, Fratacci M D, Wain J C Jr et al 1991 Inhaled nitric oxide: a selective pulmonary vasodilator reversing hypoxic pulmonary vasoconstriction. Circulation 83: 2038–2047

Furchgott R F, Zawadzki J V 1980 The obligatory role of endothelial cells in the relaxation of arterial smooth muscle by acetylcholine. Nature 288: 373–376

Gammon R B, Shin M S, Buchalter S E 1992 Pulmonary barotrauma in mechanical ventilation. Chest 102: 568–572

Garnier P, Strâmbu I, Dessanges J F et al 1994 Endogenous nitric oxide in expired air increases on exercise and isocapnic hyperventilation in normal subjects (abstract). Am J Respir Crit Care Med 149: 4778

Gattinoni L, Agostini A, Damia G et al 1980 Hemodynamics and renal function during low frequency positive pressure ventilation with extracorporeal CO_2 removal. Intensive Care Med 6: 155–161

Gattinoni L, Pesenti A, Caspani M L et al 1984 The role of total static lung compliance in the management of severe ARDS unresponsive to conventional treatment. Intensive Care Med 10: 121–126

Gattinoni L, Pesenti A, Mascheroni D et al 1986 Low-frequency positive-pressure ventilation with extracorporeal CO_2 removal in severe acute respiratory failure. JAMA 256: 881–886

Gattinoni L, Pesenti A, Bombino M et al 1988 Relationship between lung computed tomographic density, gas exchange and PEEP in acute respiratory failure. Anesthesiology 69: 824–832

Gerlach H, Pappert D, Lewandowski K et al 1993 Long-term inhalation with evaluated low doses of nitric oxide for selective improvement of oxygenation in patients with adult respiratory distress syndrome. Intensive Care Med 19: 443–449

Gurewitch M J, Van Dyke J, Young E S, Jackson K 1986 Improved oxygenation and lower peak airway pressure in severe adult respiratory distress syndrome. Chest 89: 211–213

Gustafsson L E, Leone A M, Persson M G et al 1991 Endogenous nitric oxide is present in the exhaled air of rabbits, guinea pigs and humans. Biochem Biophys Res Commun 181: 852–857

Hernandez L A, Cocjer P J, May S et al 1990 Mechanical ventilation increases microvascular permeability in oleic acid-injured lungs. J Appl Physiol 69: 2057–2061

Hickling K G, Henderson S J, Jackson R 1990 Low mortality associated with low volume pressure limited ventilation with permissive hypercapnia in severe adult respiratory distress syndrome. Intensive Care Med 16: 372–377

Higenbottam T W, Pepke-Zaba J, Scott J P et al 1988 Inhaled endothelium-derived relaxing factor in primary pulmonary hypertension (abstract). Am Rev Respir Dis 137 (Suppl): 107

High K M, Snider M T, Richard R et al 1992 Clinical trials of an intravenous oxygenator in patients with adult respiratory distress syndrome. Anesthesiology 77: 856–863

Högman M, Frostell C G, Hedenström H, Hedenstierna G 1993 Inhalation of nitric oxide modulates adult human bronchial tone. Am Rev Respir Dis 148: 1474–1478

Ignarro L J, Buga G M, Wood K S et al 1987 Endothelium-derived relaxing factor produced and released from artery and vein is nitric oxide. Proc Natl Acad Sci USA 84: 9265–9269

Isaacson T C, Hampl V, Weir E K et al 1994 Increased endothelium-derived NO in hypertensive pulmonary circulation of chronically hypoxic rats. J Appl Physiol 76: 933–940

Kinsella J P, Neish S R, Shaffer E, Abman S H 1992 Low-dose inhalational nitric oxide in persistent pulmonary hypertension of the newborn. Lancet 340: 819–820

Kolobow T, Gattinoni L, Tomlinson T, Pierce J E 1978 An alternative to breathing. J Thorac Cardiovasc Surg 75: 261–266

Koul B, Vesterqvist O, Egberg N, Steen S 1992 Twenty-four hour heparin-free veno-right ventricular ECMO: an experimental study. Ann Thorac Surg 53: 1046–1051

Liu S F, Crawley D E, Barnes P J, Evans T W 1991 Endothelium-derived relaxing factor inhibits hypoxic pulmonary vasoconstriction in rats. Am Rev Respir Dis 143: 32–37

Marini J J, Kelsen S G 1992 Re-targeting ventilatory objectives in adult respiratory distress syndrome. Am Rev Respir Dis 146: 2–3

Martin W, Smith J A, White D G 1986 The mechanisms by which haemoglobin inhibits the relaxation of rabbit aorta induced by nitrovasodilators, nitric oxide or bovine retractor penis inhibitory factor. Br J Pharmacol 89: 563–571

Mira J P, Monchi M, Brunet F et al 1994 Lack of efficacy of inhaled nitric oxide in ARDS (letter). Intensive Care Med 20: 532

Moncada S, Higgs E A 1993 The L-arginine-nitric oxide pathway. N Engl J Med 329: 2002–2012

Moncada S, Palmer R M J, Higgs E A 1991 Nitric oxide: physiology, pathophysiology, and pharmacology. Pharmacol Rev 43: 109–142

Monchi M, Brunet F, Dinh-Xuan A T 1993 Inhaled nitric oxide for the adult respiratory distress syndrome (letter). N Engl J Med 329: 206–207

Morris A H, Wallace C J, Clemmer T P et al 1990 Extracorporeal CO_2 removal therapy for adult respiratory distress syndrome patients. Respir Care 35: 224–231

Morris A H, Wallace C J, Menlove R L et al 1994 Randomized clinical trial of pressure-controlled inverse ratio ventilation and extracorporeal CO_2 removal for adult respiratory distress syndrome. Am J Respir Crit Care Med 149: 295–305

Mortensen J D 1987 An intravenacaval blood gas exchange device: a preliminary report. Trans Am Soc Artif Intern Organs 33: 570–573

Murad F 1986 Cyclic guanosine monophosphate as a mediator of vasodilation. J Clin Invest 78: 1–5

Nathan CF, Hibbs JB Jr 1991 Role of nitric oxide synthesis in macrophage antimicrobial activity. Curr Opin Immunol 3: 65–70

Palmer R M J, Ferrige A G, Moncada S 1987 Nitric oxide release accounts for the biological activity of endothelium-derived relaxing factor. Nature 327: 524–526

Payen D M, Gatecel C, Plaisance P 1993 Almitrine effect on nitric oxide inhalation in adult respiratory distress syndrome (letter). Lancet 341: 1664

Pepke-Zaba J, Higenbottam T W, Dinh-Xuan A T et al 1991 Inhaled nitric oxide as a cause of selective pulmonary vasodilatation in pulmonary hypertension. Lancet 338: 1173–1174

Pesenti A, Kolobow T, Buckhold D K 1982 Prevention of hyaline membrane disease in premature lambs by apneic oxygenation and extracorporeal carbon dioxide removal. Crit Care Med 8: 11–17

Pesenti A 1990 Target blood gases during ARDS ventilatory management. Intensive Care Med 16: 349–351

Petros A, Bennett D, Vallance P 1991 Effect of nitric oxide synthase inhibitors on hypotension in patients with septic shock 338: 1557–1558

Petty T L, Ashbaugh D G 1971 The adult respiratory distress syndrome: clinical features, factors influencing prognosis and principles of management. Chest 60: 233–239

Roberts J D, Polaner D M, Lang P, Zapol W M 1992 Inhaled nitric oxide in persistent pulmonary hypertension of the newborn. Lancet 340: 818–819

Rossaint R, Falke K J, López F et al 1993 Inhaled nitric oxide for the adult respiratory distress syndrome. N Engl J Med 328: 399–405

Shapiro B A, Cane R D, Harrison R A 1983 Positive end-expiratory pressure in acute lung injury. Chest 83: 558–563

Slutsky A S 1994 Consensus conference on mechanical ventilation. Intensive Care Med 20: 64–79

Stamler J S, Jaraki O, Osborne J et al 1992a Nitric oxide circulates in mammalian plasma primarily as an S-nitroso adduct of serum albumine. Proc Natl Acad Sci USA 89: 7674–7677

Stamler J S, Singel D J, Loscalzo J 1992b Biochemistry of nitric oxide and its redox-activated forms. Science 258: 1898–1902

Suchyta M R, Clemmer T P, Elliott C G et al 1992 The adult respiratory distress syndrome: a report of survival and modifying factors. Chest 101: 1074–1079

Venegas J G, Yamada Y, Hales C A 1991 Contribution of diffusion jet flow and cardiac activity to regional ventilation in CFV. J Appl Physiol 71: 1540–1553

Walmrath D, Schneider T, Pilch J et al 1993 Aerosolised prostacyclin in adult respiratory distress syndrome. Lancet 342: 961–962

Wetterberg T, Steen S 1991 Total extracorporeal lung assist: a new clinical approach. Intensive Care Med 17: 73–77

Zapol W M, Snider M T, Hill J D et al 1979 Extracorporeal membrane oxygenation in severe acute respiratory failure. JAMA 242: 2193–2196

Zwischenberger J B, Cox C S, Minifee P K et al 1993 Pathophysiology of ovine smoke inhalation injury treated with extracorporeal membrane oxygenation. Chest 103: 1582–1586

2. Acute lung injury: new concepts in ventilatory support

K.G. Hickling

[handwritten: High Vt and high PIP may exacerbate ARDS]
[handwritten: barotrauma / volutrauma / release of cytokines etc.]

INTRODUCTION

Until recently most studies of different strategies of ventilatory support for adult patients with acute respiratory distress syndrome (ARDS) have investigated only their immediate effects on gas exchange and haemodynamics, the assumption being that the ventilatory approach has no influence on the natural history of the pulmonary disease. There is now, however, compelling evidence from animal studies to suggest that the techniques of mechanical ventilation which have traditionally been employed in ARDS, particularly the use of a large tidal volume (Vt) and the resulting high peak inspiratory pressure (PIP), may cause additional lung injury, and may possibly result in the release of inflammatory mediators. A disseminated inflammatory response resulting from ventilator-induced lung injury in patients with ARDS might augment or perpetuate multiple organ dysfunction and respiratory failure and could contribute to the poor prognosis of this condition. Thus, for example, ventilator-induced lung injury in rabbits impairs bacterial clearance from the lung after instillation of *E. coli*, and results in an increased incidence of positive blood cultures (Parker et al 1991). This could have very important clinical implications if it occurs in patients. Concerns about possible ventilator-induced lung injury have prompted the evaluation of alternative ventilatory strategies for ARDS.

EVIDENCE FOR VENTILATOR-INDUCED LUNG INJURY

This section includes some evidence concerning mechanisms.

Animals commencing with normal lungs

Many studies of ventilator-induced lung injury have recently been reviewed (Parker et al 1993, Hickling 1990, 1992), and only a selection will be discussed here. Sheep ventilated with a PIP of 50 cmH$_2$O (resulting in a Vt of 50–70 ml/kg) developed progressive hypoxaemia, falling compliance and lung consolidation, and all died within 48 hours. At autopsy the lungs were 'highly abnormal' (Kolobow et al 1987). Mechanical ventilation with a PIP of 30 cmH$_2$O (and Vt of approximately 30 ml/kg) for 48 hours still caused lung injury, but this was less severe and no animals died (Tsuno et al 1990). Progressive hypoxaemia developed when baby pigs were ventilated with a PIP of 40 cmH$_2$O, and animals sacrificed after 22 hours showed extensive hyaline membranes, neutrophil infiltration, thickening of the alveolar septa with capillary congestion, and proliferation of alveolar macrophages and type II pneumocytes (Tsuno et al 1991). Six animals were supported by continued ventilation with a Vt of 14 ml/kg for 3–6 days following the initial period of high PIP ventilation. At autopsy the lungs showed severe pathological changes; most alveolar spaces were replaced by proliferating fibroblasts and type II pneumocytes (Fig. 2.1). In another study lung injury was induced in sheep by ventilation with a PIP of 50 cmH$_2$O. Subsequent management involved the use of extracorporeal CO$_2$ removal (ECCO$_2$R) and apnoeic oxygenation; or controlled mechanical ventilation (CMV), with a Vt of 10–15 ml/kg (Borelli et al 1988). In sheep with mild lung injury, 3 of 11 managed with CMV survived, whereas 9 of 11 managed with ECCO$_2$R survived, suggesting that the 'lung rest' associated with ECCO$_2$R and apnoeic oxygenation was beneficial. All the sheep with severe lung injury (following 27 hours of high PIP ventilation) died in both groups, from severe hypotension and oliguria unresponsive to fluid therapy, suggesting that in these animals high PIPs had induced cardiovascular injury in addition to respiratory failure.

High pressures / volumes → (mechanical? inflammatory?) pulmonary injury (+ 2° CCF)

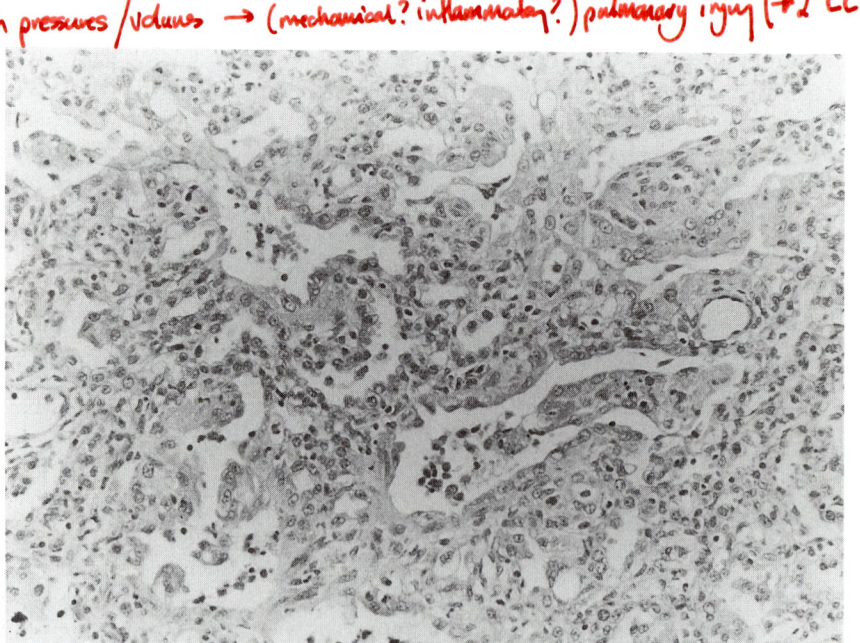

Fig. 2.1 Section of lung from a pig ventilated with a PIP of 40 cmH$_2$O for 24 hours, and then for 6 days with a Vt of 14 ml/kg. Most alveolar spaces are collapsed and replaced with marked proliferation of type II pneumocytes and fibroblasts. Reproduced from Tsuno et al 1991 with permission.

Dreyfuss (1988): "VOLUTRAUMA" : PEEP protective (pulmonary redema).
'critical' end-inspiratory volume → pathology
VENTILATORY SUPPORT IN ACUTE LUNG INJURY   23

Dreyfuss and colleagues have conducted an elegant series of studies examining the effect of ventilation with high PIP in rats. Ventilation with a PIP of 45 cmH$_2$O resulted in pulmonary oedema, hyaline membranes and increased vascular permeability to albumin (Dreyfuss et al 1985). They stressed that this lung injury was a result of overdistension rather than the high PIP per se: thus, negative pressure ventilation using an 'iron lung' ventilator with a high Vt also resulted in lung injury, whereas when thoraco-abdominal strapping prevented lung overdistension high PIP ventilation did not cause injury (Dreyfuss et al 1988). They therefore suggest the use of the term 'volutrauma' rather than barotrauma (Dreyfuss & Saumon 1992). The pulmonary oedema was markedly attenuated and the ultrastructural changes in alveolar epithelial and endothelial cells substantially reduced by the application of 10 cmH$_2$O of PEEP (Dreyfuss et al 1988). The protective effect of PEEP in this model may be related at least in part to its haemodynamic effects; animals ventilated with PEEP sustained similar increases in vascular permeability to those without PEEP at the same PIP, but the amount of pulmonary oedema was less with PEEP (Dreyfuss et al 1993). The end-inspiratory lung volume is critical in determining lung injury rather than mean lung volume or the amplitude of phasic distension (Dreyfuss and Saumon, 1993). Lung injury occurred with a normal Vt if PEEP was sufficiently high, and moderate increases in Vt or PEEP which were innocuous when applied alone caused lung injury when combined. Immature lungs appear to be more susceptible to overdistension injury at any PIP; probably because they contain less elastic tissue and collagen producing higher lung and chest wall compliance, and possibly a reduced tensile strength of lung tissue (Nardell and Brody 1982). Parker and colleagues (1993) have also conducted an extensive series of investigations of ventilator-induced lung injury.

Models of surfactant depletion

The effect of various forms of ventilatory support has been compared in many studies in rabbits following repeated saline lavage of the lungs to remove surfactant. This process results in some injury to the bronchiolar epithelium, but does not cause major morphological changes at alveolar level, so any such changes can be attributed to subsequent ventilatory management (Lachmann et al 1980). Dorrington and colleagues showed that CMV with a PIP of 20 cmH$_2$O in this model produced progressive hypoxaemia and hyaline membrane formation, but this did not occur with extracorporeal CO$_2$ removal and apnoeic oxygenation (Dorrington et al 1989). Bryan and colleagues compared CMV with a PIP of 25 cmH$_2$O with high frequency oscillation (HFO) in this model, with a mean airway pressure of 15 cmH$_2$O in both groups (Hamilton et al 1983). Animals in

Interaction of PIP + surfactant depletion → hypoxaemia

– severity of lung pathology limited by – ↓PIP
– apnoeic oxygenation
– HFO
– granulocyte depletion

the CMV group developed progressive hypoxaemia and all 5 died within 20 hours (3 from hypoxia and acidosis and 2 from tension pneumothorax). In contrast, oxygenation remained unchanged in the HFO group, and 4 of the 5 animals survived the 20-hour protocol, the fifth dying from a pneumothorax. Hyaline membranes were much more prominent in the CMV group. Because granulocyte infiltration of the alveolar septa was prominent in some animals, the effect of granulocyte depletion by pretreatment with nitrogen mustard was studied (Kawano et al 1987). The granulocyte-depleted animals maintained normal oxygenation and vascular permeability during 4 hours of CMV with a Vt of 12 ml/kg, and had relatively normal lung histology. By contrast the normal rabbits became hypoxaemic and 2 of 6 animals died. They showed a marked increase in pulmonary and systemic vascular permeability to albumin, and at autopsy there was extensive hyaline membrane formation and infiltration of the alveoli and interstitium with granulocytes. It was subsequently demonstrated (Burger et al 1990) that thromboxane A2 receptor blockade or indomethacin prevented the pulmonary hypertension which otherwise occurs with CMV in this model. Indomethacin reduced the degree of hypoxaemia, but neither drug prevented the increase in vascular permeability.

Studies examining the effect of lung recruitment using PEEP in saline-lavaged rabbits have consistently shown a substantial reduction of lung injury when adequate recruitment is achieved. When PEEP was set above the inflection point of the pressure-volume curve during CMV, little lung injury occurred, whereas animals ventilated with the same mean and peak airway pressure using low PEEP and increased I:E ratio showed more severe lung injury (Sandhar et al 1988). Even high-frequency ventilation resulted in lung injury in this model when ventilation occurred at low lung volumes, whereas when adequate recruitment was achieved lung injury was markedly reduced (McCulloch et al 1988). Slutsky and colleagues recently studied ventilation at different levels of PEEP in excised rabbit lungs following in vivo saline lavage (Muscedere et al 1992). PEEP greater than the pressure at the inflection point of the pressure-volume curve was as effective in minimizing lung injury as a constant distending pressure with no ventilation. Lower levels of PEEP were related to the site of injury; with no PEEP the injury was predominantly in respiratory bronchioles, whereas with 4 cmH$_2$O PEEP the respiratory bronchioles were relatively normal and the injury affected mainly alveolar ducts. The lung injury in this model may be related to shear stresses occurring during repetitive opening of closed airways; as the PEEP level is increased, the small airways remain open throughout the respiratory cycle and the site of repetitive opening moves distally.

[handwritten annotation:] TxA₂ inhibition / indomethacin may reduce PHT in animal models of ARDS c̄ surfactant depletion.

Ventilation at low lung volumes more damaging than ventilate w̄ PEP in surfactant depletion? shear stress in periodically open airways?

MECHANISMS OF VENTILATOR-INDUCED LUNG INJURY

Normal lungs

overdistension (end-inspiratory volume) ?cumulative ($\overline{Paw}$)

The mechanism of lung injury probably differs in normal animals and in immature or surfactant-depleted lungs (Coker et al 1992). In normal animals considerable overdistension of the lung is required to produce injury, and the end-inspiratory volume appears to be the critical determinant (Dreyfuss & Saumon 1993). The cumulative duration of exposure to high lung volume also appears to be important. Prolongation of the inspiratory time (resulting in higher mean airway pressure) caused a greater increase in vascular permeability than a shorter inspiratory time (Johnson et al 1990). Similarly, 20 minutes of high PIP ventilation in rats caused greater injury than 5 or 10 minutes (Dreyfuss et al 1985). Lung injury occurred after only 2 minutes' exposure to high PIP, but resolved after 45 minutes of normal ventilation (Dreyfuss et al 1992).

Rabbit lungs exposed to elevated vascular distending pressures (Fu et al 1992) developed an increased incidence of 'stress failure' of the capillaries at high lung volumes (Fig. 2.2). Preliminary observations in our laboratory suggest that similar lesions may occur during high-volume ventilation in rabbits with normal vascular pressures. (Fig. 2.3), but further work is required to confirm that the lesions are not artifactual. This may be one explanation for the increase in vascular permeability following high-volume ventilation. Separation of the endothelium from epithelium and basement membrane has also been demonstrated to develop within minutes of exposure to high distending pressures (Dreyfuss et al 1985), and rupture of alveolar walls can also occur (Rouby et al 1993).

Surfactant-depleted lungs

shear stress in airways closed at end-expiration
alveolar rupture related to high insp^y flow rates?

Surfactant-depleted lungs are injured at lower inspiratory pressures than normal lungs and probably through different mechanisms. After surfactant inactivation, isolated, perfused rabbit lungs developed increased vascular permeability during ventilation with a PIP of 15 or 30 cmH$_2$O, whereas without surfactant inactivation a PIP of 45 cmH$_2$O was required (Coker et al 1992). Following surfactant depletion lung injury results from ventilation at low lung volumes with derecruitment following each lung inflation. The detailed mechanisms are not understood, but it is thought that as the airway pressure rises with each ventilator cycle the collapsed terminal airways snap open from the proximal to the distal end. A pressure wave moves down the airway, and at the junction between the open and closed airway large shear stresses occur in the airway wall which may be responsible for the epithelial injury seen in the terminal airways (Robertson 1984). In surfactant-depleted lungs, surface tension does not decrease at low lung volumes, and the pressure gradient required to maintain alveolar patency

Outcome: Resultant compliance or P_aO_2 following IPPV

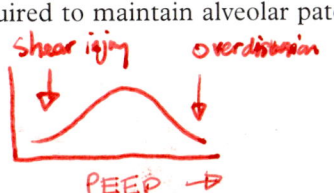

Shear injury   overdistension
↓   ↓
PEEP →

increases according to LaPlace's law. Alveoli become unstable, and once collapsed require high inflation pressures to achieve re-expansion; ventilation is likely to be distributed preferentially to aerated lung. The pressure required to re-expand collapsed alveoli is higher than that required to distend the terminal bronchioles, and bronchiolar dilatation is common following ventilation of surfactant-depleted lungs (Slavin et al 1982, Rouby et al 1993). It has also been suggested that large stresses may occur on

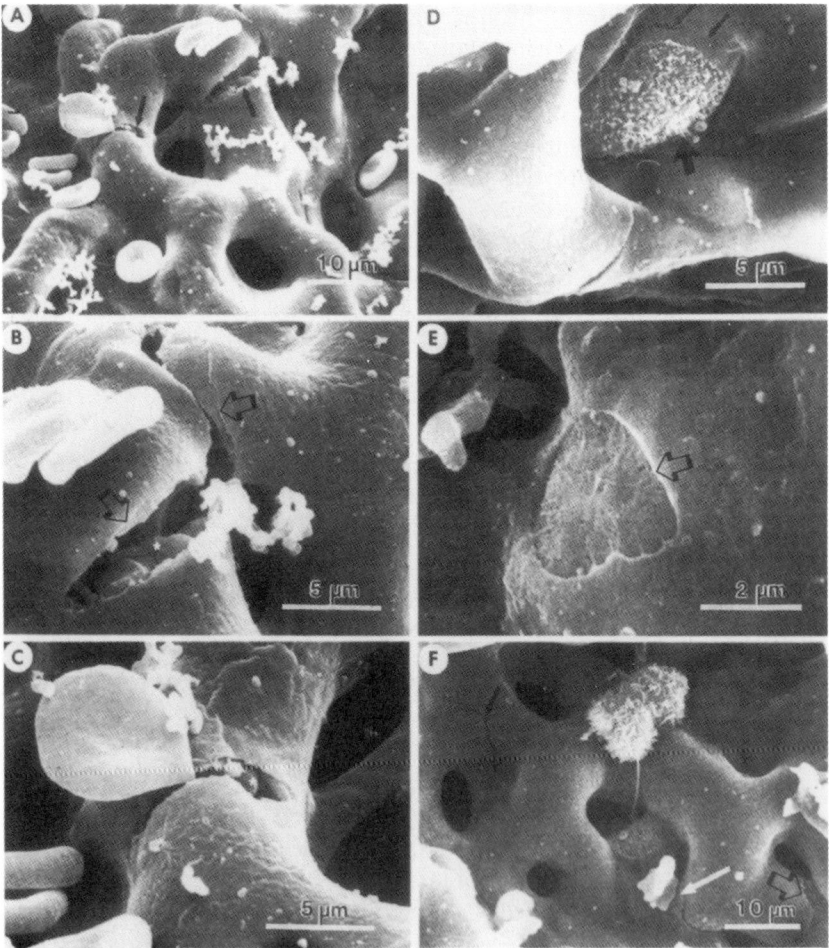

Fig. 2.2 Scanning electron micrographs showing examples of disruptions of blood-gas barrier in rabbit lungs inflated to a transpulmonary pressure of 20 cmH$_2$O and perfused with a transmural pressure of 52.5 cmH$_2$O. A: adjacent capillaries with complete rupture of blood gas barrier (solid arrows) at various angles to the capillary axis. Higher magnifications are shown in B and C. RBCs and proteinaceous material are seen on alveolar surface. D–F show lesions involving only the epithelium. Reproduced from Fu et al 1992 with permission.

alveolar walls sited between expanded and collapsed lung regions (Mead et al 1970; Lachmann 1992) and this may result in rupture of alveolar walls. If such stresses are important in the development of lung injury, then the rate of expansion of the airways and lung (i.e. the inspiratory flow rate) may be important; a high flow rate increased lung injury at a similar Vt in saline lavaged rabbits (Peevy et al 1990). Repeated collapse and re-expansion of alveoli also results in surfactant depletion (Lachmann 1992). The injury to lung tissue resulting from ventilation at low lung volumes appears to recruit granulocytes into the lung (Kawano et al 1987) and to induce an inflammatory response, which could possibly affect other organs (Kawano et al 1987, Burger et al 1990, Marini and Kelsen 1992).

The pressure required to maintain alveolar patency in surfactant-depleted lungs is less than that required to achieve re-expansion following collapse (Lachmann 1992). If alveolar recruitment can be maintained throughout the respiratory cycle with PEEP, the alveolar and airway collapse and the associated stresses as well as further surfactant depletion can be avoided (Lachmann 1992, Bos and Lachmann 1992). Surfactant-depleted lungs

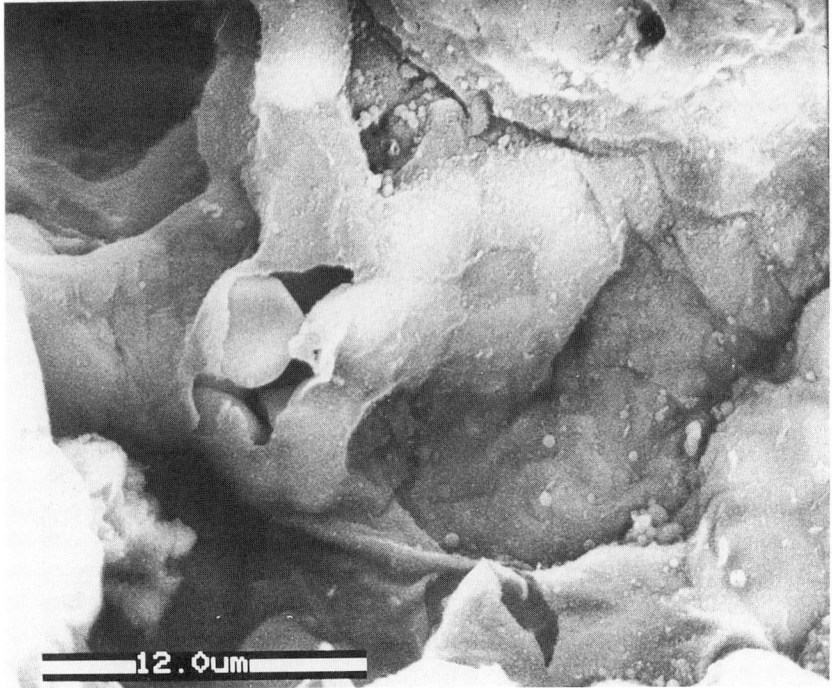

Fig. 2.3 Scanning electron micrograph showing an example of disruption of the blood gas barrier in a normal rabbit ventilated with a PIP of 40 cmH$_2$O for 4 h. Similar lesions were not observed in saline-lavaged rabbits ventilated with a PIP of 20–25 cmH$_2$O. (Preliminary observations in our laboratory: further work is in progress to confirm that the lesions are not artefactual.)

presumably remain susceptible to overdistention injury if ventilated with high Vt; thus it is probable that two distinct types of ventilator-induced lung injury may occur in surfactant-deficiency states.

CLINICAL STUDIES DEMONSTRATING VOLUTRAUMA IN ARDS

Although it has not been definitely established that the ventilator-induced lung injury demonstrated in animal models occurs in man, at present it seems reasonable to assume that it does. Rouby and colleagues recently described pathological changes in the lungs of 30 patients who died with ARDS (Rouby et al 1993). Many had intraparenchymal pseudocysts in inflammatory and fibrotic lung, which appeared to have formed from dilated alveolar ducts and terminal bronchioles (Fig. 2.4). In non-inflammatory (usually anterior) lung many areas of alveolar overdistension and rupture were seen (Fig. 2.5). These lesions were more common in patients who had been ventilated with a high PIP. Others have also described bronchiolar dilatation following mechanical ventilation (Slavin et al 1982), and emphysematous cysts in the anterior lung regions have been described in patients with ARDS even during pressure-limited ventilation (Toth et al 1992). A retrospective study of patients receiving extracorporeal support

Bronchiolar dilatation + emphysematous cysts suggestive of overdistension + pulmonary trauma in patients dying with ARDS? evidence of volutrauma?

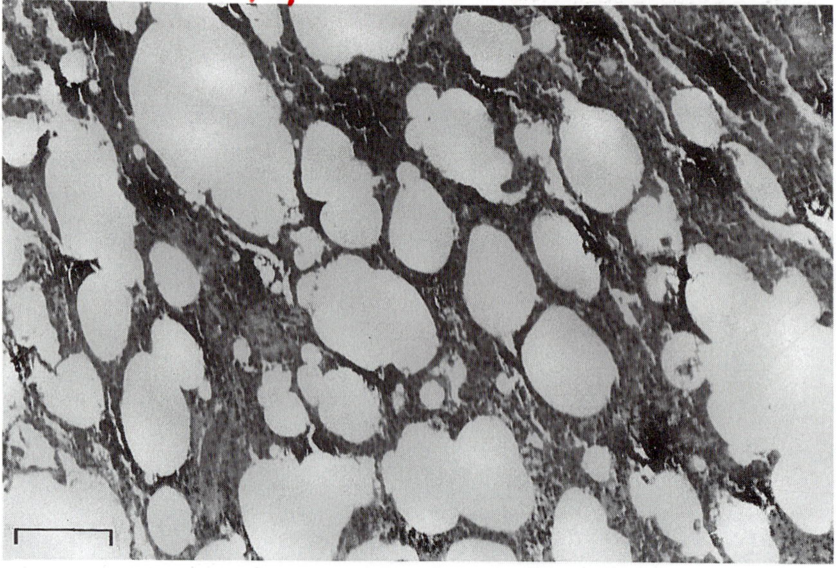

Fig. 2.4   Lung section from an inflammatory lung area of the left lower lobe of a patient with ARDS who died afer 7 days of ventilation with Vt of 650 ml, PIP of 45 cmH$_2$O and PEEP of 10 cmH$_2$O. Intraparenchymal pseudocysts are seen. Reproduced from Rouby et al 1993 with permission.

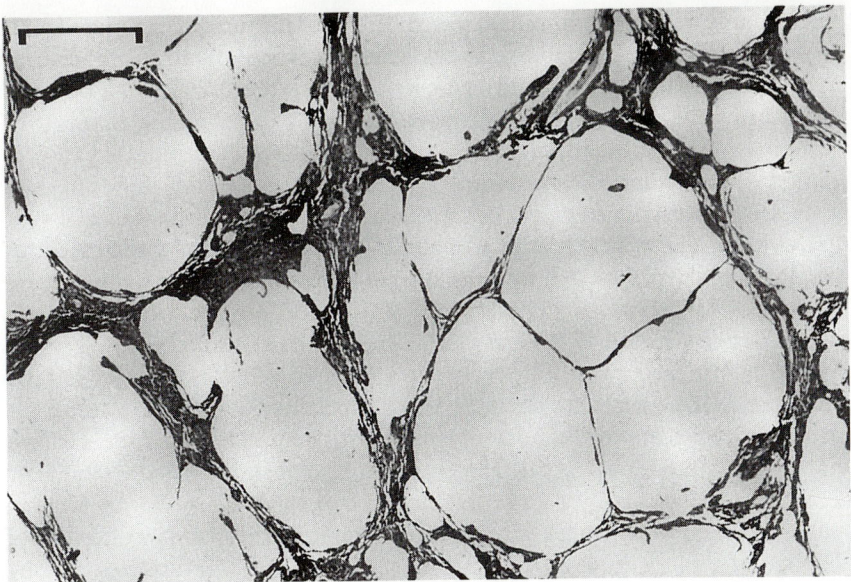

Fig. 2.5   Lung section from a non-inflammatory lung area from the left upper lobe of the same patient as Fig. 2.3. Severe airspace enlargement resulted from alveolar overdistension and destruction of alveolar septa. Reproduced from Rouby et al 1993 with permission.

for severe ARDS suggested that survival was inversely related to the prior duration of maximum ventilator support with high airway pressures and FiO_2 (Pranikoff et al 1994). Maximum support for > 5 days was associated with 21% survival, whereas with 1–2 days' maximum support survival was 75%. This observation may simply reflect the severity or evolution of the underlying illness, but most deaths were due to end-stage pulmonary fibrosis, suggesting a possible relationship to ventilator-induced injury.

THE LUNG IN ARDS

Gattinoni, Pesenti and colleagues in Milan have made substantial contributions to our understanding of lung mechanics and the effects of PEEP in ARDS. Using CT scans, they demonstrated that reduced compliance in early ARDS is not a result of a uniform increase in elastic recoil of lung tissue, but rather is due to a reduction in the volume of aerated lung; the remaining lung is non-aerated and does not contribute to ventilation. The amount of aerated lung may be only half to one-third of normal, but its specific compliance (defined as compliance per unit volume of aerated lung tissue) usually appears to be relatively normal (Gattinoni et al 1987). The lung can be divided into regions which are aerated and ventilated, those which are non-aerated but recruitable by PEEP, and those which are non-aerated and non-recruitable with PEEP (Gattinoni et al 1987). The non-

Early ARDS - volume of aerated lung falls → overall compliance ↓
- lung aerated + ventilated
Gattinoni : - lung non-aerated, but recruitable ī PEEP
- lung non-aerated and NOT recruitable

aerated lung occurs predominantly in the dependent regions (i.e. posteriorly in supine patients) and redistributes rapidly when patients are placed in the prone position (Gattinoni et al 1991, Langer et al 1988). The non-aeration of the dependent lung regions appears to be mainly a result of compression by the overlying lung; the amount of PEEP required to prevent end-expiratory collapse at any lung level is equal to the superimposed hydrostatic pressure from the lung above this level (Gattinoni et al 1993, Pelosi et al 1994). The lung thus behaves like a wet sponge; the distribution of water is relatively uniform throughout, but the lower regions are compressed by those above. The amount of PEEP required to recruit lung which is non-aerated as a result of this mechanism should be equal to the hydrostatic pressure resulting from the overlying lung. The density of lung tissue in ARDS varies from 0.5 to 0.8 g/ml, and the antero-posterior dimension of the chest in adults varies from 12 to 25 cm; thus the amount of PEEP required may vary from 6 cmH$_2$O (12 cm × 0.5 g/ml) to 20 cmH$_2$O (25 cm × 0.8 g/ml) in a large patient with severe ARDS; in an average patient it would not normally be more than 15 cmH$_2$O (Gattinoni et al 1993). A small amount of additional recruitment may sometimes be achieved with higher levels of PEEP, but this represents lung which is non-aerated as a result of different processes. An important implication of these findings is that if sufficient PEEP is applied to maximally recruit dependent lung regions, the non-dependent regions will be overdistended; the use of conventional Vt may then result in overdistension injury (see below).

IMPLICATIONS FOR CLINICAL MANAGEMENT

From the evidence reviewed so far, it appears that there are two important principles which should be followed to minimize ventilator-induced lung injury in early ARDS (1) maximize lung recruitment, and (2) limit PIP or P$_{PL}$, although such management has not yet been adequately evaluated in controlled clinical studies (Slutsky 1993). In the later stages of ARDS lung mechanics change and it is less clear whether pressure-limited strategies are important.

1. Maximize lung recruitment

Maximum lung recruitment should be obtained by the use of an appropriate level of PEEP (Lachmann 1992), and possibly other recruitment manoeuvres (see below). In early ARDS the thoracopulmonary pressure-volume curve usually shows a lower as well as an upper 'inflection point', and marked hysteresis. The lower inflection is a curved region over which the slope (i.e. compliance) increases, representing recruitment of previously collapsed alveoli. It has been suggested that PEEP should be set at a pressure above that of the lower inflection point (Bentio and Lemaire

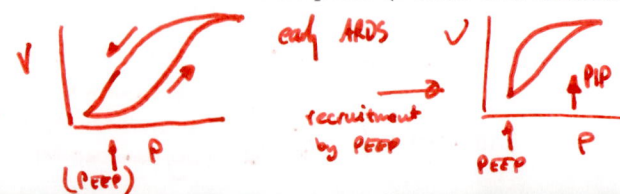

a) set PEEP above lower inflection point (of deflation curve?)
b) set PIP below upper inflection point (regulate Vt)

VENTILATORY SUPPORT IN ACUTE LUNG INJURY   31

(PEEP may be greater than 'best Peep' & FiO₂ <0.6, and co ↓?)

1990). Much of the hysteresis of the pressure-volume curve is thought to be due to lung recruitment, and the deflation curve may give a better indication of the pressure required to prevent end-expiratory collapse than the opening pressures shown by the inflation curve (Kolton et al 1982). Maximum recruitment is probably indicated by the elimination of the lower inflection point and a marked reduction of hysteresis (Bentio & Lemaire 1990). A simpler bedside approach is to determine the level of PEEP which minimizes the difference between end-expiratory and plateau pressure (P_{PL}) during ventilation (Suter et al 1975), whilst using a low Vt to ensure that the upper inflection point is not reached before end-inspiration; if this occurs the measured 'best compliance' will be less, and a lower PEEP level will be selected. The relationship between the level of PEEP selected using approaches designed to maximize recruitment and that chosen using oxygenation criteria (e.g. minimum PEEP for $FiO_2 < 0.6$ or the level of PEEP giving maximum oxygen delivery) has not been adequately determined. The best method for selecting PEEP is still not clear (Slutsky 1993), but fortunately in practice the level of PEEP chosen when attempting to maximize lung recruitment does not usually differ greatly from that which optimizes oxygenation; maximum recruitment may, however, require slightly higher PEEP and may have greater haemodynamic consequences.

2. Limit PIP or P_{PL}

c) P_{PL} unaffected by airway + breathing system resistance:
PIP overestimates Paw. $P_{PL} ≤ 30$ cm H₂O ? PIP ≤ 40 cm H₂O
d) Vt ≤ 7 ml/kg

The second principle is to use a sufficiently low Vt to avoid lung over-distension at end-inspiration; this goal may sometimes conflict with that of achieving adequate oxygenation. Because of the gravitational compression of dependent lung described above (Gattinoni et al 1993), the use of sufficient PEEP to prevent end-expiratory collapse of lung units in dependent regions will result in non-dependent regions operating at much higher lung volume, indeed some may be close to the upper inflection point of the pressure-volume curve at the beginning of inspiration (Bone 1993). If a Vt of 10–15 ml/kg is then delivered into a greatly reduced volume of aerated lung which is already almost fully distended this may result in considerable overdistension. There is evidence from autopsy studies and CT scan studies (Toth et al 1992) that much overdistension of non-dependent regions does occur (Rouby et al 1993). Such overdistension will be indicated by a high PIP and P_{PL}; because the specific compliance of aerated lung in early ARDS is usually relatively normal (Gattinoni et al 1987) the degree of distension of aerated lung will be similar to that of normal lung at the same P_{PL}. PIP is affected by the resistance of the endotracheal tube and the airways; P_{PL} gives a better indication of peak alveolar pressure and end-inspiratory lung distension. In sheep ventilation with a PIP of only 30 cmH_2O (and therefore P_{PL} less than this) for 48 hours resulted in lung injury (Tsuno et al 1990). However, the levels of PIP or P_{PL} required to induce lung injury cannot easily be extrapolated between species because of variations in lung and chest wall compliance (which affect the degree of lung distension at any airway pressure), and possible inter-species variation in susceptability to lung injury at a given distension (Parker et al 1993). P_{PL} should always be limited to <35 cmH$_2$O when possible (ACCP Consensus Committee 1994), but the safe upper limit for P_{PL} in ARDS is not known, and it may well be less than this. When it is possible to do so without compromising oxygenation or causing severe respiratory acidosis, it may be preferable to limit P_{PL} to 30 cmH$_2$O. A Vt of 6–7 ml/kg can be used initially in ARDS, and this should be reduced further if a high PIP or P_{PL} results. Vt of 4–7 ml/kg will often be required (Hickling et al 1994). Tidal volumes of 6 ml/kg have been shown to be safe and well tolerated in ARDS (Lee et al 1990, Kiiski et al 1992, Hickling et al 1994, Thomsen et al 1994).

Permissive hypercapnia

e) gradual increase in PaCO$_2$ better tolerated (catecholamines ↑)
f) inhaled NO reduces PHT + ②V dysfunction

These objectives can frequently not be achieved whilst maintaining normocapnia but if PaCO$_2$ is allowed to rise it is usually possible to maintain satisfactory oxygenation with a low Vt and PIP limited to 30–40 cmH$_2$O (Hickling et al 1990, 1994), or P_{PL} to 30–35 cmH$_2$O. A slightly higher level of PEEP may be required, as the mean airway pressure falls when Vt is reduced. Hypercapnia appears to be remarkably well tolerated even in critically ill patients, but is clearly contraindicated in patients with raised intracranial pressure, and should be introduced cautiously in patients with ischaemic heart disease or severely impaired left ventricular function. Most of the physiological effects of hypercapnia appear to be due to the resulting intracellular acidosis, and this is compensated relatively rapidly during sustained hypercapnia (at least in experimental models). In an isolated cat papillary muscle preparation (Foex & Fordham 1972), 75% of the reduction in force of contraction following an abrupt increase in PCO$_2$ of the perfusing fluid was corrected spontaneously over 60 minutes. It is likely that other physiological effects of hypercapnia could be minimized by ensuring that PCO$_2$ rises slowly. In normal man and animals cardiac output increases during hypercapnia as a result of increased sympathetic activity and catecholamine release, and myocardial contractility is increased (Cullen & Eger 1974). Splanchnic and renal blood flow also increase during hypercapnia in ewes (Tzouanakis et al 1993). Even severe acute hypercapnia (PaCO$_2$ 155–269 mmHg) was remarkably well tolerated in children with adequate oxygenation, and did not result in detectable residual neurological deficit (Goldstein et al 1990). In patients with severe impairment of ventricular function, however, myocardial depression from acute hypercapnia is a possibility, and it may therefore be sensible to avoid a sudden rise of $PaCO_2$. However, even critically ill patients tolerate marked acute respiratory acidosis well (Hickling et al 1994). In a randomized cross-over study of 10 patients with ARDS during neuromuscular blockade, cardiac output was higher during pressure-limited hypercapnic ventilation than during normocapnic ventilation, even in patients requiring inotropic drug infusions (Henderson S, personal communication). Pulmonary artery pressure rose minimally during hypercapnia (Fig. 2.6). Capellier and colleagues also found permissive hypercapnia to be well tolerated with a rise in car-

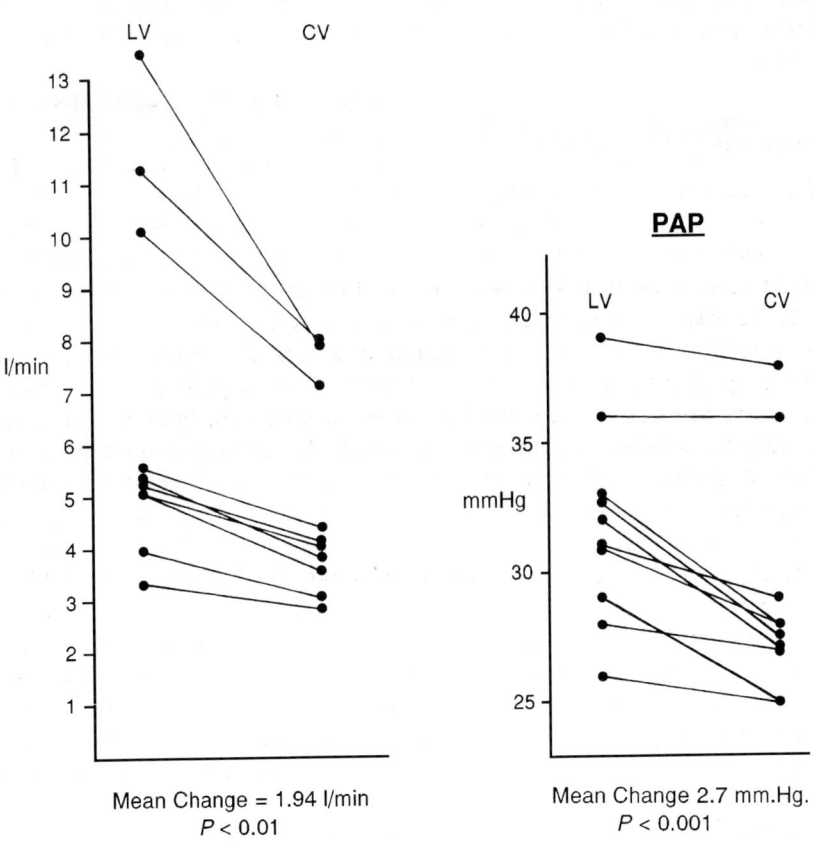

Fig. 2.6 Comparison of cardiac output and pulmonary artery pressure (PAP) in 10 patients with ARDS during a period of controlled hypoventilation (LV) and a period of conventional ventilation with normocapnia (CV), administered in random order with neuromuscular blockade during both periods. Mean $PaCO_2$ increased from 38.5 to 57.8 mmHg, cardiac output from 4.93 to 6.87 l/min ($P < 0.01$), and mean PA pressure from 29.1 to 31.8 mmHg ($P < 0.01$) from the CV to LV period. Drawn from data provided by Henderson S, personal communication.

diac output and only a modest increase in pulmonary artery pressure (Capellier et al 1992). Inhaled nitric oxide effectively reverses the pulmonary hypertension and right ventricular dysfunction resulting from permissive hypercapnia (Wysocki et al 1993).

Because of the potentially adverse effects of hypercapnia it has been suggested that pH should not be allowed to fall below 7.2 or 7.3. However, intracellular pH is compensated much more rapidly than extracellular pH during sustained hypercapnia. In addition many critically ill patients have a metabolic acidosis, and hydrogen ions, unlike CO_2, diffuse only slowly across cell membranes (Tang et al 1991). Furthermore, inadequate tissue perfusion is associated with marked intracellular hypercapnic acidosis which is not reflected in the arterial blood (Johnson & Weil 1991). For these reasons, arterial pH may not reflect intracellular pH, especially during the gradual onset of hypercapnia. The use of pH as a guide to the safe limit for hypercapnia may therefore not be entirely valid; our approach has been to allow hypercapnia as required in order to limit PIP and P_{PL}, provided cardiac output and oxygenation are satisfactory.

The use of bicarbonate or other agents to correct pH during permissive hypercapnia has not been adequately evaluated. Some issues and controversies relating to pressure-limited ventilation with permissive hypercapnia in ARDS have recently been reviewed (Hickling 1992). We have reported two uncontrolled series of patients (Hickling et al 1990, 1994) managed using this approach who had mortality rates lower than those predicted by APACHE II (16% vs 39.6% and 26.4% vs 53.3%). This ventilatory approach also reduced mortality and lung injury in saline-lavaged rabbits (Epton et al 1993). Controlled trials are being conducted to determine whether this ventilatory strategy does improve outcome in ARDS, but at present it seems justified to allow hypercapnia if this is necessary to limit P_{PL} (ACCP Consensus Committee 1994).

Tracheal gas insufflation   *h) flushing deadspace (tracheal catheter)*

Insufflation of air/O_2 through a tracheal catheter with the tip situated close to the carina can significantly improve CO_2 elimination during mechanical ventilation by flushing out the anatomical deadspace of the upper airway, as well as by causing some gas mixing distal to the catheter tip. The magnitude of $PaCO_2$ reduction is related mainly to the catheter flow rate; catheter position is less critical providing the tip is within a few centimetres of the carina (Nahum et al 1992). This technique is particularly effective with very low Vt, when anatomical deadspace is higher in proportion to Vt. Thus it may be useful in association with permissive hypercapnia, allowing a moderate reduction of $PaCO_2$ or a further reduction of Vt. Clinical experience in severe ARDS is limited, however, and several technical and safety issues remain (Ravenscraft et al 1993).

Spont. breathing — respiratory workload , PCV high transpulmy pressures
— pressure fluctuations , VCV low transpulmy pressures

VENTILATORY SUPPORT IN ACUTE LUNG INJURY   35

Neuromuscular blockade — neuromuscular dysfunction (critical illness polyneuropathy, myopathy)

SPONTANEOUS BREATHING VERSUS NEUROMUSCULAR BLOCKADE

If only limited ventilatory support is provided in ARDS, using intermittent mandatory ventilation (IMV) with a low Vt and limited PIP, the work of breathing is frequently high. An increase in cardiac output is then required to supply increased blood flow to the respiratory muscles, and respiratory muscle fatigue may occur. Respiratory drive during permissive hypercapnia with spontaneous breathing appears to be variable between patients, and the rate of adaptation to hypercapnia may vary (Hickling et al 1994). Some patients with quite severe hypercapnia have only moderately increased work of breathing, whereas others maintain a much lower $PaCO_2$ and a high work of breathing. Most patients, however, appear to tolerate spontaneous breathing well, even when the respiratory muscle workload is high (Hickling et al 1994). Patient discomfort does not usually occur, as patients becoming hypercapnic using this approach are usually unconscious or obtunded as a result of their underlying illness and hypercapnia. Work of breathing can be reduced by increasing ventilatory support (thus risking more ventilator-induced lung injury), by reducing respiratory drive with opiates, or by neuromuscular blockade. If pressure support ventilation (PSV) or pressure control ventilation (PCV) are used to reduce respiratory work, Vt should be monitored; high transpulmonary pressure (and regional lung distension) can occur with only moderate levels of airway pressure as a result of inspiratory effort. We limit pressure support to a level producing a Vt no greater than that achieved by a PIP of 30–40 cmH_2O during a mandatory breath with no respiratory muscle activity (Hickling 1992). During volume control ventilation (VCV) inspiratory effort will reduce the PIP, and transpulmonary pressure may be underestimated. PIP will then rise if inspiratory effort is abolished.

There has been increasing concern about the occurrence of neuromuscular dysfunction causing prolonged weakness following even relatively short-term use of neuromuscular blockade. A severe myopathy with elevated creatine kinase concentration appears to be associated with combined use of neuromuscular blockade (particularly with pancuronium and vecuronium) and steroids, but may occur with either (Hirano et al 1992, Barrett et al 1993, Hansen-Flaschen et al 1993) and a neuropathy may also develop. Prolonged neuromuscular blockade has also been widely recognized following continuous infusions of pancuronium or vecuronium, usually in patients with renal failure, probably due to accumulation of metabolites. Critical illness polyneuropathy is also increasingly recognized in a majority of patients with sepsis and multiple organ failure and may also be associated with myopathy (Coakley et al 1993). It therefore seems desirable to avoid the use of muscle relaxants if possible, and preferably to limit their use to short periods in patients who can not be managed adequately otherwise.

SPECIFIC VENTILATORY SUPPORT STRATEGIES

Many new ventilatory modes and variations of inspiratory flow profiles have been developed over the past decade, but there is little evidence to demonstrate any clear advantage for the newer forms of support.

Pressure control (PCV) or volume control ventilation (VCV)

The popularity of PCV has increased following the demonstration of ventilator-induced lung injury associated with high PIP. PCV allows continuous limitation of PIP whereas with VCV PIP will vary with changing lung mechanics. Because it appears to be the degree of lung distension that determines injury, it is, however, questionable whether transient increases in PIP associated with variable lung and chest wall mechanics during VCV are of great importance. Conversely, PCV allows Vt to increase as a result of a greater inspiratory effort as discussed above; this could potentially increase lung injury. In the absence of inspiratory muscle activity PCV results in a lower PIP than VCV at the same Vt. This is largely a result of the reduction of inspiratory flow at end-inspiration during PCV, which is associated with a lower pressure drop across the airways and endotracheal tube. Peak alveolar pressure (indicated by P_{PL}) and lung distension are similar with each mode. PCV results in a higher mean airway pressure than VCV with same Vt and I:E ratio because of the different inspiratory pressure and flow profile. Combined with more uniform distribution of ventilation, this could result in better oxygenation at the same levels of Vt and PEEP. Two recent studies failed to demonstrate a substantial difference in oxygenation or haemodynamics between PCV and VCV with equivalent ventilator settings (Lessard et al 1992, Davis et al 1994). Thus it is difficult to demonstrate major advantages of PCV, and it has the potential to be more injurious than VCV as a result of the more rapid 'ripping open' of airways and alveoli in early inspiration (Peevy et al 1990). Further studies are required to determine whether PCV has any real advantage over VCV. During extended or reverse I:E ratio ventilation there are considerable differences between the two modes in relation to the effects of intrinsic PEEP (see below).

(A) PCV results in a lower PIP th VCV at a given Vt but Vt = f (compliance) PCV

Extended and inverse ratio ventilation *ideal strategy - volume-limited PCV?*

Extended and inverse ratio ventilation have been widely used as a means of improving oxygenation in severe ARDS. As the duration of inspiration increases in proportion to the length of the respiratory cycle, mean airway pressure and mean alveolar pressure increase, and this is usually associated with improved oxygenation at the same level of PIP and PEEP (Marcy & Marini 1991). Thus a given mean airway pressure can be achieved at lower

Prolonged I/E : MAP↑, PIP↓
recruitment → best PEEP↓ *} +*
: gas trapping — EEV↑
— intrinsic PEEP↑ } —

VCV + intrinsic PEEP : PIP↑ V_T, MV → (↓V_T to reduce over-distension)

PCV + intrinsic PEEP : PIP → V_T, MV ↓ → $PaCO_2$ ↑

levels of PIP and PEEP, thereby reducing peak lung distension. The longer inspiration may be effective in recruiting some lung units which would not otherwise be re-expanded; some alveoli may need sustained traction for recruitment (Marcy & Marini 1991). The improvement in oxygenation is often time dependent and the maximum benefit may not occur for several hours (Marcy & Marini 1991). The distribution of ventilation may also improve with prolonged inspiratory time, contributing to improved oxygenation. As the expiratory time is progressively shortened, gas trapping occurs (i.e. incomplete expiration) resulting in increased end-expiratory volume and intrinsic PEEP. This is another important mechanism resulting in improved oxygenation. It has been suggested that there may be theoretical advantages to creating intrinsic PEEP in this way rather than using applied PEEP in ARDS (Lachmann 1992), but a real benefit has not been demonstrated. Indeed there is no clear evidence that inverse ratio ventilation improves outcome, although encouraging results have been reported (Andersen 1989, Thomsen et al 1994). There are probably advantages in achieving adequate oxygenation and lung recruitment by using PEEP to prevent end-expiratory collapse when this can be achieved with levels of PEEP up to 15 or occasionally 20 cmH$_2$O (i.e. levels equivalent to the superimposed pressure from the overlying lung). When satisfactory oxygenation can not be achieved at these levels of PEEP however, it may be preferable to increase mean airway pressure further by extending the I:E ratio rather than increasing PEEP further (ACCP Consensus Committee 1994). This usually requires heavy sedation or paralysis.

When intrinsic PEEP occurs during inverse I:E ratio ventilation, the consequences differ depending on whether VCV or PCV is used. During VCV, as intrinsic PEEP increases PIP rises and Vt and minute ventilation remain constant. To prevent potentially dangerous lung overdistension, usually either Vt should be reduced or the expiratory time increased; hypercapnia should be accepted (ACCP Consensus Committee 1994). In contrast during PCV, as intrinsic PEEP increases PIP remains constant and Vt and minute ventilation decrease, resulting in increased PaCO$_2$. Either technique is acceptable provided that PIP or P$_{PL}$ and Vt are carefully monitored. With either approach the haemodynamic consequences of the increased mean airway pressure and intrinsic PEEP must be carefully monitored.

Ⓑ extend I:E if PaO_2 ↓ at PEEP = 15-20 a H$_2$O

Monitor PIP/P, V_T and haemodynamics

Other support strategies

Clinical trials of high frequency ventilation (HFV) in both ARDS and neonatal RDS have been disappointing and have failed to demonstrate an improved outcome. However, the implementation of HFV in some of these studies has been criticised because recruitment manoeuvres were not routinely used and mean airway pressure may not have been sufficiently high (Bryan & Froese 1991). During HFV it is possible to take advantage of the

? HFV
? HFO
NB recruitment

hysteresis seen in surfactant-depleted lungs by using a sustained inflation to achieve maximum recruitment, and then maintaining the lung at a pressure above that at which de-recruitment occurs (Kolton et al 1982). Sufficient ventilation can be achieved with very small oscillations of airway pressure, in contrast to conventional ventilation which requires large phasic changes in airway pressure allowing de-recruitment of the lung at end expiration. It has been demonstrated in saline-lavaged rabbits that even HFV resulted in lung injury if sufficient recruitment of lung volume was not achieved (McCulloch et al 1988). Further controlled trials of HFV are being conducted using protocols designed to optimize lung recruitment. A number of other ventilatory approaches have been developed including pressure-release ventilation, proportional-assist ventilation and various servo-controlled modes of ventilation, but there is at present no evidence that they have any advantage over alternative modes (ACCP Consensus Committee 1994). Prone positioning and 'kinetic therapy' (frequent body position changes using a rotating bed) have been shown to improve gas exchange in ARDS, although the benefit may be transient (Langer et al 1988, Gattinoni et al 1991, Hormann et al 1994). An improvement in outcome has not been demonstrated.

Intra-tracheal instillation of perfluorocarbon is an exciting new technique. In saline-lavaged rabbits ventilated with an FiO_2 of 1, the instillation of 15 ml/kg of intra-tracheal perfluorocarbon resulted in an increase of PaO_2 from 75 to 420 mmHg, and a reduction of $PaCO_2$ and airway pressures (Tutuncu et al 1993). This technique appears to improve lung compliance and facilitate gas exchange, and may reduce shear stresses on the lung; it clearly deserves further evaluation. Exogenous surfactant administration has also been evaluated in preliminary studies in sepsis-induced ARDS, showing improvement in oxygenation and a non-significant reduction in mortality (Wiedemann et al 1992). It is very expensive in adults, however, and further evaluation is required (Lewis & Jobe 1993).

CLINICAL STUDIES OF PRESSURE-LIMITED VENTILATION STRATEGIES

No controlled trials have yet to determine whether the ventilatory approaches described above improve the outcome in ARDS, but a number of uncontrolled studies suggest that this may be the case. A survival rate of 45% was achieved in 51 patients meeting the 1979 ECMO study entry criteria (Suchyta et al 1991). Most were managed using low Vt (5–8 ml/kg) with pressure-limited ventilation, and $PaCO_2$ was allowed to rise moderately providing pH remained $\geq$ 7.3 (Morris A, personal communication). Control group patients in the randomized trial of $ECCO_2R$ at the same institution had a similar survival rate (42%); the better than expected outcome may in part be due to pressure limitation and permissive hypercapnia

(Morris et al 1992). More recently the same group have reported a survival rate of 60% in 53 patients with ARDS using a similar strategy (Thomsen et al 1994). Falke and colleagues reported 76% survival in 49 patients with severe ARDS who were referred for consideration of extracorporeal support. In patients not receiving such support survival was 92% (Lewandowski et al 1993). These patients were initially managed with pressure-limited ventilation and permissive hypercapnia and frequent body position changes. The patient population was selected and none were immunocompromised, but nevertheless the results are impressive. Andersen and colleagues have also reported a survival rate of 49% in patients with very severe ARDS using a pressure-limited strategy with pressure control inverse ratio ventilation (Andersen 1989). Hickling et al reported survival rates of 84% and 74% in 2 series of patients with ARDS managed with pressure limitation and permissive hypercapnia (Hickling et al 1994).

It is not possible to conclude that the improved outcome in these studies results from altered ventilatory strategies; many other changes in management have occurred in recent years, and the patient populations in these studies may differ from those of earlier series with respect to age, comorbidities and varying definitions of ARDS. Randomized trials will be required to determine whether outcomes can be improved by modified ventilatory strategies; satisfactory studies will be difficult to conduct. Preliminary results have been reported of the first 19 patients with severe ARDS (Murray Score > 3.0) in a randomized trial comparing pressure-limited ventilation (Vt < 6 ml/kg, PIP < 49 cmH_2O, permissive hypercapnia, PEEP above inflection point, PCIRV if required) with conventional ventilation (Vt 12 ml/kg, normocapnia, PEEP to maintain PaO_2 > 60 mmHg and FiO_2 ≤ 0.6). The mean APACHE II Score was 26 in the pressure-limited group and 18 in the control group. PaO_2/FiO_2 ratio and compliance were initially similar but both improved in the pressure-limited group and became significantly higher. Overall mortality was similar, but 4 deaths from respiratory failure occurred in the control group and none in the pressure-limited group (Amato et al 1993). Other randomized trials are commencing or being designed, and their results are awaited with great interest.

KEY POINTS FOR CLINICAL PRACTICE

- Animal studies have consistently demonstrated that ventilation of normal lungs with high end-inspiratory volume induces acute lung injury histologically indistinguishable from ARDS. In sheep this occurs with PIP as low as 30 cmH_2O.
- In animal studies of surfactant-depleted lungs, ventilation at low end expiratory lung volume, allowing repeated end expiratory collapse, also induces severe injury even when very low Vt and PIP are used. If ventilation is continued for a sufficient period of time, severe respiratory failure and death occur in both models.

- In severe ARDS, the amount of aerated lung contributing to ventilation is reduced, and may be only one-third to one-half of normal. This aerated lung may often have a relatively normal specific compliance. A Vt of 10–15 ml/kg and adequate PEEP frequently results in overdistension of this aerated lung, indicated by high PIP and P_{PL}.
- It seems reasonable at present to assume that such ventilator-induced lung injury occurs in patients with ARDS, although this has not been definitely established. Strategies to avoid such ventilator-induced injury include:
- Obtain maximum lung recruitment using PEEP. If satisfactory oxygenation is not achieved with PEEP of 15 cmH_2O (perhaps 20 cmH_2O for large patients) extended or inverse ratio ventilation should usually be used rather than further increases in PEEP. PIP (VCV) or Vt and minute ventilation (PCV), haemodynamics and intrinsic PEEP should be monitored during inverse ratio ventilation.
- Limit P_{PL} to 30 or 35 cmH_2O by reducing Vt (VCV) or setting appropriate pressure (PCV).
- In order to achieve these goals $PaCO_2$ may be allowed to rise to quite high levels if necessary, providing pH remains at an acceptable level. A pH of 7.1 (perhaps even lower) is probably acceptable providing cardiovascular function remains satisfactory and no adverse effects occur.
- Permissive hypercapnia should not be used in the presence of intracranial hypertension, and should be introduced cautiously and gradually in patients with severe ischaemic heart disease, hypotension or arrhythmias.

REFERENCES

ACCP Consensus Committee (Chairman, A S Slutsky) 1994 Report of American College of Chest Physicians Consensus Conference on Mechanical Ventilation. Intensive Care Med 20:
64–79 (Part 1): 150–162 (Part 2), Crit Care Med 1994 (in press) and Chest 1993; 104: 1833–1859
Amato M B P, Barbas C S V, Medelros D M et al 1993 A new approach to mechanical ventilation in ARDS: Preliminary results of a prospective randomized protocol. Intensive Care Med 19: S42
Andersen J B 1989 Ventilatory strategy catastrophic lung disease. Inversed ratio ventilation (IRV) and combined high frequency ventilation (CHFV). Acta Anaesthesiol Scand 33 (Suppl 90): 145–148
Barrett S, Mourani S, Villareal C et al 1993 Rhabdomyolysis associated with status asthmaticus. Crit Care Med 21: 151–153
Bentio S, Lemaire F 1990 Pulmonary pressure-volume relationship in acute respiratory distress syndrome in adults: Role of positive end expiratory pressure. J Crit Care 15: 27–34
Bone R C 1993 The ARDS Lung — New insights from computed tomography (Editorial). JAMA 269: 2134–2135
Borelli M, Kolobow T, Spatola R et al 1988 Severe acute respiratory failure managed with continuous positive airway pressure and partial extracorporeal carbon dioxide removal by an artificial membrane lung. Am Rev Respir Dis 138: 1480–1487
Bos J A H, Lachmann B 1992 Effects of artificial ventilation on surfactant function. In: Rugheimer E (ed) New aspects on respiratory failure. Springer, Berlin, pp 194–208
Bryan A C and Froese A B 1991 Reflections on the HIFI trial. Paediatrics 87: 565–567

Burger D, Fung D, Bryan A C 1990 Lung injury in a surfactant-deficient lung is modified by indomethacin. J Appl Physiol 69: 2067–2071

Capellier G, Toth J L, Walker P et al 1992 Haemodynamic effects of permissive hypercapnia. Am Rev Respir Dis 146: A527

Coakley J H, Nagendran K, Honavar M et al 1993 Preliminary observations on the neuromuscular abnormalities in patients with organ failure and sepsis. Intensive Care Med 19: 323–328

Coker P J, Hernandez L A, Peevy K J et al 1992 Increased sensitivity to mechanical ventilation after surfactant inactivation in young rabbit lungs. Crit Care Med 20: 635–640

Cullen D J, Eger E I 1974 Cardiovascular effects of carbon dioxide in man. Anesthesiology 41: 345–349

Davis K, Branson R, Porembka D 1994 Pressure control vs volume control: is flow waveform the difference? Crit Care Med 22: A89

Dorrington K L, McRae K M, Gardaz J P et al 1989 A randomised comparison of total extracorporeal CO_2 removal with conventional mechanical ventilation in experimental hyaline membrane disease. Intensive Care Med 15: 184–191

Dreyfuss D, Saumon G 1992 Barotrauma is volutrauma, but which volume is the one responsible? Intensive Care Med 18: 139–141

Dreyfuss D, Saumon G 1993 Role of tidal volume, FRC, and end-inspiratory volume in the development of pulmonary edema following mechanical ventilation. Am Rev Respir Dis 148: 1197–1203

Dreyfuss D, Soler P, Saumon G 1992 Spontaneous resolution of pulmonary edema caused by short periods of cyclic overinflation. J Appl Physiol 72(6): 2081–2089

Dreyfuss D, Soler P, Basset G, Saumon G 1988 High inflation pressure pulmonary edema. Respective effects of high airway pressure, high tidal volume and positive end-expiratory pressure. Am Rev Respir Dis 137: 1159–1164

Dreyfuss D, Basset G, Soler P, Saumon G 1985 Intermittent positive-pressure hyperventilation with high inflation pressures produces pulmonary microvascular injury in rats. Am Rev Respir Dis 132: 880–884

Epton M, Neil A, Graham P et al 1993 The effects of low volume pressure limited ventilation on acute lung injury in surfactant depleted rabbits. Am Rev Respir Dis 148: A890

Foex P, Fordham R M M 1972 Intrinsic myocardial recovery from the negative inotropic effects of acute hypercapnia. Cardiovasc Res 6: 257–262

Fu Z, Costello M, Tsukimoto K et al 1992 High lung volume increases stress failure in pulmonary capillaries. J Appl Physiol 73: 123–133

Gattinoni L, Pesenti A, Avalli L et al 1987 Pressure-volume curve of total respiratory system in acute respiratory failure. Computed tomographic study. Am Rev Respir Dis 136: 730–736

Gattinoni L, Pelosi P, Vitale G et al 1991 Body position changes redistribute lung computed-tomographic density in patients with acute respiratory failure. Anesthesiol 74: 15–23

Gattinoni L, D'Andrea L, Pelosi P et al 1993 Regional effects and mechanism of positive end-expiratory pressure in early adult respiratory distress syndrome. JAMA 269: 2122–2127

Goldstein B, Shannon D C, Todres D 1990 Supercarbia in children: clinical course and outcome. Crit Care Med 18: 166–168

Hamilton P P, Onayemi A, Smith J A et al 1983 Comparison of conventional and high frequency ventilation: oxygenation and lung pathology. J Appl Physiol 55: 131–138

Hansen-Flaschen J, Cowen J, Raps E 1993 Neuromuscular blockade in the intensive care unit — more than we bargained for. Am Rev Respir Dis 147: 234–236

Hickling K G 1990 Ventilatory management of ARDS: can it affect the outcome? Intensive Care Med 16: 219–226

Hickling K G 1992 Low volume ventilation with permissive hypercapnia in the adult respiratory distress syndrome. Clinical Intensive Care 3: 67–78

Hickling K G, Henderson S J, Jackson R 1990 Low mortality associated with low volume pressure limited ventilation with permissive hypercapnia in severe adult respiratory distress syndrome. Intensive Care Med 16: 372–377

Hickling K G, Henderson S, Walsh J et al 1994 Low mortality using low volume pressure limited ventilation with permissive hypercapnia in ARDS: a prospective study. Crit Care Med 22: 1568–1578

Hirano M, Ott B, Raps E et al 1992 Acute quadriplegic myopathy: a complication of treatment with steroids, nondepolarising blocking agents, or both. Neurology 42: 2082–2087

Hormann C, Baum M, Putensen C et al 1994 Effect of kinetic therapy in patients with severe adult respiratory distress syndrome. Crit Care Med 22: A87

Johnson BA and Weil MH 1991 Redefining ischaemia due to circulatory failure as dual defects of oxygen deficits and of carbon dioxide excesses. Crit Care Med 19: 1432–1438

Johnson W H, Young J A, Parker J C et al 1990 High mean airway pressure exacerbates barotrauma induced microvascular injury in isolated perfused rabbit lungs. FASEB J 4: A970

Kawano T, Mori S, Cybulsky M et al 1987 Effect of granulocyte depletion in a ventilated surfactant-depleted lung. J Appl Physiol 62:27–33

Kiiski R, Takala J, Kari A, Milic-Emili J 1992 Effect of tidal volume on gas exchange and oxygen transport in the adult respiratory distress syndrome. Am Rev Respir Dis 146: 1131–1135

Kolobow T, Moretti M P, Fumagali R et al 1987 Severe impairment in lung function induced by high peak airway pressure during mechanical ventilation. An experimental study. Am Rev Respir Dis 135: 312–315

Kolton M, Cattran C, Kent C et al 1982 Oxygenation during high-frequency ventilation compared with conventional mechanical ventilation in two models of lung injury. Anesth Analg 61:323–332

Lachmann B 1992 Open up the lung and keep the lung open. Intensive Care Med 18: 319–321

Lachmann B, Robertson B, Vogel J 1980 In vivo lung lavage as an experimental model of the respiratory distress syndrome. Acta Anaesthesiol Scand 24: 231–236

Langer M, Mascheroni D, Marcolin R, Gattinoni L 1988 The prone position in ARDS patients: A clinical study. Chest 94: 103–107

Lee P C, Helsmoortel C M, Cohn S M, Fink M P 1990 Are low tidal volumes safe? Chest 97: 425–429

Lessard M, Guerot E, Mariette C et al 1992 Pressure controlled versus volume-controlled ventilation in patients with adult respiratory distress syndrome (ARDS). Am Rev Respir Dis 146: A454

Lewandowski K, Falke K J, Rossaint R et al 1993 Low mortality associated with advanced treatment including V-V ECMO for severe ARDS. Intensive Care Med 19: S42

Lewis J F, Jobe A H 1993 Surfactant and the adult respiratory distress syndrome. Am Rev Respir Dis 147: 218–233

McCulloch P R, Forkert P G, Froese A B 1988 Lung volume maintenance prevents lung injury during high frequency oscillation in surfactant-deficient rabbits. Am Rev Respir Dis 137: 1185 1192

Marcy T W, Marini J J 1991 Inverse ratio ventilation in ARDS — Rationale and implementation. Chest 100: 494–504

Marini J J, Kelsen S G 1992 Re-targeting ventilatory objectives in adult respiratory distress syndrome: New treatment prospects — persistent questions. (Editorial) Am Rev Respir Dis 146: 2–3

Mead J, Takishima T, Leith D 1970 Stress distribution in lungs: a model of pulmonary elasticity. J Appl Physiol 28: 596–608

Morris A H, Wallace C J, Clemmer T P et al 1992 Final Report: Computerised protocol controlled clinical trial of new therapy which includes $ECCO_2R$ for ARDS. Am Rev Respir Dis 146: A184

Muscadere J G, Mullen J B M, Gan K et al 1992 Tidal ventilation at low airway pressures can cause pulmonary barotrauma. Am Rev Respir Dis 146: A454

Nahum A, Ravenscraft S A, Nakos G et al 1992 Tracheal gas insufflation during pressure-control ventilation. Am Rev Respir Dis 146: 1411–1418

Nardell E A, Brody J S 1982 Determinants of mechanical properties of rat lung during postnatal development. J Appl Physiol 53: 140–148

Parker J C, Roohparvar S, Foster J et al 1991 High peak inspiratory pressures (PIP) affect the rate of bacterial clearance from rabbit lungs. Am Rev Respir 143: A570

Parker J C, Hernandez L A, Peevy K J 1993 Mechanisms of ventilator-induced lung injury. Crit Care Med 21: 131–143

Peevy K J, Hernandez L A, Moise A A et al 1990 Barotrauma and microvascular injury in lungs of nonadult rabbits: Effect of ventilation pattern. Crit Care Med 18: 634–637

Pelosi P, D'Andrea L, Vitale G et al 1994 Vertical gradient of regional lung inflation in adult respiratory distress syndrome. Am J Respir Crit Care Med 149: 8–13

Pranikoff T, Steimle C N, Anderson H L et al 1994 What is the LD50 of mechanical ventilation in severe ARF?: Evidence from the ECLS experience. Crit Care Med 22: A206

Ravenscraft S A, Burke W C, Nahum A et al 1993 Tracheal gas insufflation augments CO_2 clearance during mechanical ventilation. Am Rev Respir Dis 148: 345–351

Robertson B 1984 Lung surfactant. In: Robertson B, Van Golde L, Battenburg J (eds) Pulmonary surfactant. Elsevier, Amsterdam.

Rouby J J, Lherm T, Lassale E et al 1993 Histologic aspects of pulmonary barotrauma in critically ill patients with acute respiratory failure. Intensive Care Med 19: 383–389

Sandhar B K, Niblett D J, Argiras E P et al 1988 Effects of positive end-expiratory pressure on hyaline membrane formation in a rabbit model of the neonatal respiratory distress syndrome. Intensive Care Med 14: 538–546

Slavin G, Nunn J F, Crow J, Dore C 1982 Bronchiolectasis — a complication of artificial ventilation. Br Med J 285: 931–935

Slutsky A S 1993 Barotrauma and alveolar recruitment. Intensive Care Med 19: 369–371

Suchyta M R, Clemmer T P, Orme J F et al 1991 Increased survival of ARDS patients with severe hypoxemia (ECMO criteria). Chest 99: 951–955

Suter P, Fairley B, Isenberg M 1975 Optimum end-expiratory airway pressure in patients with acute pulmonary failure. N Engl J Med 292: 284–289

Tang W, Weil M H, Gazmuri R J et al 1991 Reversible impairment of myocardial contractility due to hypercarbic acidosis in the isolated perfused rat heart. Crit Care Med 19: 218–224

Thomsen G E, Morris A H, Pope D et al 1994 Mechanical ventilation of patients with adult respiratory distress syndrome using reduced tidal volumes. Crit Care Med 22: A205

Toth J L, Capellier G, Walker P et al 1992 Lung emphysematous changes in ARDS. Am Rev Respir Dis 145: A184

Tsuno K, Miura K, Takeya M et al 1991 Histopathologic pulmonary changes from mechanical ventilation at high peak airway pressures. Am Rev Respir Dis 143: 1115–1120

Tsuno K, Prato P, Kolobow T 1990 Acute lung injury from mechanical ventilation at moderately high airway pressures. J Appl Physiol 69: 956–961

Tutuncu A, Faithfull N, Lachmann B 1993 Intratracheal perfluorocarbon administration combined with mechanical ventilation in experimental respiratory distress syndrome: Dose-dependent improvement of gas exchange. Crit Care Med 21: 962–969

Tzouanakis A E, Nguyen T, Tao W et al 1993 Effect of permissive hypercapnia on renal and mesenteric blood flow in an ovine model. Am Rev Respir Dis 148: A891

Wiedemann H, Baughman R, deBoisblanc B et al 1992 A multi-censored trial in human sepsis-induced ARDS of an aerosolised human surfactant (Exosurf). Am Rev Respir Dis 145: A184

Wysocki M, Vignon E, Roupie E et al 1993 Improvement in right ventricular function with inhaled nitric oxide in patients with the adult respiratory distress syndrome and permissive hypercapnia. Am Rev Respir Dis 148: A350

Principles of ventilatory support:

1) Avoid high PIP
2) Avoid low end-expiratory volumes (airway collapse)
3) Avoid high V_T (> 10 ml/kg) $\dot{=}$ ARDS
   - specific compliance of aerated-ventilated lung compartment is near-normal

4) a) Maximize recruitment with PEEP up to 15cm H_2O (? 20cm H_2O in large individuals?)

   b) further recruitment manoeuvres include
      i) $\uparrow$ I/E
      ii) IRV ($\uparrow\uparrow$ I/E!)

   c) Monit PIP (VCV) or V_T, MV (PCV)

   d) Monitor intrinsic PEEP and haemodynamics

5) Limit P_{PL} to 30-35cm H_2O: $\downarrow V_t$ (VCV)
   set appropriate PIP (PCV)

6) Permissive hypercapnia: pH$_a$ of 7.1 acceptable if stable haemodynamics
   - risk factor - space-occupying intracranial lesion
     IHD
     hypotension
     dysrhythmias

3. Exogenous surfactant administration for ARDS

J. F. Lewis   R. A. W. Veldhuizen

[handwritten annotation: Exogenous surfactant - novel (experimental) treatment ∴ adults]

[handwritten annotation: Dipalmitoyl phosphatidylcholine + phosphatidylglycerol + others]

INTRODUCTION   *[handwritten annotation: Surfactant associated protein (SP-A – D)]*

Exogenous surfactant administration is a relatively novel therapeutic approach for adult patients with acute respiratory distress syndrome (ARDS). Over the last four years, basic research efforts have proved sufficiently successful that this treatment modality is currently being tested in clinical trials. In this chapter, a brief overview of the pulmonary surfactant system will be given, followed by a rationale for administering exogenous surfactant to patients with ARDS. Subsequently, various factors felt to be important in the design of optimal surfactant treatment strategies for these patients will be outlined. Finally, a specific approach to treating patients with ARDS will be proposed, with the goal of optimizing responses to exogenous surfactant administration.

Pulmonary surfactant

[handwritten annotation: Surface tension reduced by monomolecular phospholipid layer.]

Pulmonary surfactant prevents alveolar collapse by reducing the surface tension at the air–liquid interface of the alveoli (King & Clements 1972). The composition of surfactant is highly conserved among species and consists of a mixture of 90% lipids and 10% proteins (Possmayer et al 1984, Shelley et al 1984). Phosphatidylcholine (PC) represents 70% of the surfactant lipid, with a high percentage present as the disaturated species, dipalmitoylphosphatidylcholine (DPPC). The second most abundant lipid is phosphatidylglycerol (10%). Phosphatidylethanolamine, sphingomyelin, phosphatidylinositol, lysophosphatidylcholine and neutral lipids are present in lower amounts. Surfactant also contains 4 different proteins designated as surfactant-associated protein A (SP-A), SP-B, SP-C and SP-D (Persson et al 1988, Possmayer 1988).

Surface tension reduction by surfactant is accomplished by the formation of a monomolecular phospholipid layer enriched in DPPC at the air–liquid interface. The other components of surfactant are felt to be necessary for the generation and maintenance of this DPPC monolayer. For example, the two hydrophobic proteins SP-B and SP-C, have been shown to have an important role in generating the monolayer (Yu & Possmayer 1990,

1992), while SP-A, a hydrophilic protein, has a biophysical role in enhancing the effects of SP-B (Possmayer 1988). Furthermore, SP-A has other
important functions within the lung including the regulation of surfactant
reuptake and secretion by Type II cells (Wright & Dobbs 1991); the formation of a unique alveolar structural form of surfactant called tubular
myelin (Suzuki et al 1989); counteracting inhibition of surfactant by blood
proteins (Cockshutt et al 1990); and modulating host defence mechanisms
(Van Iwaarden et al 1990). The fourth surfactant-associated protein, SP-
D, has not been shown to contribute to the surface tension reducing properties of surfactant, but rather appears to be involved in host defence
(Hawgood & Shiffer 1991, Van Iwaarden et al 1992).

Surfactant cellular metabolism involves synthesis within the endoplas-
mic reticulum of Type II pneumocytes, storage in lamellar bodies and subsequent secretion into the alveolar space (Wright & Clements 1987,
Wright & Dobbs 1991). Within the alveoli, the newly secreted lamellar
bodies are converted into the lattice-like, tubular myelin structures which
are thought to be precursors of the phospholipid monolayer. Small vesicular lipid structures are then formed from the monolayer which, in turn,

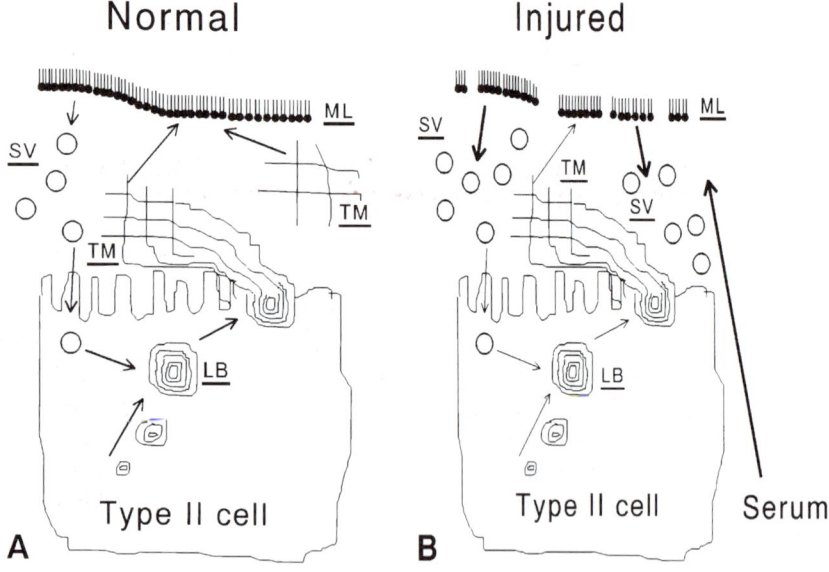

Fig. 3.1   Schematic of the metabolic life cycle of surfactant. A. In normal lungs surfactant
is synthesized in the Type II cells, secreted into the alveolar space, converted to tubular
myelin which is thought to be the precursor of the monolayer. During respiration small
vesicles are formed which are taken up and recycled or degraded. B. In injured lungs
synthesis and secretion of surfactant is decreased (thin arrows), the ability to form a
monolayer is impaired and the formation of small vesicles is enhanced (thick arrows). In
addition serum proteins leak into the airspace and further decrease surfactant activity (thick
arrows). LB = Lamellar body; ML = Monolayer; SV = Small vesicles; TM = Tubular
myelin.

may be taken up by the Type II cell for degradation or recycling (Fig. 3.1A) (Wright & Clements 1987, Wright & Dobbs 1991). Surfactant obtained from the lungs, either by whole lung lavage or bronchoalveolar lavage, can be separated via differential centrifugation into large surfactant aggregates (LA) consisting of lamellar bodies, tubular myelin and large vesicular structures; and small surfactant aggregates (SA) or small vesicular structures (Baritussio et al 1984, Gross & Narine 1989). Analysis of these fractions obtained from normal lungs reveals that phospholipid composition is similar for LA and SA, but SA contain less surfactant-associated proteins. The major difference between LA and SA is, however, their functional activity. LA are very surface active when tested in vitro and in vivo whereas SA are inactive (Yamada et al 1990, Veldhuizen et al 1993).

An area of surfactant research which has recently attracted considerable *Host defence* interest is the role of the surfactant system in host defence and immunity. In vitro studies have demonstrated the effects of surfactant and its components on alveolar macrophage functions (Hoffman et al 1987, Hayakawa et al 1989), alveolar and peripheral blood lymphocyte functions (Ansfield et al 1980a,b), inflammatory cell cytokine release (Speer et al 1991, Thomassen et al 1992), and on bacteria and viruses themselves (LaForce et al 1973, Van Iwaarden et al 1991). Future studies, including in vivo experiments evaluating the effects of exogenous surfactant on the host's inflammatory response, are warranted.

RATIONALE FOR EXOGENOUS SURFACTANT THERAPY IN ACUTE RESPIRATORY DISTRESS SYNDROME (ARDS)

There are several reasons to be optimistic about the use of exogenous surfactant for the treatment of patients with ARDS. First, it is highly effective in neonatal respiratory distress syndrome (nRDS), a condition in which there is a primary deficiency of surfactant. Secondly, surfactant alterations have been observed in bronchoalveolar lavage (BAL) samples obtained from patients with ARDS and are felt to contribute to the lung dysfunction associated with this disease. Thirdly, exogenous surfactant administration has proven effective in several animal models of ARDS, and finally, initial clinical evaluation of exogenous surfactant therapy in patients with ARDS has been promising.

Exogenous surfactant therapy in nRDS

In 1959, Avery and Mead implicated a deficiency of endogenous surfactant in the development of nRDS (Avery & Mead 1959). Since then, over 35 randomized controlled clinical trials evaluating exogenous surfactant therapy have been performed as a result of which surfactant supplementation for nRDS has become routine (Jobe & Ikegami 1987, Jobe 1993). Treating

Surfactant supplementation effective in neonatal RDS

surfactant-deficient neonates with exogenous surfactant has decreased the mortality associated with nRDS by 50%, and has reduced the incidence of associated complications such as barotrauma and interventricular haemorrhage. Because of its efficacy in these infants, administration of exogenous surfactant has been proposed as a treatment modality for patients with ARDS.

Surfactant alterations in ARDS

Impaired surfactant function was implicated in patients with ARDS even in the original description of this condition by Ashbaugh and colleagues (Ashbaugh et al 1967). In contrast to nRDS, the surfactant impairment in ARDS was not due to a deficiency, but rather to alterations in surfactant metabolism and inactivation by serum proteins present within the airspace of the injured lungs (Lewis & Jobe 1993). These alterations have not only been observed in patients with ARDS (Petty et al 1977, Pison et al 1987, Hallman et al 1989, Pison et al 1990, Gregory et al 1991), but have been extensively studied in a variety of animal models of acute lung injury (Holm et al 1985b, Berry et al 1986, Lewis et al 1990, Gross 1991, Lewis & Jobe 1993, Veldhuizen et al 1993). Interestingly, the changes that occur to the surfactant system in lung injury appear to be independent of the underlying cause, and are remarkably consistent between different species. As schematically shown in Figure 3.1B, proposed alterations of surfactant metabolism include abnormal phospholipid synthesis, a decreased ability to form an effective phospholipid monolayer, and an increase in small surfactant aggregate formation. An influx of serum proteins into the airspace also disrupts surfactant function (Jobe 1989). Analysis of lung lavage samples obtained from animal models of lung injury reflect these alterations in surfactant metabolism; the phospholipid composition of surfactant is changed (phosphatidylcholine and phosphatidylglycerol are decreased whereas sphingomyelin and lysophophatidylcholine are increased)(Lewis & Jobe 1993), there is an increased ratio of small to large surfactant aggregates (Lewis et al 1990, Veldhuizen et al 1993), the surface tension lowering ability of large aggregates is impaired (Lewis et al 1990), and there is an increased amount of serum protein recovered in the lavage (Lewis & Jobe 1993).

In patients with ARDS, alterations in the endogenous surfactant system have been measured post mortem (Petty et al 1977) and in BAL samples obtained at various stages of lung injury (Hallman et al 1989, Pison et al 1989, Gregory et al 1991). Gregory and co-workers (Gregory et al 1991) analysed BAL samples obtained from patients with ARDS, from patients at risk of developing ARDS and from normal control subjects. Their results (summarized in Figure 3.2) not only demonstrated the alterations of recovered surfactant described above in the patients with ARDS, but similar, albeit less pronounced changes in 'at risk' patients. Moreover, recent

Impared surfactant function : ARDS - defective monolayer function ass. c̄ alvealar transudates of serum proteins observations have confirmed that the ratio of small to large surfactant aggregates was increased in patients with ARDS, similar to previously reported animal data (Veldhuizen et al 1995). Since secondary alterations of the endogenous surfactant system contributed to lung dysfunction, exogenous surfactant administration was felt to be a rational therapeutic approach.

Ratio of Small surfactant aggregates / large surfactant aggregates = SA/LA ↑ in ARDS

Exogenous surfactant administration in animal models of ARDS

Animal models of acute lung injury that mimic clinical ARDS have been used extensively to evaluate the efficacy of exogenous surfactant administration, which has been shown to improve lung function. Some of these models include: N-nitroso-N-methylurethane (NNMU) induced injury in rabbits (Lewis et al 1990) and rats (Harris et al 1989), hyperoxic injury in rabbits (Matalon et al 1987) and baboons (Simonsen et al 1992), and repetitive saline, lung-lavage injury in several species (Berggren et al 1986, Oetomo et al 1988, Lewis et al 1991b, Lewis et al 1993b). The beneficial effects of exogenous surfactant in these models has prompted clinical studies evaluating surfactant therapy in patients with ARDS.

Animal models of surfactant depletion mimicly ARDS respond to exogenous surfactant.

Surfactant therapy in patients with ARDS

Surfactant supplementation in patients with ARDS has been reported in several anecdotal cases and a number of clinical studies (Table 3.1). In

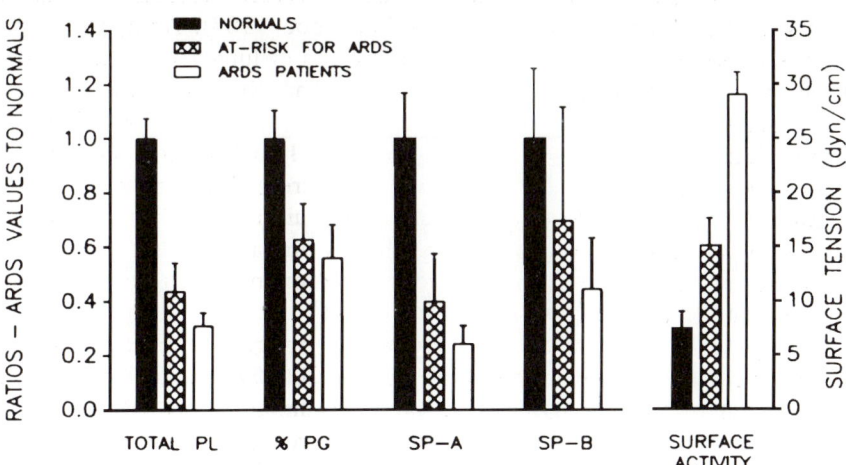

Fig. 3.2 Alterations in surfactant recovered from BAL samples obtained from normal subjects (solid bars), patients at risk of ARDS (cross hatched bars) and patients with ARDS (open bars). Total phospholipid (PL), % phosphatidylglycerol (PG), SP-A and SP-B are expressed as a ratio of control subjects. Surface activity, measured in vitro, is expressed as dynes/cm at the minimum surface area. Redrawn from Gregory et al 1991.

most, an increase in ventilation efficiency and oxygenation was demonstrated in response to exogenous surfactant therapy. Initial reports from a large randomized controlled trial suggested that aerosolized exogenous surfactant (Exosurf ®, Burroughs Wellcome, Research Triangle Park, NC, USA) had beneficial effects on gas exchange and shunt fraction (Weg et al 1991, Wiedemann et al 1992). However, this study has recently been terminated due to non-significant improvements in lung function (Anzueto et al 1994). In a more recent, controlled clinical trial reported by Gregory and colleagues (Gregory et al 1994), a dramatic decrease in mortality from 44 to 17% was demonstrated. In this study, exogenous surfactant (Survanta®, Ross Laboratories, Columbus, OH, USA) was instilled into the lungs of patients via the endotracheal tube, with several doses administered over the treatment period in some cases.

Randomized trial: aerosolized surfactant ineffective. Instilled via ETT effective?

Table 3.1   Clinical experience using exogenous surfactant administration for patients with ARDS

Authors (ref)	Number of patients	Surfactant preparation	Delivery method	Dose
Richman et al 1989	3	Curosurf ®	Lobar instillation	4 grams (divided doses)
Lachmann 1989	1	Surfactant Extract®	Tracheal instillation	300 mg/kg
Nosaka et al 1990	2	Surfactant TA®	Tracheal instillation	240 mg/dose (4-15 doses)
Weg et al 1991 Wiedemann et al 1992	52	Exosurf ®	Aerosol	6-12 mg/kg/day (deposition ?)
Spragg et al 1994	6	Curosurf ®	Lobar instillation	4 grams (divided doses)
Lewis et al 1994	7	bLES®	Tracheal instillation	100 mg/kg (1-4 doses)
Gregory et al 1994	59	Survanta®	Tracheal instillation	50-100 mg/kg (1-8 doses)

IMPORTANT ISSUES RELATED TO EXOGENOUS SURFACTANT THERAPY

Although the results of both animal and clinical studies evaluating exogenous surfactant therapy give cause for optimism, this treatment is far from becoming standard clinical practice in ARDS. Data from animal studies and preliminary clinical experience indicate that several factors require further investigation. These include the best means of delivery, the optimal dose and timing of surfactant administration, and the specific preparation to use for patients with ARDS. Moreover, due to the significant differences between the pathophysiology of ARDS and nRDS, various aspects of surfactant supplementation for patients with ARDS cannot be directly extrapolated from the nRDS experience and need to be thoroughly investigated. Subsequent sections will describe the current state of knowledge on each of these issues.

Exogenous surfactant delivery techniques

Currently, there are two distinct methods used to administer exogenous surfactant, both of which have proved effective in acute lung injury. Tracheal instillation is the traditional method of delivery used in neonates, and has recently been shown to significantly improve lung function in patients with ARDS. Aerosolized exogenous surfactant has also been shown to be effective in several animal models of acute lung injury. The advantages and disadvantages of both delivery methods will be discussed.

Bolus instillation — large does administered rapidly

Instillation

Instilling a liquid bolus of exogenous surfactant directly into the lungs via the endotracheal tube is the current method of delivery used to treat preterm infants with nRDS (Hallman et al 1985, Jobe & Ikegami 1987, Collaborative European Multicenter Study Group 1988, Fujiwara et al 1990, Halliday et al 1993). A variety of bolus injection schemes have been adopted, all with the ultimate goal of improving surfactant distribution within the lung in order to maximize efficacy. Current clinical practices generally include either disconnecting the infant from the ventilator during the instillation procedure (Zola et al 1993), or manually injecting the surfactant during inspiration through a side-port adaptor of the endotracheal tube (Phibbs et al 1991). Treatment procedures may also involve moving the infant into various positions during instillation in order to optimize distribution. Despite these variations in methods of administration, clinical studies have not shown any differences between the techniques with respect to efficacy or incidence of air leak and death from nRDS (Soll & McQueen 1992). A recent animal study, however, did demonstrate differences between specific delivery techniques. Ueda and colleagues (Ueda et al 1994) showed that exogenous surfactant instilled into preterm lamb lungs using an infusion technique was less uniformly distributed than surfactant delivered in separate boluses. These distribution differences correlated with differences in measured physiological parameters between groups, suggesting that in some circumstances, the specific technique of instillation may be relevant.

Most studies evaluating exogenous surfactant therapy in adult animal models of acute lung injury, and anecdotal reports in humans with ARDS (Table 3.1), have also utilized the instillation technique (Berggren et al 1986, Matalon et al 1987, Oetomo et al 1988, Harris et al 1989, Lewis et al 1990, Lewis et al 1991a, Van Daal et al 1992, Lewis et al 1993b). The major advantage of this method for patients with severe ARDS is that large quantities of surfactant can be administered over a relatively short period of time. This factor may be important in order to overcome the surfactant

> $>100 mg/kg$
> $>4 ml/kg$
>
> foaming?
> $PaCO_2 \uparrow$
> $Paw \uparrow$
>
> COST!

inhibitory effects of serum proteins present within the airspace of injured lungs (Holm et al 1988, Jobe 1989). On the other hand, the doses (≥ 100 mg lipid/kg) and volumes (≥ 4 ml/kg) currently used would be expected to obstruct airways and create foaming when the surfactant mixes with gas within the lung. In fact, in a recent study using a lung lavage model of lung injury in adult sheep, significant increases in $PaCO_2$ and peak airway pressures were documented shortly after an exogenous surfactant preparation (Survanta®, Ross Laboratories, Columbus, OH, USA) was instilled through the endotracheal tube into the lungs (Lewis & McCaig 1993). The long-term adverse effects of these changes are unknown, but it is reasonable to assume that in these animals the ventilatory impairment associated with this particular instillation procedure compromised any subsequent benefi-cial effects. Another potential disadvantage of instilling surfactant through the endotracheal tube in adult patients is the need for appropriate posi-tioning in order to optimize distribution. Although the impact of body positioning on surfactant distribution in adults is unknown, at the present time it is recommended that the subject be moved between the administra-tion of aliquots (Gregory et al 1994, Lewis et al 1994a). This may be a cumbersome and somewhat impractical manoeuvre to perform in some larger, critically ill patients. An additional limitation to this delivery tech-nique may be cost and availability. If a minimum dose of 100 mg lipid/kg is required for adults with ARDS, and if several doses per patient are ad-ministered, it is possible that resources and cost will eventually limit the use of natural surfactant preparations.

Aerosolization

Although a seemingly attractive method of surfactant delivery, aerosolized exogenous surfactant administration has received relatively little attention over the past four years. Initial studies evaluating exogenous surfactant therapy for neonates included trials which demonstrated that delivering surfactant as an aerosol was disappointing (Robilliard et al 1964, Chu et al 1967). This was due to a combination of the ineffective surfactant prepa-rations used and the inadequate and inefficient nebulizers available at that time. Recently, aerosolized exogenous surfactant has been shown to be effective in a preterm lamb model of nRDS (Lewis et al 1991b) and in several adult animal models of acute lung injury (Lewis et al 1991a, Simonsen et al 1992, Lewis et al 1993a, Lewis et al 1993b, Lewis & McCaig 1993, Li et al 1994). Not only have significant short-term improvements in lung function been demonstrated, but aerosolized surfactant also de-layed the onset of lung dysfunction and decreased the shunt fraction asso-ciated with oxygen toxicity in adult baboons (Simonsen et al 1992).

Aerosolization of exogenous surfactant has several potential advantages over the tracheal instillation technique. Firstly, a number of animal studies utilizing different models of lung injury in various species, have confirmed the finding that significant physiological improvements occurred with very small quantities of aerosolized surfactant deposited in lung tissue (Lewis et al 1991a,b, Lewis & McCaig 1993, Lewis et al 1993a,b). In fact, in adult rabbits with lung injury induced by subcutaneous NNMU (Lewis et al 1991a) and in adult sheep with repetitive saline lavage induced lung injury (Lewis & McCaig 1993), improvements in lung function with aerosolized surfactant were actually *superior* to instilled surfactant. In these studies, only 3–5 mg lipid/kg of aerosolized surfactant was deposited in lung tissue. This was approximately one-twentieth the total quantity of surfactant administered by instillation (100 mg lipid/kg). One potential explanation for this provocative observation is that the small dose of aerosolized surfactant deposited within the lung had a superior distribution pattern compared to the instilled surfactant. Indeed, in adult sheep with a uniform lung injury induced by whole-lung saline lavage, surfactant distribution was superior when delivered as an aerosol compared to instillation (Lewis et al 1993b).

Encouragingly, recent studies have also shown this delivery method to be relatively efficient. In an initial study using the lavage sheep model, 0.5 mg lipid/kg of aerosolized surfactant was recovered in lung tissue (~ 6% of the total surfactant nebulized), resulting in a 50% improvement in oxygenation over three hours of treatment (Lewis et al 1993b). Using the same animal model but an improved nebulization system, ~5 mg lipid/kg of aerosolized surfactant was recovered in lung tissue (~31% of total nebulized) (Lewis & McCaig 1993). This resulted in a 230% improvement in oxygenation. With continued improvements in aerosol technology, this delivery technique may well prove to be cost-effective for this patient population.

Despite these promising results, there are several disadvantages associated with the use of aerosolization. One very important issue that has been studied and shown to influence the efficacy of aerosolized exogenous surfactant is the effect of the underlying pattern of lung injury prior to surfactant administration (Lewis et al 1993a, Lewis & McCaig 1993). As noted previously, adult sheep with a *uniform* pattern of lung injury had a relatively *homogenous* distribution of aerosolized exogenous surfactant across all lobes of lung. As expected, these animals also had significant improvements in physiological parameters in response to the surfactant treatment. On the other hand, when a single lobe of lung was protected and the remaining lung was injured, over 50% of the total ventilation (and the aerosolized surfactant) was deposited in the normal lobe (Lewis et al 1993a). Consequently, significantly less surfactant was deposited in areas of the lung that needed it most, and virtually no physiological improvements were noted in response to this therapy. Given that the pattern of lung injury in patients with severe ARDS can be quite *heterogenous* (Gattinoni et al 1988), some variability in response to aerosolized surfactant could be expected in this patient population due to this phenomenon.

- Aerosol may preferentially deposit surfactant in normal area of lung, and not in diseased lung.
- Inhibitory effect of serum protein significant at low surfactant doses

Table 3.2   Exogenous surfactant delivery techniques

	Instillation	Aerosolization
Advantages	• Large dose	• Distribution (if uniform injury)
	• Rapid delivery	• 'Gentle' delivery of drug
	• Rapid response	• Standardized technique
Disadvantages	• Distribution	• Distribution (if non-uniform injury)
	• Liquid bolus	• Slow delivery
	• Variable technique	• Slower response

Summary

Both instilled and aerosolized exogenous surfactant have proved effective in several animal models of lung injury and in patients with ARDS. The advantages and disadvantages of each method of administration (summarized in Table 3.2) may dictate which delivery technique is appropriate for an individual patient. Further investigations are required to understand better the limitations of each method so that optimal treatment strategies can be designed for patients with ARDS.

Exogenous surfactant dosing and timing of administration

Dose

The optimal dose of exogenous surfactant for patients with acute lung injury is unknown. In preterm animal models of nRDS, it has been shown that at least 50 mg lipid/kg of surfactant was required for optimal response when surfactant was delivered via tracheal instillation (Jobe & Ikegami 1987). Based on this data, most animal studies of acute lung injury have used 100 mg lipid/kg/dose, and even larger doses have been used in anecdotal reports of surfactant instillation in patients with ARDS (≥200 mg/kg/dose) (Table 3.1). The rationale for these large doses is not only to overcome the inhibitory effects of serum proteins on surfactant function (Holm et al 1988, Jobe 1989), but also to optimize surfactant distribution, since this is felt to influence the efficacy of exogenously instilled surfactant. To address this particular issue, Gilliard and co-workers (Gilliard et al 1990) compared the effect of surfactant volume versus surfactant concentration on distribution patterns in normal and injured rabbit lungs. They found that in normal lungs, volume was more critical than concentration in optimizing distribution. However, in oleic acid injured lungs, the distribution was volume independent. In this latter case, the flooded alveoli associated with severe injury was felt to enhance surfactant distribution, just as the fluid-filled lungs of preterm newborns facilitate surfactant distribution (Jobe & Ikegami 1987). These studies imply that with less severe lung injury where relatively smaller quantities of surfactant may be effective, larger volumes of material may be required for optimal distribution. Unfortunately, as noted previously, this approach is limited by the impairment of lung function which can result from the instillation of large volumes of surfactant into the lungs. To complicate the dosing issue further, it has been observed that aerosolized exogenous surfactant was effective with very small quantities of surfactant deposited in lung tissue compared to even the minimum instilled doses utilized. Since these small quantities of surfactant are presumably insufficient to overcome protein inhibitory effects within the airspace, the exact mechanism of aerosolized surfactant efficacy remains unknown.

Dose difficult to determine – depends on mode of administration – distribut

Timing   *better ÷ flooded alveoli (neonates)*

The optimal timing of surfactant administration over the course of the lung injury in patients with ARDS has not been formally studied. Neonatal studies have shown that in surfactant-deficient lungs, earlier administration was associated with a better outcome (Dunn et al 1991, Dunn 1993). This advantage was somewhat balanced, however, by the number of infants receiving exogenous surfactant who would not have developed nRDS. Data available from animal models of acute lung injury would suggest that in patients with ARDS, earlier administration of exogenous surfactant is also superior to later treatment. For example, exogenous surfactant administered *at the start* of hyperoxic exposure limited the subsequent progression of lung injury, decreased histological evidence of alveolar damage and improved overall survival in hyperoxia-injured adult rabbits (Matalon et al 1987, Engstrom et al 1989) and baboons (Simonsen et al 1992) compared to a group of non-surfactant treated, injured animals. In contrast, if surfactant was administered *after* hyperoxic exposure, it had a minimal effect on these variables. Similarly, in the repetitive lavage model of lung injury, exogenous surfactant was more effective when administered to animals immediately after the final lavage procedure compared to those receiving surfactant one hour after the final lavage, when the lung injury was more severe due to the period of high pressure ventilation prior to treatment (Berggren et al 1986, Lewis & McCaig 1993, Lewis et al 1993b). Based on this evidence, early administration of exogenous surfactant to patients with ARDS would be ideal. Progressive lung dysfunction would potentially be prevented and the significant morbidity and mortality associated with ARDS might be decreased. Unfortunately, it is very difficult not only to identify patients at an early stage of lung injury, but to predict which patients would benefit from this particular intervention. Clinical scoring systems based on physiological impairment may not be sufficiently sensitive for this purpose (Murray et al 1988). Recent evidence would suggest that altered alveolar surfactant aggregate ratios may be an earlier and sensitive marker of acute lung injury (Lewis et al 1994b). Further investigation is required to test the reliability and practicality of sensitive markers of acute lung injury that would serve to identify which patients would benefit most from early exogenous surfactant therapy.

Early administration best – but no good

indicator of patients at risk [ARDS

?? alveolar surfactant aggregate ratios??

Although unambiguous guidelines for the optimal timing of surfactant therapy and surfactant dosing schedules are not available, it is clear that administration of exogenous surfactant very late in the course of lung injury is not effective. In a recent clinical pilot study in paediatric patients with ARDS, exogenous surfactant therapy was administered to patients with an established diagnosis of ARDS (Lewis et al 1994a). Those who did not respond had been treated at least four days after the diagnosis of ARDS was made. In contrast, patients who responded favourably were usually treated within 48 hours of diagnosis. A lung in the fibro-proliferative stage of injury would not be expected to respond to exogenous surfactant and this should be recognized when considering the timing of therapy for individual patients with ARDS (Bitterman 1992).

Patients seen to respond to surfactant given within 48h of ∆ ARDS

Summary

To date, clinical studies evaluating exogenous surfactant therapy have considered its effect in patients with established ARDS. Although results are promising, the specific dose and dosing interval is unknown. Further studies are required to determine how much and how often surfactant should be given to these patients. An alternative approach would be to administer surfactant very early in the course of lung injury, thereby preventing progressive lung dysfunction, although it has yet to be determined which patients will benefit in these circumstances.

Exogenous surfactant preparations

There are four categories of surfactant preparations currently being used for patients with nRDS and ARDS: (1) natural surfactant extracts, (2) modified minced-lung surfactant extracts, (3) synthetic surfactants and (4) human surfactant.

Natural surfactant extracts

Natural surfactant extracts   -   cost
                                -    lacks SP-A
                                -    low yield per animal

Natural surfactant extracts are produced by chloroform extraction of lung lavage material that has undergone differential centrifugation to isolate the large surfactant aggregate fraction (Yu et al 1983). These preparations contain the surfactant lipids as well as the hydrophobic proteins SP-B and SP-C, but do not contain SP-A. In general, these preparations have excellent surface tension reducing ability when tested both in vitro and in vivo. A potential drawback to their widespread use is the long-term availability and cost. These limitations might become significant if large doses prove necessary for adult patients with ARDS. Examples of some natural surfactant extracts currently used include: Infasurf® (ONY, Buffalo NY, USA), bLES® (Bovine lipid extract surfactant, BLES Biochemicals, London Ont, Canada) and Alveofact® (Thomea GmbH, Biberach, Germany).

Modified minced lung surfactant extracts   [handwritten: Pigs, cattle extract. Added DPPC + palmitate]

Modified minced lung extracted surfactants are obtained from either por-   [handwritten: — lacks SP-A]
cine or bovine sources. After chloroform extraction, DPPC and palmitic   [handwritten: — low SP-B]
acid are added to the minced lung extract to enhance biophysical activity.   [handwritten: " SP-C]
Compared to the natural surfactant extracts, these preparations contain
smaller quantities of the proteins SP-B and SP-C. This is, in part, why
modified minced lung extracts reduce the surface tension at a slower rate
than natural surfactant preparations (Ikegami et al 1987, Cockshutt et al
1991). However, the surfactant yield per animal is higher, making availability somewhat less of a problem compared to the natural extracts. Examples of minced lung surfactants currently used include: Survanta® (Ross
Laboratories, Chicago, IL, USA), Surfactant TA® (Tokyo Tanabe, Tokyo,
Japan) and Curosurf® (Chiesi Farmaceutici, Parma, Italy).

Synthetic surfactants   [handwritten: Protein-free. Reduced efficacy due to absence of SP-B + SP-C]

The importance of SP-B and SP-C in surfactant function have made the
generation of protein-free synthetic products difficult (Hall et al 1992).
Currently, there are three different synthetic surfactant compounds in use:
(1) ALEC® (Artificial Lung Expanding Compound, Britannia Pharmaceu-
ticals, Surrey, UK), a lipid mixture of DPPC and PG (Morley 1989), (2)
Exosurf® (Burroughs Wellcome, Research Triangle Park, NC, USA), composed of DPPC and two spreading/adsorption agents, hexadecanol and
tyloxapol (Durand et al 1985), and (3) KL4® (R.W. Johnson, Pharmaceu-
tical Research Institute, New Jersey, USA), a mixture of lipid and a synthetic peptide based on the structure of SP-B (Cochrane & Revak 1991).
Advantages of synthetic products include future availability as well as the
absence of surfactant-associated proteins, which have antigenic potential
(Strayer et al 1989). The information on surface tension reducing ability
varies between these different preparations and direct comparison studies
are lacking.

Human surfactant   [handwritten: from amniotic fluid. Limited availability.]

The fourth type of preparation, human natural surfactant, is obtained by
purification of surfactant isolated from amniotic fluid collected from
caesarean sections (Hallman et al 1983), which contains all the surfactant
lipids and proteins including SP-A. Although human surfactant would
obviously be the ideal exogenous preparation to use in patients with ARDS,
the future availability and the extensive purification protocols necessary
for clinical use of this material limit the commercial viability of this option.

Comparison of surfactant preparations

All four types of surfactant preparations have been shown to be effective in the treatment of infants with nRDS (Enhorning et al 1985, Kwong et al 1985, Konishi et al 1988, Shapiro & Notter 1988, Morley 1989, Soll et al 1990, Dunn et al 1991, Long et al 1991, Merritt et al 1991, Phibbs et al 1991, Deng et al 1992, Speer et al 1992, Halliday et al 1993). Studies directly comparing the efficacy of the various exogenous surfactant preparations are limited, however (Ikegami et al 1987, Notter & Shapiro 1987, Levine et al 1991, Cummings et al 1992). Using a preterm lamb model of nRDS, Cummings and colleagues (Cummings et al 1992) compared the effects of four different preparations on physiological parameters and survival (Fig. 3.3). In these experiments, the natural surfactant extract, Infasurf®, was superior to the minced lung extract, Survanta®. Interestingly, the artificial surfactant preparation, Exosurf®, did not improve lung function and resulted in poor survival similar to the control, non-treated animals. An additional, unexplained observation was that the natural, unextracted surfactant product which one would assume would have superior function due to the presence of all three surfactant proteins, was less effective than the natural extract.

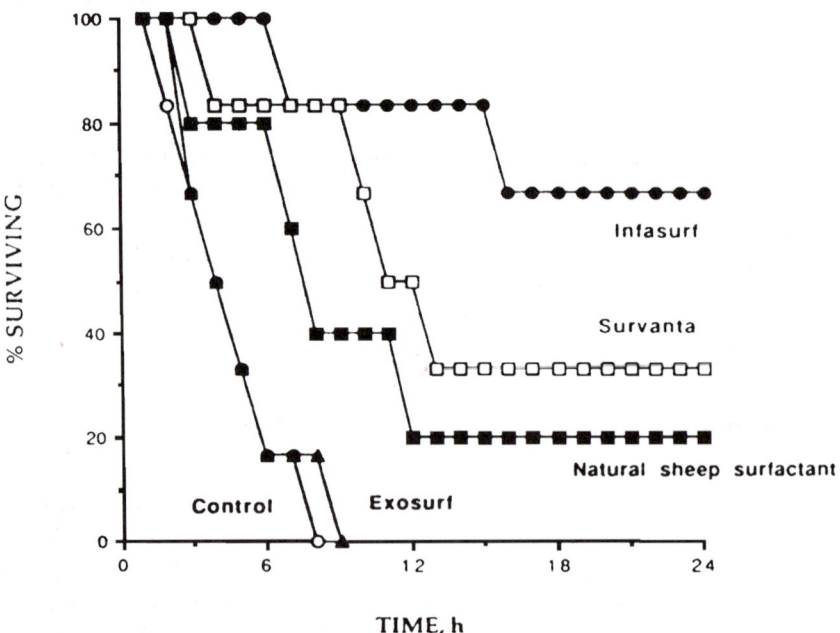

Fig. 3.3 Percentage survival of preterm lambs delivered at time 0 h and treated by tracheal instillation with different surfactant preparations. Reproduced from Cummings et al 1992 with permission.

To date, there have been no direct comparisons of exogenous surfactant preparations in animal models of ARDS. Since the underlying aetiology and pathophysiology of ARDS is complex and distinct from nRDS, it is probable that the efficacy of different products will be very different in patients with ARDS. For example, in the lungs of neonates with nRDS, surface tension reducing activity is the most crucial property of the exogenously administered surfactant. In patients with ARDS, other inherent properties such as the role of the exogenous surfactant in down-regulating the function of alveolar macrophages (Speer et al 1991, Thomassen et al 1992), and its susceptibility to protein inhibition (Holm et al 1985a) may be of greater importance. The alveolar metabolism of the exogenous surfactant is also likely to be different in adults with ARDS compared to neonates (Lewis et al 1992, Ikegami et al 1993). Finally, the interaction of the exogenous substance with the endogenous surfactant pool at various stages of lung injury may influence the efficacy of a particular preparation.

In the absence of direct comparisons, it is difficult to reach a conclusion as to which surfactant preparation is optimal for patients with ARDS. Generally, however, data from animal experiments and the limited clinical studies performed to date (Table 3.1) suggest that the natural surfactant extracts and the modified minced lung extracts are more effective than the most commonly used synthetic preparation, Exosurf®. Since other synthetic surfactants have not yet been tested in patients with ARDS, no firm conclusions should be drawn regarding synthetic preparations as a whole.

Summary

Several different exogenous surfactant preparations are currently available, all of which are effective in neonates with nRDS. In patients with ARDS, lung injury is complex and the effectiveness of exogenous preparations may vary significantly. With an increased understanding of the pathophysiology of the lung injury in ARDS, and with continued evaluation studies, it should be possible to develop optimal exogenous surfactant preparations for patients with ARDS.

PROPOSED EXOGENOUS SURFACTANT TREATMENT STRATEGIES

From information available to date, it is obvious that no single treatment protocol will be appropriate for all patients with ARDS. Early recognition and treatment of high-risk patients would seem ideal, although a number of patients will present at later stages of lung injury, when pulmonary dysfunction is severe. Since several factors influence the host's response to exogenous surfactant at any particular time over the course of their dis-

Early recognition of "high risk" patients

ease, it will be necessary to characterize the patient's illness before deciding on a specific therapeutic approach. The two extremes will involve an
'early' treatment regiment and/or a 'late' treatment regiment (Fig. 3.4).

'Early' surfactant administration

As noted previously, the major goal of administering exogenous surfactant
at an early stage of lung injury is to prevent progressive lung dysfunction.
The advantages of this approach are several. Firstly, due to the role of the
surfactant system in lung defence and modulating the inflammatory response, early administration of exogenous surfactant would potentially
downregulate the inflammatory cascade and mitigate against the development of multiple organ failure (MOF) (Sluiter et al 1988, Speer et al 1991,
Hayakawa et al 1992, Manz Keinke et al 1992, Thomassen et al 1992).
Secondly, with earlier administration of surfactant to a less severely injured
lung and a more 'preserved' endogenous surfactant environment, metabolic interactions may be enhanced. Exogenous and endogenous surfactant
components have been shown to interact, resulting in some circumstances
in an enhanced activity of the exogenous preparation (Lewis et al 1992,
Ikegami et al 1993). These interactions could potentially obviate the need
for further therapy. Finally, since less protein would be present within the

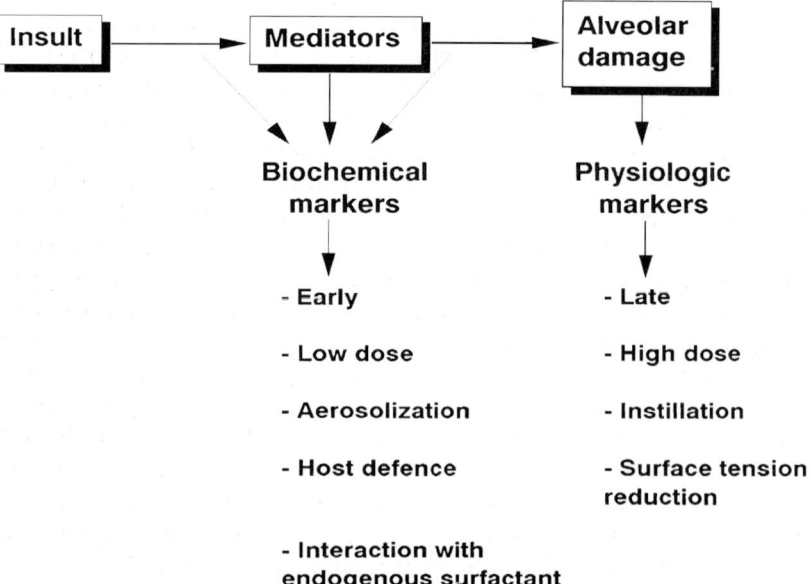

Fig. 3.4 Outline of the proposed design of two possible exogenous surfactant treatment
strategies for patients with ARDS.

airspace at an early stage of injury, smaller quantities of exogenous surfactant would be required to overcome protein inhibitory effects (Jobe 1989, Holm et al 1985a). These factors, together with the assumption that the pattern of lung injury is more uniform in less severely injured lungs, suggests that aerosolization of exogenous surfactant would be an ideal delivery technique to use at this stage of lung injury (Lewis et al 1993a). Moreover, in patients with mild lung dysfunction, a relatively 'gentle' administration of exogenous surfactant would be more appropriate than instilling liquid boluses into the lungs (Lewis & McCaig 1993). Finally, a specific exogenous surfactant preparation for this situation could be chosen based on its ability to impact host defence, interact with endogenous surfactant components and be efficiently deposited within the lung by aerosol. As noted previously, however, the major factor limiting the design of 'early' surfactant treatment strategies is patient recognition. At this stage of the illness, it is probable that a biochemical marker, perhaps the ratio of small to large surfactant aggregates in BAL samples, will be most reliable (Lewis et al 1994b).

?? Early aerosol administration of surfactant ??
Not proven — ? Biochemical marker SA/LA ÷ BAL?

'Late' surfactant administration

Exogenous surfactant administration has been shown to be effective in patients with established ARDS (Table 3.1). Expectations in this situation, however, should be different from those of earlier surfactant treatment protocols with regards to prevention of lung dysfunction. Specific indications for surfactant therapy at this stage of injury will be based on physiological impairments such as hypoxaemia, shunt fraction and decreased compliance, rather than biochemical markers. As such, optimal exogenous surfactant preparations used in these patients should have superior biophysical properties, rather than interactive potential. Also, larger quantities of surfactant would be required to overcome the protein inhibition phenomenon and a more acute physiological improvement with surfactant therapy would be expected due to the severity of the illness. In this situation, instillation of larger doses of exogenous surfactant would be appropriate, with potential selective instillation into more severely damaged areas of lung in non-uniform injuries (Richman et al 1989, Spragg et al 1994). The number of doses required for an individual patient would be dictated by the response to the first dose and subsequent changes in physiological parameters (Nosaka et al 1990, Gregory et al 1994, Lewis et al 1994a). The impact of this treatment strategy on morbidity may be more impressive than mortality. It may also be possible that patients not responding to exogenous surfactant at this stage of injury are in the fibrotic stage of lung injury and have irreversible lung damage (Bitterman 1992). Further studies are required to assess whether the response to exogenous surfactant administration at this stage of injury may reflect short-term prognosis.

?? Late bolus administration of high-dose surfactant ??
? Instillation into (dependent) more severely damaged areas ?
? Indications — PaO$_2$ ↓ Q$_s$/Q$_t$ ↑ ΔV/ΔP ↓ ?

Summary

In summary, several factors will dictate the nature of exogenous surfactant treatment protocols for individual patients with ARDS. The method of delivery, timing, dosage and specific surfactant preparation used should all be considered before exogenous surfactant is administered to patients with lung injury. Failure to optimize any one of these factors may result in a poor response to therapy in an individual patient, or to significant variability of responses in clinical trials. Future clinical studies evaluating this therapy should be designed so that each of these factors is optimized.

FUTURE DIRECTIONS

As surfactant treatment protocols are tested in patients with ARDS, it is imperative that basic research efforts continue. The endogenous surfactant system represents an important aspect of lung homeostasis and over the past four years basic research has provided important information that has influenced our approach to the management of lung disease. For example, studies investigating the effects of surfactant on lung defence have extended surfactant-related research from a purely biophysical viewpoint to an area involving inflammatory mediators. The impact of these findings will be enormous and future studies should focus on characterizing the surfactant system in other inflammatory lung diseases, including pneumonia and asthma. Furthermore, with this knowledge, optimal preparations can be designed and delivered to patients in order to optimize outcome. Other future areas of surfactant research should include its evaluation as a delivery vehicle for other medications such as antibiotics, antioxidants and the selective vasodilator, nitric oxide. The future of exogenous surfactant administration is exciting and will involve a wide spectrum of lung disease.

ACKNOWLEDGEMENTS

This work was supported in part by the Medical Research Council of Canada and the Ontario Ministry of Health.

KEY POINTS FOR CLINICAL PRACTICE

- Endogenous pulmonary surfactant is altered in patients with ARDS and these alterations contribute, in part, to lung dysfunction.
- Exogenous surfactant administration has proven effective in several animal models of acute lung injury. Clinical experience in patients with ARDS is promising.
- Several factors require further investigation prior to the routine use of exogenous surfactant for patients with ARDS.

- Advantages of tracheal instillation of surfactant include the ability to deliver large quantities over relatively short periods of time to overcome protein inhibitory effects. Disadvantages include delivering a liquid bolus into injured lungs and variable surfactant distribution depending on the specific instillation technique used.
- Advantages of aerosolized exogenous surfactant include a more 'gentle' delivery technique and a uniform distribution of surfactant if the lung injury is uniform. Disadvantages include the time required to administer the material and an inferior surfactant distribution if the lung injury is non-uniform.
- The optimal dose of exogenous surfactant is unknown but may depend on the severity and nature of the injury. Aerosolized exogenous surfactant is effective with very small quantities of material deposited in lung tissue compared to instilled doses (approximately 1:20). 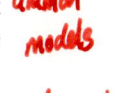 *animal models*
- Earlier administration of exogenous surfactant in the course of lung injury would be ideal; however, identifying which patients would benefit most from this therapy requires further study. *SA/LA ratio*
- Various exogenous surfactant preparations are available, and differ in their efficacy. Therefore, the choice of an exogenous preparation may influence acute physiological response, course of lung dysfunction and patient outcome.
- Optimal exogenous surfactant treatment strategies may include an 'early' approach where surfactant is administered to patients at risk of ARDS in the hope of preventing progression. Alternatively, later treatments for patients with established ARDS would entail instilling large doses of surfactant into severely injured lungs in order to improve gas exchange acutely.
- Future studies will focus on optimizing surfactant treatment strategies for patients with ARDS, as well as evaluating exogenous surfactant as a novel therapeutic intervention for other inflammatory lung diseases such as pneumonia and asthma.

REFERENCES

Ansfield M J, Kaltreider H B, Benson B J et al 1980a Immunosuppressive activity of canine pulmonary surface active material. J Immunol 122: 1062–1066

Ansfield M J, Kaltreider H B, Benson B J et al 1980b Canine surface active material and pulmonary lymphocyte function studies with mixed-lymphocyte culture. Exp Lung Res 1: 3–11

Anzueto A, Baughman R, Guntupalli K et al 1994 An international, randomized, placebo-controlled trial evaluating the safety and efficacy of aerosolized surfactant in patients with sepsis-induced ARDS. Am J Respir Crit Care Med 149: A567.

Ashbaugh D G, Bigelow D B, Petty T L et al 1967 Acute respiratory distress in adults. Lancet 2: 319–323

Avery M E, Mead J 1959 Surface properties in relation to atelectasis and hyaline membrane disease. Am J Dis Child 97: 517–523

Baritussio A, Bellina L, Carraro R et al 1984 Heterogeneity of alveolar surfactant in the rabbit: composition, morphology, and labelling of subfractions isolated by centrifugation of lung lavage. Eur J Clin Invest 14: 24–29

Berggren P, Lachmann B, Curstedt T et al 1986 Gas exchange and lung morphology after surfactant replacement in experimental adult respiratory distress syndrome induced by repeated lung lavage. Acta Anaesthesiol Scand 30: 321–328

Berry D, Ikegami M, Jobe A 1986 Respiratory distress and surfactant inhibition following vagotomy in rabbits. J Appl Physiol 61: 1741–1748

Bitterman P B 1992 Pathogenesis of fibrosis in acute lung injury. Am J Med 92 (suppl 6A): 39S–43S

Chu J, Clements J A, Cotton E K et al 1967 Neonatal pulmonary ischemia: clinical and physiological studies. Pediatrics 40: 709–782

Cochrane C G, Revak S D 1991 Pulmonary surfactant protein B (SP-B): structure-function relationships. Science 254: 566–568

Cockshutt A M, Absolom D R, Possmayer F 1991 The role of palmitic acid in pulmonary surfactant: enhancement of surface activity and prevention of inhibition by blood proteins. Biochem Biophys Acta 1085: 248–256

Cockshutt A M, Weitz J, Possmayer F 1990 Pulmonary surfactant-associated protein A enhances the surface activity of lipid extract surfactant and reverses inhibition by blood proteins in vitro. Biochemistry 29: 8424–8429

Collaborative European Multicenter Study Group 1988 Surfactant replacement therapy for severe neonatal respiratory distress syndrome: an international randomized clinical trial. Pediatrics 82: 683–691

Cummings J J, Holm B A, Hudak M L et al 1992 A controlled clinical comparison of four different surfactant preparations in surfactant-deficient preterm lambs. Am Rev Respir Dis 145: 999–1004

Deng H H, Kuo M C, Chung K H et al 1992 Clinical use of single-dose surfactant TA therapy for premature infants with severe respiratory distress syndrome. Acta Paediatr Sin 33: 408–416

Dunn M S 1993 Surfactant replacement therapy: prophylaxis or treatment? Pediatrics 92: 148–150

Dunn M S, Shennan A T, Zayack D et al 1991 Bovine surfactant replacement therapy in neonates of less than 30 weeks' gestation: a randomized controlled trial of prophylaxis versus treatment. Pediatrics 87: 377–386

Durand D J, Clyman R I, Heymann M A et al 1985 Effects of a protein-free, synthetic surfactant on survival and pulmonary function in preterm lambs. J Pediatr 107: 775–780

Engstrom P C, Holm B A, Matalon S 1989 Surfactant replacement attenuates the increase in alveolar permeability in hyperoxia. J Appl Physiol 67: 688–693

Enhorning G, Shennan A, Possmayer F et al 1985 Prevention of neonatal respiratory distress syndrome by tracheal instillation of surfactant: a randomized clinical trial. Pediatrics 76: 145–153

Fujiwara T, Konishi M, Chida S et al 1990 Surfactant replacement therapy with a single postventilatory dose of a reconstituted bovine surfactant in preterm neonates with respiratory distress syndrome: final analysis of a multicenter, double-blind, randomized trial and comparison with similar trials. The Surfactant-TA Study Group. Pediatrics 86: 753–764

Gattinoni L, Pesenti A, Bombino M et al 1988 Relationships between lung computed tomographic density, gas exchange, and PEEP in acute respiratory failure. Anesthesiology 69: 824–832

Gilliard N, Richman P M, Merritt T A et al 1990 Effect of volume and dose on the pulmonary distribution of exogenous surfactant administered to normal rabbits or to rabbits with oleic acid lung injury. Am Rev Respir Dis 141: 743–747

Gregory T J, Longmore W J, Moxley M A et al 1991 Surfactant chemical composition and biophysical activity in acute respiratory distress syndrome. J Clin Invest 88: 1976–1981

Gregory T J, Gadek J E, Weiland J E et al 1994 Survanta supplementation in patients with acute respiratory distress syndrome (ARDS). Am J Respir Crit Care Med 149: A124.

Gross N J 1991 Surfactant subtypes in experimental lung damage: radiation pneumonitis. Am J Physiol 260: L302–L310

Gross N J, Narine K R 1989 Surfactant subtypes of mice: metabolic relationships and conversion in vitro. J Appl Physiol 67: 414–421

Hall S B, Venkitaraman A R, Whitsett J A et al 1992 Importance of hydrophobic apoproteins as constituents of clinical exogenous surfactants. Am Rev Respir Dis 145: 24–30

Halliday H L, Tarnow Mordi W O, Corcoran J D et al 1993 Multicentre randomised trial comparing high and low dose surfactant regimens for the treatment of respiratory distress syndrome (the Curosurf 4 trial). Arch Dis Child 69: 276–280

Hallman M, Maasilta P, Sipila I et al 1989 Composition and function of pulmonary surfactant in adult respiratory distress syndrome. Eur Respir J Suppl 3: 104s–108s

Hallman M, Merritt T A, Jarvenpaa A L et al 1985 Exogenous human surfactant for treatment of severe respiratory distress syndrome: a randomized prospective clinical trial. J Pediatr 106: 963–969

Hallman M, Merritt T A, Schneider H et al 1983 Isolation of human surfactant from amniotic fluid and a pilot study of its efficacy in respiratory distress syndrome. Pediatrics 71: 473–482

Harris J D, Jackson F, Jr, Moxley M A et al 1989 Effect of exogenous surfactant instillation on experimental acute lung injury. J Appl Physiol 66: 1846–1851

Hawgood S, Shiffer K 1991 Structures and properties of the surfactant-associated proteins. Annu Rev Physiol 53: 375–394

Hayakawa H, Giridhar G, Myrvik Q N et al 1992 Pulmonary surfactant phospholipids modulate priming of rabbit alveolar macrophages for oxidative responses. J Leukoc Biol 51: 379–385

Hayakawa H, Myrvik Q N, St Clair R W 1989 Pulmonary surfactant inhibits priming of rabbit alveolar macrophage. Evidence that surfactant suppresses the oxidative burst of alveolar macrophage in infant rabbits. Am Rev Respir Dis 140: 1390–1397

Hoffman R M, Claypool W D, Katyal S L et al 1987 Augmentation of rat alveolar macrophage migration by surfactant protein. Am Rev Respir Dis 135: 1358–1362

Holm B A, Enhorning G, Notter R H 1988 A biophysical mechanism by which plasma proteins inhibit lung surfactant activity. Chem Phys Lipids 49: 49–55

Holm B A, Notter R H, Finkelstein J N 1985a Surface property changes from interactions of albumin with natural lung surfactant and extracted lung lipids. Chem Phys Lipids 38: 287–298

Holm B A, Notter R H, Siegle J et al 1985b Pulmonary physiological and surfactant changes during injury and recovery from hyperoxia. J Appl Physiol 59: 1402–1409

Ikegami M, Agata Y, Elkady T et al 1987 Comparison of four surfactants: in vitro surface properties and responses of preterm lambs to treatment at birth. Pediatrics 79: 38–46

Ikegami M, Ueda T, Absolom D et al 1993 Changes in exogenous surfactant in ventilated preterm lamb lungs. Am Rev Respir Dis 148: 837–844

Jobe A 1989 Protein leaks and surfactant dysfunction in the pathogenesis of respiratory distress syndrome. Eur Respir J Suppl 3: 27s–32s

Jobe A, Ikegami M 1987 Surfactant for the treatment of respiratory distress syndrome. Am Rev Respir Dis 136: 1256–1275

Jobe A H 1993 Pulmonary surfactant therapy. N Engl J Med 328: 861–867

King R J, Clements J A 1972 Surface active materials from dog lung: composition and physiological correlations. Am J Physiol 223: 707–714

Konishi M, Fujiwara T, Naito T et al 1988 Surfactant replacement therapy in neonatal respiratory distress syndrome. A multi-centre, randomized clinical trial: comparison of high versus low-dose of surfactant TA. Eur J Pediatr 147: 20–25

Kwong M S, Egan E A, Notter R H et al 1985 Double-blind clinical trial of calf lung surfactant extract for the prevention of hyaline membrane disease in extremely premature infants. Pediatrics 76: 585–592

Lachmann B 1989 Animal models and clinical pilot studies of surfactant replacement in adult respiratory distress syndrome. Eur Respir J Suppl 3: 98s–103s

LaForce F M, Kelly W J, Huber G L 1973 Inactivation of staphylococci by alveolar macrophages with preliminary observations on the effect of alveolar lining material. Am Rev Respir Dis 108: 784–790

Levine D, Edwards D K, Merritt T A 1991 Synthetic vs human surfactant in the treatment of respiratory distress syndrome: radiographic findings. Am J Roentgenol 157: 371–374

Lewis J F, Jobe A H 1993 Surfactant and the adult respiratory distress syndrome. Am Rev Respir Dis 147: 218–233

Lewis J F, McCaig L A 1993 Aerosolized versus instilled exogenous surfactant in a nonuniform pattern of lung injury. Am Rev Respir Dis 148: 1187–1193

Lewis J F, Ikegami M, Jobe A H 1990 Altered surfactant function and metabolism in rabbits with acute lung injury. J Appl Physiol 69: 2303–2310

Lewis J, Ikegami M, Higuchi R et al 1991a Nebulized vs instilled exogenous surfactant in an adult lung injury model. J Appl Physiol 71: 1270–1276

Lewis J F, Ikegami M, Jobe A H et al 1991b Aerosolized surfactant treatment of preterm lambs. J Appl Physiol 70: 869–876

Lewis J F, Ikegami M, Jobe A H 1992 Metabolism of exogenously adminstered surfactant in the acutely injured lungs of adult rabbits. Am Rev Respir Dis 145: 19–23

Lewis J F, Ikegami M, Jobe A H et al 1993a Physiologic responses and distribution of aerosolized surfactant (Survanta) in a nonuniform pattern of lung injury. Am Rev Respir Dis 147: 1364–1370

Lewis J F, Tabor B, Ikegami M et al 1993b Lung function and surfactant distribution in saline lavaged sheep given instilled vs nebulized surfactant. J Appl Physiol 74: 1256–1264

Lewis J, Dhillon J, Frewen T 1995 Exogenous surfactant therapy in pediatric patients with ARDS. Am J Respir Crit Care Med 149(4): A125

Lewis J F, Veldhuizen R A W, Possmayer F et al 1995 Altered alveolar surfactant aggregates is an early marker of acute lung injury in septic sheep. Am J Respir Crit Care Med 150: 123–130

Li W Z, Chen W M, Kobayashi T 1994 Aerosolized surfactant reverses respiratory failure in lung-lavaged rats. Acta Anaesthesiol Scand 38: 82–88

Long W, Corbet A, Cotton R et al 1991 A controlled trial of synthetic surfactant in infants weighing 1250 g or more with respiratory distress syndrome. The American Exosurf Neonatal Study Group I, and the Canadian Exosurf Neonatal Study Group. N Engl J Med 325: 1696–1703

Manz Keinke H, Plattner H, Schlepper Schafer J 1992 Lung surfactant protein A (SP-A) enhances serum-independent phagocytosis of bacteria by alveolar macrophages. Eur J Cell Biol 57: 95–100

Matalon S, Holm B A, Notter R H 1987 Mitigation of pulmonary hyperoxic injury by administration of exogenous surfactant. J Appl Physiol 62: 756–761

Merritt T A, Hallman M, Berry C et al 1991 Randomized, placebo-controlled trial of human surfactant given at birth versus rescue administration in very low birth weight infants with lung immaturity. J Pediatr 118: 581–594

Morly C J 1989 Prophylactic treatment of premature babies with artificial surfactant (ALEC). Dev Pharmacol Ther 13: 182–183

Murray J F, Mattham M A, Luce J M et al 1988 An expanded definition of the adult respiratory distress syndrome. Am Rev Respir Dis 138: 720–723

Nosaka S, Sakai T, Yonekura M et al 1990 Surfactant for adults with respiratory failure (letter). Lancet 336: 947–948

Notter R H, Shapiro D L 1987 Lung surfactants for replacement therapy: biochemical, biophysical, and clinical aspects. Clin Perinatol 14: 433–479

Oetomo S B, Reijngoud D J, Ennema J J et al 1988 Surfactant replacement therapy in surfactant-deficient rabbits: early effects on lung function and biochemical aspects. Lung 166: 65–73

Persson A, Rust K, Chang D et al 1988 CP4: a pneumocyte-derived collagenous surfactant-associated protein. Evidence for heterogeneity of collagenous surfactant proteins. Biochemistry 27: 8576–8584

Petty T L, Reiss O K, Paul G W et al 1977 Characteristics of pulmonary surfactant in adult respiratory distress syndrome associated with trauma and shock. Am Rev Respir Dis 115: 531–536

Phibbs R H, Ballard R A, Clements J A et al 1991 Initial clinical trial of EXOSURF, a protein-free synthetic surfactant, for the prophylaxis and early treatment of hyaline membrane disease. Pediatrics 88: 1–9

Pison U, Gono E, Joka T et al 1987 Phospholipid lung profile in adult respiratory distress syndrome — evidence for surfactant abnormality. Prog Clin Biol Res 236A: 517–523

Pison U, Seeger W, Buchhorn R et al 1989 Surfactant abnormalities in patients with respiratory failure after multiple trauma. Am Rev Respir Dis 140: 1033–1039

Pison U, Obertacke U, Brand M et al 1990 Altered pulmonary surfactant in uncompli- cated and septicemia-complicated courses of acute respiratory failure. J Trauma 30: 19–26

Possmayer F 1988 A proposed nomenclature for pulmonary surfactant-associated proteins. Am Rev Respir Dis 138: 990–998

Possmayer F, Yu S H, Weber J M et al 1984 Pulmonary surfactant. Can J Biochem Cell Biol 62: 1121–1133

Richman P S, Spragg R G, Robertson B et al 1989 The adult respiratory distress syndrome: first trials with surfactant replacement. Eur Respir J Suppl 3: 109s–111s

Robilliard E, Alerie Y, Dagenais-Perusse P et al 1964 Microaerosol administration of synthetic dipalmitoyl lecithin in the respiratory distress syndrome: a preliminary report. Can Med Assoc J 90: 55–57

Shapiro D L, Notter R H 1988 Controversies regarding surfactant replacement therapy. Clin Perinatol 15: 891–902

Shelley S A, Paciga J E, Balis J U 1984 Lung surfactant phospholipids in different animal species. Lipids 19: 857–862

Simonsen S G, Huang Y C, Fracica P J et al 1992 Exogenous surfactant improves oxygenation in hyperoxic lung injury. Am Rev Respir Dis 145: A610

Sluiter W, Van Hemsbergen Oomens L W, Elzenga Claasen I et al 1988 Effect of lung surfactant on the release of factor increasing monocytopoiesis by macrophages. Exp Hematol 16: 93–96

Soll R F, Hoekstra R E, Fangman J J et al 1990 Multicenter trial of single-dose modified bovine surfactant extract (Survanta) for prevention of respiratory distress syndrome. Ross Collaborative Surfactant Prevention Study Group. Pediatrics 85: 1092–1102

Soll R F, McQueen M C 1992 Respiratory distress syndrome. In: Sinclair J C, Bracken M B (eds) Effective care of the newborn infant. Oxford University Press, Oxford, pp. 325–358

Speer C P, Gotze B, Curstedt T et al 1991 Phagocytic functions and tumor necrosis factor secretion of human monocytes exposed to natural porcine surfactant (Curosurf). Pediatr Res 30: 69–74

Speer C P, Robertson B, Curstedt T et al 1992 Randomized European multicenter trial of surfactant replacement therapy for severe neonatal respiratory distress syndrome: single versus multiple doses of Curosurf. Pediatrics 89: 13–20

Spragg R G, Gilliard N, Richman P et al 1994 Acute effects of a single dose of porcine surfactant on patients with the adult respiratory distress syndrome. Chest 105: 195– 202

Strayer D S, Merritt T A, Hallman M 1989 Surfactant replacement: immunological considerations. Eur Respir J Suppl 3: 91s–96s

Suzuki Y, Fujita Y, Kogishi K 1989 Reconstitution of tubular myelin from synthetic lipids and proteins associated with pig pulmonary surfactant. Am Rev Respir Dis 140: 75–81

Thomassen M J, Meeker D P, Antal J M et al 1992 Synthetic surfactant (Exosurf) inhibits endotoxin-stimulated cytokine secretion by human alveolar macrophages. Am J Respir Cell Mol Biol 7: 257–260

Ueda T, Ikegami M, Rider E D et al 1994 Distribution of surfactant and ventilation in surfactant-treated preterm lambs. J Appl Physiol 76: 45–55

Van Daal G J, Bos J A, Eijking E P et al 1992 Surfactant replacement therapy improves pulmonary mechanics in end-stage influenza A pneumonia in mice. Am Rev Respir Dis 145: 859–863

van Iwaarden F, Welmers B, Verhoef J et al 1990 Pulmonary surfactant protein A enhances the host-defence mechanism of rat alveolar macrophages. Am J Respir Cell Mol Biol 2: 91–98

Van Iwaarden J F, Van Strijp J A, Ebskamp M J et al 1991 Surfactant protein A is opsonin in phagocytosis of herpes simplex virus type 1 by rat alveolar macrophages. Am J Physiol 261: L204–L209

Van Iwaarden J F, Shimizu H, Van Golde P H et al 1992 Rat surfactant protein D enhances the production of oxygen radicals by rat alveolar macrophages. Biochem J 286: 5–8

Veldhuizen R A, Lee J, Sandler D et al 1993 Alterations in pulmonary surfactant composition and activity after experimental lung transplantation. Am Rev Respir Dis 148: 208–215

Veldhuizen R A W, McCaig L A, Akino T et al 1995 Pulmonary surfactant subfractions in patients with the acute respiratory distress syndrome (ARDS). Am J Respir Critical Care Med 152(6): 1867–1871

Weg J, Reines H, Balk R et al 1991 Safety and efficacy of an aerosolized surfactant (Exosurf) in human sepsis induced ARDS. Chest 100: 137S

Wiedemann H, Baughman R, deBoisblanc B et al 1992 A multicenter trial in human sepsis induced ARDS of an aerosolized synthetic surfactant (Exosurf). Am Rev Respir Dis 145: A184

Wright J R, Clements J A 1987 Metabolism and turnover of lung surfactant. Am Rev Respir Dis 136: 426–444

Wright J R, Dobbs L G 1991 Regulation of pulmonary surfactant secretion and clearance. Annu Rev Physiol 53: 395–414

Yamada T, Ikegami M, Jobe A H 1990 Effects of surfactant subfractions on preterm rabbit lung function. Pediatr Res 27: 592–598

Yu S, Harding P G, Smith N et al 1983 Bovine pulmonary surfactant: chemical composition and physical properties. Lipids 18: 522–529

Yu S H, Possmayer F 1990 Role of bovine pulmonary surfactant-associated proteins in the surface-active property of phospholipid mixtures. Biochem Biophys Acta 1046: 233–241

Yu S H, Possmayer F 1992 Effect of pulmonary surfactant protein B (SP-B) and calcium on phospholipid adsorption and squeeze-out of phosphatidylglycerol from binary phospholipid monolayers containing dipalmitoylphosphatidylcholine. Biochem Biophys Acta 1126: 26–34

Zola E M, Gunkel J H, Chan R K et al 1993 Comparison of three dosing procedures for administration of bovine surfactant to neonates with respiratory distress syndrome. J Pediatr 122: 453–459

4. The endothelium and the vascular response to sepsis

Nicholas P. Curzen   Timothy W. Evans

INTRODUCTION

The endothelium is an intimal layer of simple squamous cells which provides a continuous, fluent surface for circulating blood. It is not the passive, metabolically inert permeability barrier that was once thought, and is now known to be a metabolically and physiologically dynamic tissue with multiple functions. This chapter discusses the clinical syndromes associated with sepsis, the pathogenesis of the inflammatory response to sepsis, and in particular focuses on the damage to the endothelium caused by the mediators of inflammation and its role in orchestrating and modulating the response of the vasculature to sepsis.

Table 4.1 The clinical 'SEPSIS' syndromes (Definitions from Chest 1992; 101: 1644–1655)

SEPSIS The systemic response to infection

Includes two or more of the following:
- Temperature >38°C or <36°C
- Heart rate >90/min
- Respiratory rate >20/min or $PaCO_2$ <4.3 kPa
- White cell count >12 000/mm³ <4000/mm³, or >10% band (immature) forms

SEPSIS SYNDROME Sepsis with evidence of altered organ perfusion

Altered organ perfusion includes one or more of the following:
- PaO_2/FiO_2 ≤280 (without other cardiopulmonary disease) [mm Hg]
- Elevated lactate level (> upper limit of normal for the lab)
- Oliguria <0.5 ml/kg body weight

SYSTEMIC INFLAMMATORY RESPONSE SYNDROME The response to a variety of severe clinical insults (not necessarily infective), which is indistinguishable from sepsis.

SEPTIC SHOCK Sepsis with hypotension (sustained decrease in systolic blood pressure <90 mmHg, or drop >40 mmHg, for at least 1 h) despite adequate fluid resuscitation, in the presence of perfusion abnormalities that may include, but are not limited to lactic acidosis, oliguria or an acute alteration in mental status. Patients who are on inotropic or vasopressor agents may not be hypotensive at the time that perfusion abnormalities are measured.

[Handwritten margin annotations: Sepsis: ↓CO₂ or RR↑, WBC↑or↓, or >10% band forms, T↑or↓, HR↑; Sepsis syndrome; [mm Hg]; SIRS; Septic shock]

SEPSIS: THE CLINICAL PROBLEM

Sepsis and its associated syndromes represents a potentially devastating systemic inflammatory response estimated to occur in 1% of hospitalized patients, 10–20% of whom die. Mortality approaches 60–90% in those who develop septic shock (Bone et al 1989, Vincent & Bihari 1992), a figure that has changed little since intensive care was first developed, despite improvements in monitoring and supportive techniques. Attempts to classify the patterns of response seen in septic patients has lead to the identification of a constellation of typical clinical and haematological findings (Table 4.1). These syndromes are associated with the positive identification of an infecting causative agent in less than 50% of cases (Balk & Bone 1989). The term 'systemic inflammatory response syndrome' (SIRS) has therefore emerged as a useful definition of the resulting clinical state (ACCP Consensus Conference 1992), which avoids the requirement for identifiable infection. Recent clinical investigations have also emphasized the central role of sepsis-induced, endothelium-mediated circulatory failure in the pathophysiology of multiple organ failure (MOF), which carries an especially poor prognosis (Bone et al 1992).

The effects of failure of the functional and structural integrity of the endothelium that characterize SIRS are most obvious in the adult respiratory distress syndrome (ARDS), which complicates up to 25% of cases of SIRS (Macnaughton & Evans 1992), and has a mortality approaching 65%. ARDS is characterized by non-hydrostatic pulmonary oedema and refractory hypoxia. Pulmonary hypertension is a common complication of acute lung injury, and is associated with an increased mortality. Pulmonary vascular resistance is increased, even after correction for arterial hypoxaemia, and this results from both functional (vasoconstriction) and structural (embolization and vascular remodelling) changes in the pulmonary vasculature (Griffiths & Evans 1994). It has become increasingly apparent that acute lung injury can produce a spectrum of clinical presentations, only the most severe of which can be classified as ARDS. This spectrum reflects, among other factors, the variety of initiating insult, and with this in mind it is not surprising that lung injury is now considered to represent only the pulmonary manifestation of a wide-ranging vascular insult (Fig. 4.1), with equally variable clinical sequelae.

PATHOGENESIS OF SEPSIS

The initiating factor in the complex cascade of inflammatory events leading to clinical sepsis is the release of endotoxin or certain other comparable substances derived from yeasts, viruses, fungi, or Gram-positive bacteria (Bone 1991). Endotoxin is a lipopolysaccharide component of the cell wall of Gram-negative bacteria. The presence of endotoxin in the circulation can result from exogenous bacteria or via translocation of intestinal flora

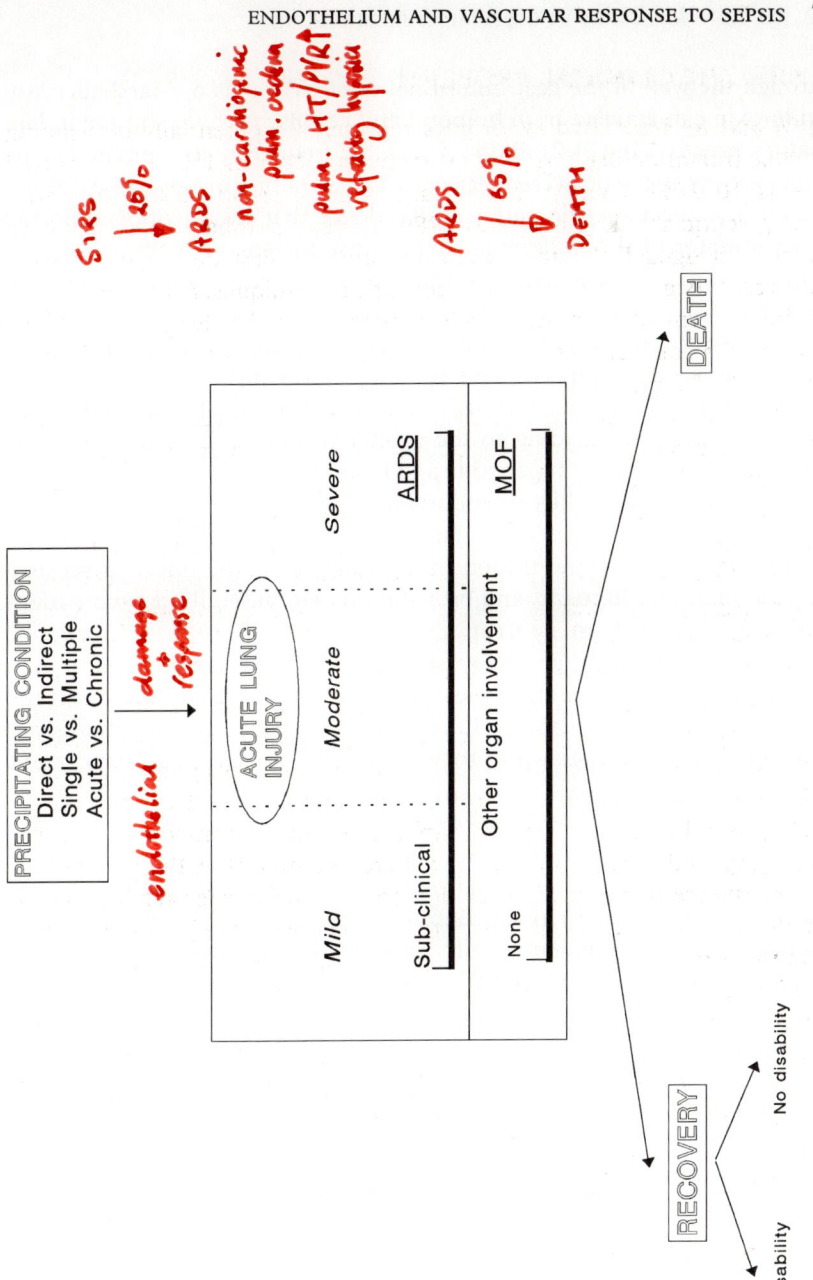

Fig. 4.1   The spectrum of disease: injury to the lung and other organs. A range of aetiological insults cause a spectrum of clinical illness whose severity is determined to a large extent by the damage to the vascular endothelium and the course of the resulting inflammatory response. ARDS = Acute respiratory distress syndrome; MOF = Multiple organ failure.

through the wall of the gastrointestinal tract (Meakins & Marshall 1986). Endotoxin can activate both humoral and cellular pathways in the inflammatory process (Fig. 4.2) and is detectable frequently in the blood of patients with septic shock (Danner et al 1991), whether or not blood cultures are positive for a specific pathogen. Evidence that endotoxin is important as an initiator of the inflammatory response to sepsis is compelling, as it produces similar haemodynamic changes in humans to those observed in experimental septic shock (Suffredini et al 1989). Animal studies suggest that endotoxin stimulates the release of tumour necrosis factor alpha (TNF), interleukins (IL-1, -6, -8) and platelet activating factor (PAF) from macrophages (Tabor et al 1988). TNF is a 17-kd polypeptide that can activate neutrophils leading to the production of elastase, as well as the reactive oxygen species superoxide and hydrogen peroxide. It promotes the attachment of neutrophils to endothelium leading to endothelial cell destruction (Smedly et al 1986). Radiolabelling of neutrophils has demonstrated their rapid sequestration in the lungs after the onset of sepsis in both animals and humans, and bronchoalveolar lavage fluid from patients with ARDS is rich in neutrophils (Weiland et al 1986). Injection of endotoxin causes TNF levels to rise acutely in both animals and humans (Michie et al 1988), eventually leading to hypotension and increased pulmonary capillary permeability. Levels of TNF are elevated in patients with sepsis and may correlate with prognosis (Waage et al 1987, Calandra et al 1990).

IL-1 shares many of the properties of TNF, producing hypotension and pulmonary oedema in animal models (Curzen et al 1994a). IL-6 production is stimulated by other cytokines, acts by regulating lymphocyte function and rises later in the inflammatory response. IL-8 is a potent chemotactic agent for neutrophils, and continues to be produced during the subsequent inflammatory response by, amongst other tissues, endothelium.

Following the activation of neutrophils by TNF, platelet activating factor (PAF), leukotrienes, and prostanoids including prostacyclin (PGI$_2$) and thromboxane A$_2$ are released. Platelet activation ensues, leading to the release of numerous vasoactive, chemoattractant and endothelium-damaging substances. Endotoxin is also a potent activator of the complement cascade. In addition, there is activation of both intrinsic and extrinsic coagulation cascades by the combination of cytokines, endotoxin and activated endothelial cells and platelets. When activated, Factor XII can initiate the intrinsic coagulation cascade as well as the contact system which generates bradykinin. This pathway, as well as neutrophil-generated proteases, stimulates the fibrinolytic systems, and can result in disseminated intravascular coagulopathy (DIC).

One of the integral features of this complex inflammatory response is that it involves mediator- and endotoxin-induced endothelial damage leading to loss of function and increased capillary permeability, which has been

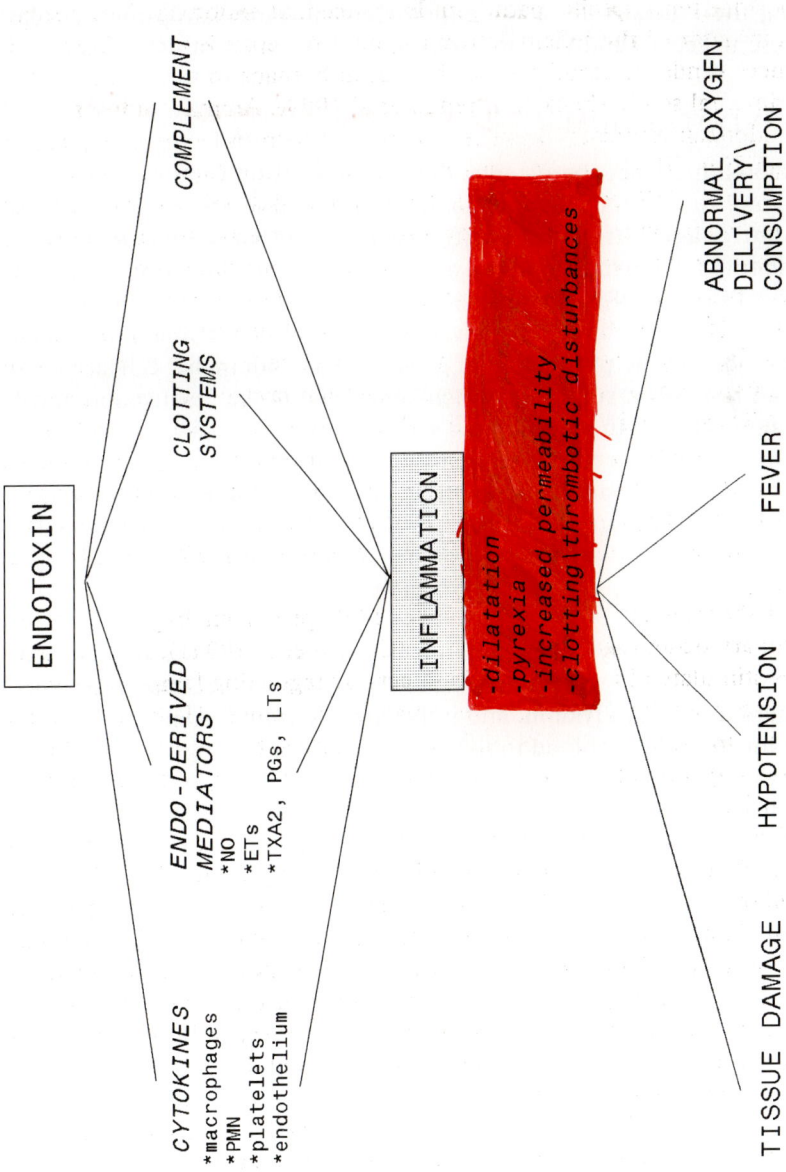

Fig. 4.2 The initiation of the inflammatory response by endotoxin. Endo-derived = Endothelium-derived; ETs = Endothelins; LTs = Leukotrienes; NO = Nitric oxide; PGs = Prostaglandins; PMN = Polymorphonuclear leucocytes; TXA₂ = Thromboxane.

shown to be due to changes in the cytoarchitecture of these cells produced by realignment of intracellular contractile proteins (Phillips & Tsan 1992). It is the investigation of the interactions between inflammatory cells and their mediators and the endothelium and its derived factors which is highlighting the crucial role of the endothelium in modulating the vascular response to sepsis, and thus in determining the extent of tissue injury.

THE ENDOTHELIUM   ① Antithrombic/anticoagulant activity

In order to maintain the patency of blood vessels and the fluidity of the circulating surface for blood, endothelial cells synthesize and release various anticoagulant and antithrombotic substances, including thrombomodulin, which binds thrombin to lower its affinity for fibrinogen (Petty & Pearson 1989). Tissue plasminogen activator (tPA) is also synthesized by the endothelium and activated by a variety of stimuli in the circulation to initiate the production of plasmin. The endothelial cell surface is also rich in heparin sulphates, which contribute to the inactivation of circulating thrombin. In addition, the synthesis and production of PGI_2 and nitric oxide are important components of its antithrombotic armoury, since both mediators are vascular smooth muscle dilators and potent inhibitors of platelet aggregation (vide infra).

Thrombomodulin
tPA
heparin sulphate
PGI_2
NO

Role in inflammation   ② Inflammation
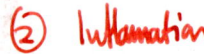

The endothelium plays an integral role in the acute inflammatory response (Ryan & Majno 1977), in responding to early (non-specific) mediators such as histamine and bradykinin, and in facilitating the adherence and subsequent migration from blood to tissue of activated neutrophils. Most of this neutrophil emigration occurs in post-capillary venules. It begins with slowing and margination of the white cells, when, under light microscopy, they can be seen rolling along the vessel wall surface because of loose tethering to the underlying endothelial cells. Subsequently, the neutrophils become more firmly adherent and their shape changes from spherical to a flatter configuration. Finally the cells migrate slowly between endothelial cells, and then through the basement membrane to the interstitium. It has become clear that this process is determined by a sequence of interactions between cell adhesion molecules (CAM) on the neutrophil and endothelial cell known as the adhesion cascade (Albelda et al 1994). The first phase of this sequence, the rolling and loose binding of the neutrophils depends upon the expression of a group of surface glycoprotein adhesion molecules, known collectively as selectins (Bevilacqua et al 1991).

HA
Bradykinin
PMN adhesion + migration

   The endothelial cell expresses two such molecules that are involved specifically in leucocyte/endothelial cell adherence: endothelial-leucocyte ad-

E-selectin
L-selectin
P-selectin

hesion molecule-1 (E-selectin), and granulocyte-associated membrane protein 140 (P-selectin). E-selectin is expressed on endothelium exposed to cytokines (including TNF and IL-1) and lipopolysaccharide. The kinetics of its production in cell culture imply that it is protein synthesis-dependent. P-selectin is found in the granules of platelets and endothelium, and expression is stimulated by thrombin and histamine (Geng et al 1990), thereby providing a mechanism by which neutrophil adhesion is initiated early in the inflammatory response before protein synthetic pathways have been activated. Simultaneously, L-selectin is expressed on neutrophils and is shed from the cell surface during this phase. Murine and rat in vivo models using antibodies directed against these molecules have demonstrated their importance in this initial phase of neutrophil emigration from the circulation (Jutila et al 1989, Ley et al 1991).

Following this slowing and rolling of neutrophils, subsequent firm adhesion and migration by the cells is dependent on the expression of another set of CAMs, known as integrins, on the neutrophil surface (Rouslahti 1991). The most important of these are the CD11\CD18 complex. The ligands for these CAMS are present on the endothelial cell surface, and the binding is promoted by cytokines including TNF, PAF and interleukins. For example, the vascular cell adhesion molecule (VCAM-1) is a member of the immunoglobulin family and is expressed in the presence of lipopolysaccharide, TNF and IL-1. The intercellular adhesion molecules (ICAM-1 and -2) are also constitutively expressed by endothelium and are therefore available for binding of neutrophils at the initiation of inflammation. Endothelial cell gene expression has been shown recently in response to various cytokines including TNF (Wolf et al 1992) and IL-1 (Maier et al 1990). The increased expression of the CD11\CD18 molecules on activated neutrophils has been demonstrated in several animal in vivo and in vitro models (Albelda et al 1994), but recently an increase in resting expression of CD11b\CD18 on granulocytes from patients with acute respiratory distress syndrome has also been shown to occur (Laurent et al 1994), and importantly appears to correlate with the hyperadhesiveness of these cells.

Following the firm binding of activated neutrophils to the endothelial surface, actual migration depends upon a chemotactic gradient, and probably also upon the expression of platelet-endothelial cell adhesion molecule-1 (PECAM-1). This is localized at the endothelial cell junctions, and recent work has demonstrated its importance both in vitro and in animal models (Muller et al 1993, Vaporciyan et al 1993).

The adhesion molecule 'cascade' thus determines the pattern of neutrophil-endothelial cell interaction in the early stage of the local inflammatory response. It represents an attractive series of targets for the application of antibody-mediated immunotherapy.

The endothelium and vascular tone

Nitric oxide

In 1980 the vascular relaxation induced by acetylcholine (ACh) was shown to be dependent on the presence of intact endothelium (Furchgott & Zawadzki 1980) and to be mediated via the release of a non-prostanoid, labile relaxant subsequently termed endothelium-derived relaxing factor (EDRF). Evidence has since accumulated that the chemical and pharmacological properties of EDRF are shared to a great extent by nitric oxide (NO).

Nitric oxide has been shown to be synthesized in vitro from the semi-essential amino acid, L-arginine, by the membrane-bound enzyme nitric oxide synthase (NOS) (Palmer et al 1988), a process that can be inhibited by the L-arginine analogues such as N^G-monomethyl-L-arginine (L-NMMA) (Johns et al 1990). Several distinct NOS genes have been identified (Lowenstein and Snyder 1992) and NOS exists in two forms (Table 4.2): a constitutive calcium- and calmodulin-dependent enzyme, which is probably responsible for basal release of NO, and an inducible calcium- and calmodulin-independent enzyme (vide infra). Both require NADPH and tetrahydrobiopterin as cofactors.

Table 4.2   Isoforms of vascular nitric oxide synthases. LPS = lipopolysaccharide; NO = Nitric oxide; NOS = Nitric oxide synthases

NOS isoforms	Type II	Type III
Response in sepsis	Constitutive	Enzyme synthesis induced by LPS and cytokines
	Immediate increase in NO activity	Massive NO production after 2–6 hours
Location	Endothelial cell Membrane-bound	Mainly smooth muscle Cytosolic
Regulation		Induction prevented by corticosteroids and inhibitors of protein synthesis
Activation	Calcium-dependent	Calcium-independent
Non-selective inhibitors		L-arginine analogues (e.g. N^G-monomethyl-L-arginine)
Selective inhibitors	None known	Aminoguanidine L-canavanine Diphenyleneiodonium

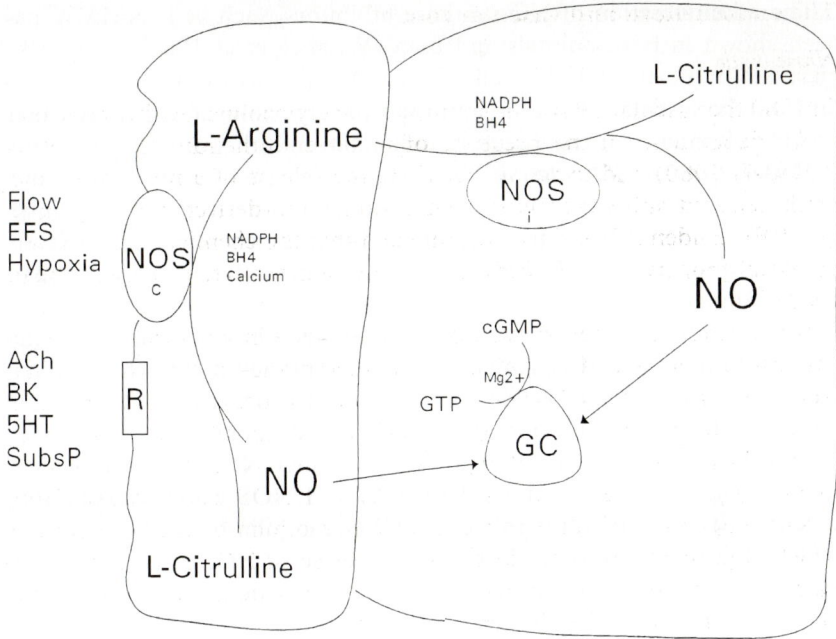

Fig. 4.3 Mechanism of action of constitutive and inducible NOS. The endothelium also contains inducible NOS, but this has been left out for clarity. ACH = Acetylcholine; BH$_4$ = Tetrahydrabiopterin; BK = Bradykinin; cGMP = cyclic guanosine monophosphate; EFS = Electrical field stimulation; GTP = guanosine triphosphate; 5HT = 5-Hydroxytryptamine; Mg^{2+} = magnesium ions; NADPH = Nicotine adenosine diphosphate; NO = Nitric oxide; NOSC = Constitutive nitric oxide synthase; NOSi = Inducible nitric oxide synthase; R = Membrane receptor; SubsP = Substance P.

NO activates soluble guanylyl cyclase, after binding to its haem moiety, which in turn causes an increase in intracellular cyclic guanine monophosphate (cGMP) content causing vascular smooth muscle to relax (Moncada et al 1991) (Fig. 4.3), a chain of events confirmed by several studies. Thus, L-arginine administration has been shown to produce vasodilatation in newborn lambs (Fineman et al 1991a,b), an effect blocked by the guanylyl cyclase inhibitor, methylene blue, or by L-NMMA. The vasodilatation was augmented, however, by a cGMP phosphodiesterase inhibitor, whose ability to raise intracellular cGMP levels has also been shown to produce vasodilatation in other models, reinforcing the importance of this mechanism as a mediator of endothelium-dependent vasodilatation. A rise in cGMP may produce vascular smooth muscle relaxation via several mechanisms which lower intracellular free calcium (Ca^{2+}) levels including: a reduction in calcium influx; a reduction in its release from intracellular stores; an increase in Ca^{2+} sequestration in intracellular stores; or by stimulation of Ca^{2+} ATPase-dependent extrusion of Ca^{2+}.

The administration of NO synthase inhibitors, such as L-NMMA, has been shown in both animals and man (Vallance et al 1989) to provoke increases in mean arterial blood pressure and decreases in regional blood flow, implying that there is a continual basal release of NO which may provide physiological regulation of tissue blood flow.

Regulation of NO release   Local blood flow is an important regulator of NO activity. Thus, increased systemic blood flow can augment agonist-evoked endothelium-dependent relaxations via an increase in NO release. The size of the hypertensive response induced by intravenous L-NMMA in animal models is dependent on basal vascular tone (Vargas et al 1990). As discussed, NO plays an important part in pulmonary vascular regulation, in that inhibitors of NOS cause dose-dependent increases in pulmonary artery pressure in awake lambs, whilst systemic arterial pressure remains unaffected. In rabbits (Wilkund et al 1990), infusion of the NOS inhibitor, L-NAME, causes an increase in respiratory rate and arterial hypoxaemia. NO is also released during exposure to acute hypoxia, may modulate hypoxic pulmonary vasoconstriction (HPV), and is capable of influencing the pulmonary vascular response to chronic hypoxia (Curzen et al 1994b). Disruption of normal regulatory mechanisms of the lung, especially HPV, is known to be a feature of sepsis-associated lung injury and these effects of NO may play a crucial role in this pathophysiology.

The release of NO has been demonstrated in response to many other pharmacological and physiological stimuli, including histamine, thrombin, adenosine triphosphate (ATP), bradykinin, calcium ionophore, and substance P.

NO release in sepsis   Patients and animals with septic shock lose peripheral vascular tone, and the responsiveness of vessels to constricting agents both in vitro and in vivo is diminished (Lorente et al 1993). The incubation of bovine aortic endothelial cells with lipopolysaccharide causes the rapid release of an NO-like factor. In patients with septic shock, the levels of NO metabolites in plasma are significantly elevated (Ochoa et al 1991), and the infusion of NOS inhibitors in such cases (Petros et al 1991) and in animal models of septic shock (Klabunde & Ritger 1991, Cobb et al 1992, Wright et al 1992) can lead to a rapid and reproducible rise in systemic vascular resistance where other vasoconstrictors are ineffective. Thus, both the synthesis and release of NO are stimulated by the inflammatory process.

Endotoxin leads to induction of a calcium-independent NO synthase (iNOS) in endothelium (Radomski et al 1990) and vascular smooth muscle (Fleming et al 1991a), as well as myocardium where its production has been shown to reduce contractility (Brady et al 1992). TNF and IL-1 can also stimulate the expression of iNOS in both endothelium and vascular smooth muscle. Patients who are treated with IL-2 chemotherapy excrete high levels of NO metabolites, implying that NO synthesis is also induced by this cytokine. L-NMMA can also inhibit TNF-induced hypotension in animals.

Further studies have demonstrated the possibility of a two-stage release of NO from the vessel wall during sepsis. In isolated endotoxin-treated rat main pulmonary arteries, NOS inhibitors reverse vascular hyporesponsiveness to phenylephrine (Griffiths et al 1993a). The NO-mediated hyporeactivity to noradrenaline starts within 60 minutes in a rat model of sepsis in vivo (Szabo et al 1993), and so is too rapid to be explained by the induction of iNOS. This implies that the endothelium responds immediately to the septic insult by releasing NO produced by the constitutive enzyme cNOS. In another study, however, the use of L-NAME after one hour in endotoxin-treated pithed rats did elevate blood pressure and enhance vascular responsiveness to both noradrenaline and sympathetic stimulation, but not to a significantly greater degree than in saline-treated animals (Guc et al 1992). This does not therefore support the hypothesis that after endotoxin insult an increase in NO release explains the early loss of vascular responsiveness in vivo, but rather suggests that some other factor(s) must be involved. From about three hours after the endotoxic insult, however, there is massive NO production as a result of induction of the inducible form of NOS (iNOS), probably mostly in the underlying vascular smooth muscle (Fleming et al 1991a). There is also evidence that endothelium is required for a maximal NO response. Thus, removal of the endothelium caused a significant delay in the onset of vascular hyporesponsiveness (6 hours compared with 4 hours) and reduced the sensitivity of rat aorta exposed to lipopolysaccharide in vitro (Fleming et al 1991b, 1993). Selective inhibitors for iNOS are now available and evidence already suggests their potential therapeutic value in sepsis (Griffiths et al 1993b, 1994).

Endothelins

In 1988 an endothelially-derived vasoconstrictor was cloned and sequenced following its isolation from the culture medium of porcine aortic endothelial cells (Yanagisawa et al 1988), and termed endothelin. This substance was found to elicit a slow-onset, sustained contraction of isolated arteries from many different species. Three similar but distinct ET-related genomic loci have now been identified which encode for three similar but distinct ET molecules (ET-1, ET-2, ET-3) (Haynes & Webb 1993), all of which are derived from prepropeptides, and consist of 21 amino acids with considerable homology. The conversion of the propeptide, Big ET-1, to ET-1 was postulated to be due to the activity of an endothelin-converting enzyme (ECE), since identified in several animal models as a phosphoramidon-sensitive neutral metalloproteinase. Two neutral proteases with ECE activity have now also been demonstrated. One is membrane-bound, phosphoramidon-sensitive and can utilize all three ETs as substrates; the other is soluble and phosphoramidon-insensitive. Three ET receptor subtypes probably exist, although so far only two have been cloned and expressed. ETA has the highest affinity for ET-1 compared with the other ETs, and although it has widespread expression in humans, in particular in vascular smooth muscle, this does not include endothelial cells. ETB is non-selective, binding all three ETs, which are equipotent in displacing ^{125}ET-I. ETB is also widespread and is expressed on endothelial cells.

ET-1 appears to act by increasing intracellular calcium (Ca^{2+}) concentration, by activating phospholipase C, which in turn leads to increases in inositol triphosphate and diacylglycerol synthesis (Fig. 4.4). Both are implicated in the initial rise in intracellular Ca^{2+} concentrations, and probably underlie the initiation of ET-1-induced vascular contraction. Protein kinase C is also implicated in a second messenger system mediating ET-1-induced contraction, particularly as staurosporine, a protein kinase C inhibitor, attenuates in vitro contractions to ET-1.

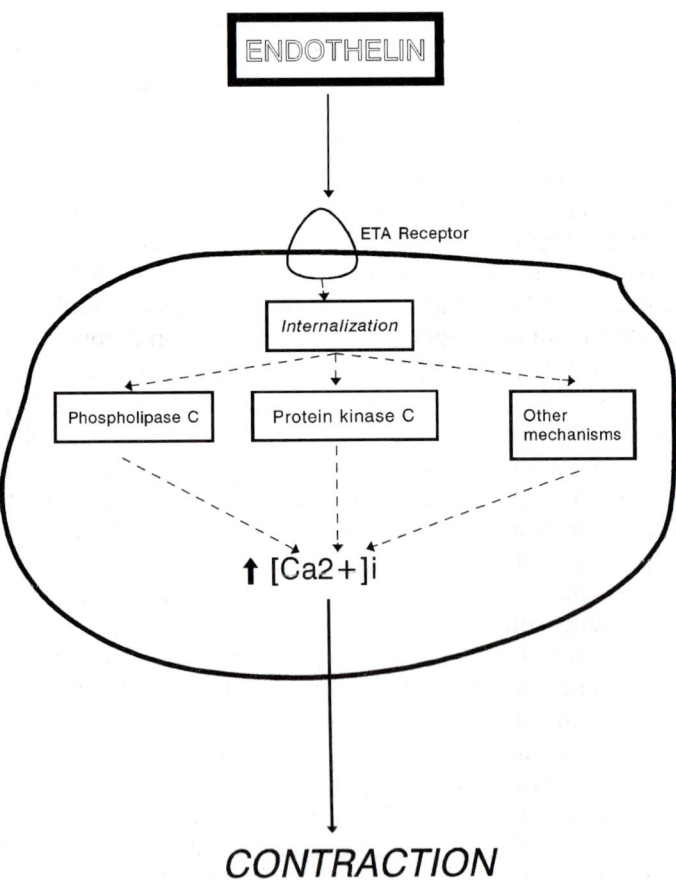

Fig. 4.4 Mechanism of action of endothelin. [Ca^{2+}]i = Free intracellular calcium ions; ETA = Endothelin A receptor.

Release of endothelins   ET-1 immunoreactivity cannot be demonstrated in homogenates of capillary endothelial cells, and release of ET from cultured endothelial cells can be prevented by the protein synthesis inhibitor cycloheximidine, suggesting that ETs are not stored but synthesized de novo in the endothelium. The factors that have been demonstrated to stimulate endothelin release in various species are diverse, and include vessel wall shear stress, hypoxia, endotoxin, TNF, interferon, adrenaline, angiotensin, thrombin, activated platelets, and some prostanoids. Release of ETs would therefore be expected in response to any disturbance to local haemodynamics and also during any inflammatory response.

Endothelins in the control of vascular tone   ET-1 is a potent vasoconstrictor in humans (Hughes et al 1989) and many animal species. The endothelium modulates the vascular response to ETs. Thus, ET-1- and ET-3-induced contraction of rat pulmonary arteries is enhanced by endothelial removal (Rodman et al 1989) and both agents elicit vasodilatation in preconstricted vessels of isolated mesentery. NO release has been demonstrated in rat mesentery in response to ET, an effect inhibited by L-NMMA (Fukuda et al 1990). ET-3 is a more potent vasodilator than ET-1, possibly because the receptor involved on the endothelium is of the ETB type, which has equal affinity for all ETs, whereas the ETA (vasoconstrictor) receptor is predominant in vascular smooth muscle and has a higher affinity for ET-1. There is a uniform haemodynamic response to ET infusion in most species, characterized by initial transient hypotension, followed by sustained hypertension (Yanagisawa et al 1988). The hypotensive response can be at least partially inhibited by NOS inhibitors (Gardiner et al 1990), but does not recur if the ET infusion is continuous rather than bolus. ET-1 and ET-3 are both coronary and pulmonary vasoconstrictors. However, ET-3 is a powerful vasodilator in isolated rat lungs under prior conditions of hypoxic vasoconstriction (Crawley et al 1992). ET-1 has been shown to have inotropic and chronotropic effects on cardiac tissue. ET-1 can induce cultured smooth muscle cell proliferation, and ET-1 and ET-3 stimulate fibroblast growth and chemotaxis (Peacock et al 1992) suggesting a role in vascular re-modelling.

Endothelins in sepsis   ETs seem to be important mediators of vascular tonic responses under physiological conditions, since they are released in response to a variety of local factors including hypoxia. Their potent effects on vascular tone and modulation of mediator release are likely to play an important role in the widespread changes associated with endotoxaemia. ET release in response to endotoxin has been confirmed by radioimmunoassay in vitro and in vivo (Sugiura et al 1989), and in endothelial cell cultures in response to TNF, interferon gamma, IL-1, transforming growth factor β (Kanse et al 1991) and free radical species. ET levels increase during endotoxaemia in many animal models and are elevated, possibly in parallel with indicators of illness severity, in patients with septic shock (Pittet et al 1991, Voerman et al 1992).

The role played by the ETs in the inflammatory response to sepsis is not yet clear. In endothelial cells and vascular smooth muscle, NO leads to the activation of soluble guanylyl cyclase with the formation of cGMP and in vascular smooth muscle this stimulates relaxation. In endothelial cells, however, cGMP can inhibit ET production (Boulanger & Luscher 1990). In human and canine models endothelin-induced contractions can also be inhibited by NO released in response to acetylcholine or bradykinin (Luscher et al 1990). The release, and subsequently high circulating levels of such a potent vasoconstrictor substance, would be expected to antagonize the observed vasodilator response, and it is possible that the interaction between ETs and NO explains this paradox. The ability of ETs to act as vasolidators under hypoxic conditions may also contribute.

Derivatives of arachidonic acid

The endothelium produces various prostanoids via the cyclo-oxygenase pathway of arachidonic acid metabolism (Fig. 4.5), principal amongst which is PGI$_2$ which activates adenylate cyclase, increasing intracellular cAMP levels and causing smooth muscle relaxation (Moncada & Vane 1979, Luscher & Vanhoutte 1990). Inhibitors of prostaglandin synthesis, such as indomethacin and meclofenamate, augment HPV (Curzen et al 1994b), implying that vasodilator prostaglandins may modulate vascular tone during hypoxic episodes. Furthermore, in a rat model of skeletal muscle microcirculation, increases in arteriolar blood flow induced an endothelium-dependent vasodilatation distal to the occlusion which could be inhibited by cyclo-oxygenase inhibitors, but not by L-NMMA. Cytokines such as TNF and IL-1 can stimulate prostanoid release, the vasodilator action of which can be augmented by the presence of endothelium (Shimakawa et al 1988).

Cyclo-oxygenase metabolism of arachidonic acid also produces vasoconstrictor agents such as thromboxane A$_2$ (TXA$_2$) and endoperoxides. TXA$_2$ is a potent constrictor of pulmonary arterioles after endotoxin infusion, and is also capable of increasing capillary permeability (Petrak et al 1989). The use of thromboxane synthase inhibition has also been shown to reduce pulmonary vasoconstriction in other animal models (Winn et al 1983).

ET-1 stimulates the release of the vasodilators PGI$_2$ and PGE$_2$, as well as the vasoconstrictor TXA$_2$, possibly via ET-induced activation of protein kinase C (Michael et al 1993). In isolated rat mesenteric arteries, ET-1 infusion produces endothelium-dependent relaxation that can be abolished by indomethacin, but not L-NMMA (Dohi & Luscher 1991). The endothelin-mediated release of these two prostanoids has also been demonstrated in other animal models. In isolated human internal mammary artery, PGI$_2$ reverses ET-1-induced vasoconstriction (Yang et al 1989). Indomethacin pretreatment of isolated rat or guinea pig lung preparations potentiates ET-induced contractions and increases ET-3-induced ET-1 formation in cultured endothelial cells (DeNucci et al 1988).

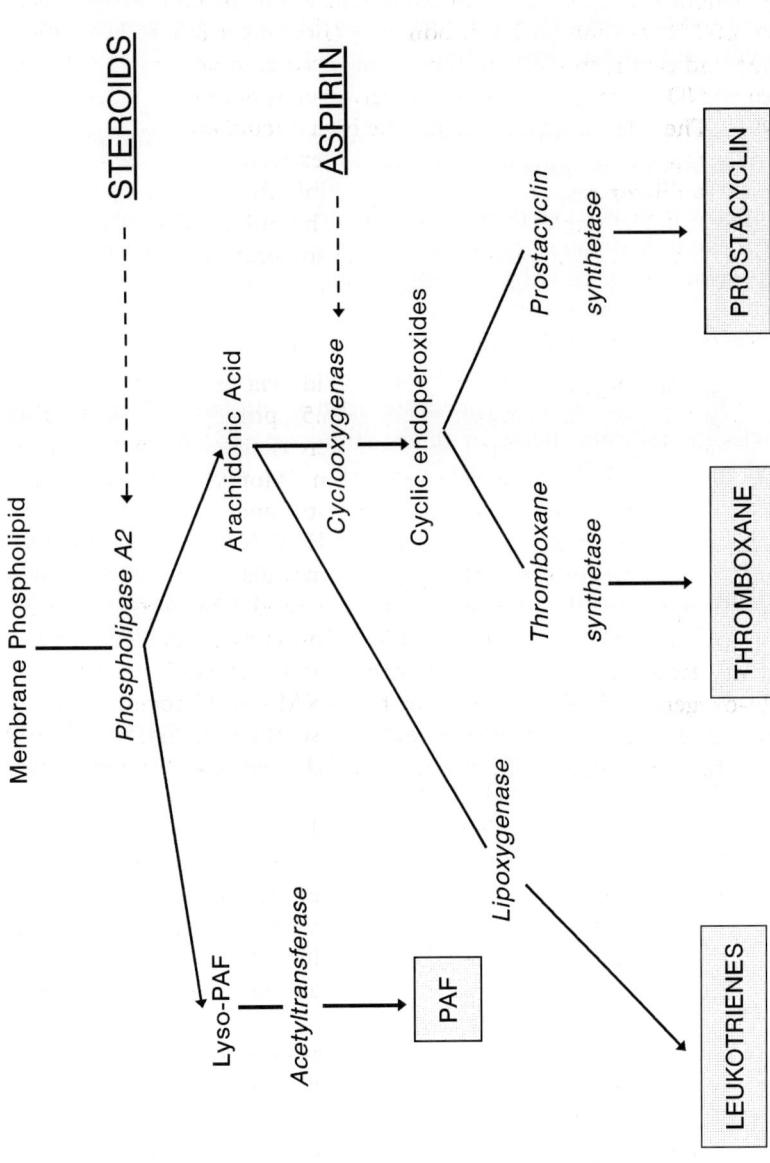

Fig. 4.5 Derivatives of membrane phospholipid. PAF = Platelet activating factor.

The role of these endothelium-derived prostanoids in the vascular response to sepsis is not fully elucidated, but evidence from animal models
of septic shock has demonstrated improved outcome from cyclo-oxygenase
inhibition (Fletcher & Ramwell 1980, Wise et al 1980). The possibility of
benefit in patients with sepsis from therapy with cyclo-oxygenase inhibitors is currently under investigation.

The interaction of endothelium-derived vasoactive mediators in the inflammatory response to sepsis

The response to sepsis can be seen as a cascade, each component of which
amplifies the inflammatory response. The interactions between individual
mediators of sepsis are highly complex, but determine the extent of
endothelial, and subsequently tissue damage (see Fig. 4.3).

After endotoxin exposure, macrophage activation leads to cytokine release. TNF and interleukins-1 and -2 are able to damage endothelial cells
and increase their permeability; activate neutrophils and endothelial cells
and facilitate adhesion between them; stimulate endothelial cells (and
macrophages) to synthesize and release NO, ETs, and prostanoids. The
activity of TNF and IL-1 to disrupt pulmonary vascular endothelium has
been shown to be synergistic. In addition, TNF administration only produces features of septic shock when PAF is present (Myers et al 1990).
The inflammatory response may then be amplified by endothelially-derived
products of arachidonic acid metabolism (Petrak et al 1989). Furthermore,
TNF, PAF and IL-1 can promote their own and each others' release from
several cells including the endothelium and macrophages. Activated platelets can stimulate the expression of ET mRNA and biosynthesis in
endothelial cell cultures, but the potency of this reaction is multiplied sev-
eral-fold by endotoxin. The ETs released can modulate the activation of
macrophages and also affect the clotting cascades via release of tPA and
von Willebrand factor from endothelial cells.

The endothelium also has a role in the down-regulation of the inflammatory response. NO, in particular, appears to have some anti-inflammatory properties, although available results are conflicting, and it is therefore
not possible to extrapolate with any confidence from one experimental
preparation to either another model or to the clinical setting. For example,
there is evidence from in vitro and in vivo studies, utilizing NO synthesis
inhibitors, that NO can modulate the increase in vascular permeability and
protein leakage that is seen during the inflammatory response (Ialenti et al
1992, Kubes & Granger 1992). It has also been shown to reduce white cell
adherence to endothelial cells (Kubes et al 1991). A further anti-inflammatory property of NO in endotoxaemia is its antithrombotic potential,
illustrated by the high rate of glomerular thrombosis in rats treated with

endotoxin and L-NMMA when compared with endotoxin without an NO-synthesis inhibitor (Schultz & Raij 1992). Finally, studies in vitro suggest a role for NO as a scavenger of superoxide radicals (Rubanyi et al 1991), which are released by activated neutrophils and are not only cytotoxic but can also alter pulmonary vascular reactivity in their own right. This remains controversial, however, since there is also evidence that NO reacts with superoxide radicals in pathological states, particularly those associated with hypoxia, to produce even more cytotoxic species such as peroxynitrites. In one rat model in vivo immune complex lung or dermal injury has been shown to be L-arginine dependent and could be prevented by L-NMMA (Mulligan et al 1991). The mechanism by which nitric oxide is able to cause tissue damage may be related to its ability to cause DNA strand breakage (Nguyen et al 1992).

The endothelium can damp down the inflammatory response in other ways. For example, PGI_2 can also inhibit TNF synthesis (Balk et al 1988). PGE_2 also inhibits the fibroblast proliferation stimulated by the cytokines and ET-1 (Elias et al 1990). In addition, PGE_2 and iloprost (a prostacyclin analogue) have been shown to inhibit LPS-stimulated induction of NO in murine macrophages (Marotta and Di Rosa 1992). Although activated platelets stimulate ET production, there appears to be regulatory negative feedback since ET can also inhibit platelet function ex vivo in the rabbit (Thiemermann et al 1988).

KEY POINTS FOR CLINICAL PRACTICE

- The endothelium is a dynamic, metabolically active layer of cells, and its ability to release anticoagulant and vasoactive substances and act as a selectively permeable barrier between the circulation and the tissues make it an integral component of all forms of vascular response.
- Sepsis is extended as a concept to include all conditions in which there is a profound systemic inflammatory response, not just those in which an infecting organism is isolated.
- The endothelium is capable of being activated during early vascular insult, such as that presented by endotoxin.
- Endothelial cell activation results in release of vasoactive mediators, expression of adhesion molecules, and anticoagulant substances. The interaction of these factors with other inflammatory cells such as polymorphs and macrophages determines the vascular response to sepsis, both at local and diverse sites. Whether the inflammatory process escalates to cause the extensive tissue damage seen in conditions such as ARDS and MOF probably depends on the balance between the pro- and anti-inflammatory mediators and the cells that produce them.

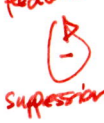

inhaled NO, PGI2
NOS inhibitors
immuno therapy

• Research is currently aimed at attempting to manipulate this inflammatory response so as to reduce tissue damage and maintain oxygenation. Interest currently centres on inhaled NO and prostacyclin, inhibitors of nitric oxide synthase such as L-NMMA and aminoguanidine, as well as immunotherapeutic agents to modulate specific parts of the response, and in particular the adhesion molecule cascade.

REFERENCES

Albelda S M, Smith C W, Ward P A 1994 Adhesion molecules and inflammatory injury. Faseb J 8:504–512

ACCP\Society of Critical Care Medicine Consensus Conference 1992 Definitions for sepsis and organ failure and guidelines for the use of innovative therapies in sepsis. Crit Care Med 20: 864–874

Balk R A, Bone R C 1989 The septic syndrome: definition and clinical implications. Crit Care Clin 5: 1–8

Balk R A, Jacobs R F, Tryka F et al 1988 Effects of ibuprofen on neutrophil function and acute lung injury in canine endotoxic shock. Crit Care Med 16: 1121–1127

Bevilacqua M, Buthcher E, Furie B et al 1991 Selectins: a family of adhesion receptors. Cell 67: 223

Bone R C 1991 The pathogenesis of sepsis. Ann Int Med 115: 457–469

Bone R C, Fisher C J, Clemmer T P et al 1989 Sepsis syndrome: a valid clinical entity. Crit Care Med 17: 389–393

Bone R C, Balk R A, Slotman G et al 1992 Adult respiratory distress syndrome sequence and importance of multiple organ failure. Chest 20: 320–326

Boulanger C, Luscher T F 1990 Endothelin is released from porcine aorta: inhibition by endothelium-derived nitric oxide. J Clin Invest 85: 587–590

Brady A J B, Poole-Wilson P A, Harding S E, Warren J B 1992 Nitric oxide production within cardiac myocytes reduces their contractility in endotoxaemia. Am J Physiol 263: H1963–1966

Calandra T, Baumgartner J D, Gray G E et al 1990 Prognosis value of TNF\cachectin, IL-1, alpha-interferon and gamma-interferon in the serum of patients with septic shock. J Infect Dis 161: 982–987

Cobb J P, Natanson C, Koev C E et al 1992 The haemodynamic effects of N^G-methyl-L-arginine, an inhibitor of nitric oxide synthase, in endotoxaemic compared to normal canines. Crit Care Med 20: S51

Crawley D E, Liu S F, Barnes P J, Evans T W 1992 Endothelin-3 is a potent vasodilator in the rat. J Appl Physiol 72: 1425–1431

Curzen N P, Griffiths M J D, Evans T W 1994a The role of the endothelium in modulating the vascular response to sepsis. Clin Sci 86: 359–374

Curzen N P, Griffiths M J D, Evans T W 1995 Pulmonary vascular control mechanisms in lung injury. In: Morice A (ed) Clinical pulmonary hypertension. Portland Press, London, pp 171–202

Danner R L, Elin R J, Hosseini J M et al 1991 Endotoxaemia in human septic shock. Chest 99: 169–175

DeNucci G, Thomas R, D'Orleans-Juste P et al 1988 Pressor effects of circulating endothelin are limited by its removal in the pulmonary circulation and by the release of prostacyclin and endothelium-derived relaxing factor. Proc Natl Acad Sci USA 85: 9797–9800

Dohi Y, Luscher T F 1991 Endothelin in hypertensive resistance arteries: intraluminal and extraluminal dysfunction. Hypertension 18: 543–549

Elias J A, Freundlich B, Kern J A, Rosenbloom J 1990 Cytokine networks in the regulation of inflammation and fibrosis in the lung. Chest 97: 1439-1445

Fineman J R, Crowley M R, Heymann M A, Soifer SJ 1991a In vivo inhibition of endothelium-dependent pulmonary vasodilatation by methylene blue in the lamb. J Appl Physiol 71: 735–741

Fineman J R, Chang R, Soifer S J 1991b L-arginine, a precursor of EDRF in vitro, produces pulmonary vasodilatation in lambs. Am J Physiol 261: H1563–1569

Fleming I, Gray G A, Schott C, Stoclet J-C 1991a Inducible but not constitutive production of nitric oxide by vascular smooth muscle cells. Eur J Pharmacol 200: 375–376

Fleming I, Julou-Schaeffer G, Gray G A, Parratt J R, Stoclet JC 1991b Evidence that an L-arginine/nitric oxide dependent elevation of cGMP content is involved in depression of vascular reactivity by endotoxin. Br J Pharmacol 103: 1047–1052

Fleming I, Gray G A, Stoclet J C 1993 Influence of the endothelium on induction of the L-arginine-NO pathway in rat aortas. Am J Physiol 264: H1200–1207

Fletcher J R, Ramwell P W 1980 Indomethacin improves survival after endotoxin in baboons. Adv Prostaglandin Thromboxane Res 7: 821–828

Fukuda N, Izumi Y, Soma M et al 1990 L-N^G-monomethyl arginine inhibits the vasodilating effects of low dose of endothelin-3 on rat mesenteric arteries. Biochem Biophys Res Commun 167: 739–745

Furchgott R F, Zawadzki J V 1980 The obligatory role of endothelial cells in the relaxation of arterial smooth muscle by acetylcholine. Nature 288: 373–376

Gardiner S M, Compton A M, Kemp P A, Bennett T 1990 Regional and cardiac haemodynamic responses to glyceryl trinitrate, acetylcholine, bradykinin and endothelin-1 in conscious rats: effects of N^G-nitro-L-arginine methyl ester. Br J Pharmacol 101: 81–88

Geng J-G, Bevilacqua M P, Moore K L et al 1990 Rapid neutrophil adhesion to activated endothelium mediated by GMP-140. Nature 343: 757–760

Griffiths M J D, Messent M, Evans T W 1993a The role of nitric oxide in the pulmonary vascular response to endotoxin. Thorax 48: 467

Griffiths M J D, Messent M, MacAllister R J, Evans T W 1993b Aminoguanidine selectively inhibits inducible nitric oxide synthase. Br J Pharmacol 110: 963–968

Griffiths M J D, Curzen N P, Sair M, Evans T W 1994 Nitric oxide inhibitors in septic shock: theoretical considerations. Clin Int Care 5: 29–36

Griffiths M J D, Evans T W 1994 Adult respiratory distress sydnrome. In: Brewis RAL, Corrin B, Geddes D M, Gibson G J (eds), Respiratory medicine, W B Saunders and Co Ltd, London, pp 605–629

Guc M O, Furman B L, Parratt J R 1992 Modification of alpha-adrenoceptor-mediated pressor responses by N^G-nitro-L-arginine methyl ester and vasopressin in endotoxin-treated pithed rats. Eur J Pharmacol 224: 63–69

Haynes W G, Webb D J 1993 The endothelin family of peptides: local hormones with diverse roles in health and disease? Clin Sci 84: 485–500

Hughes A D, Thom S A McG, Woodall N et al 1989 Human vascular responses to endothelin-1: observations *in vivo* and *in vitro*. J Cardiovasc Pharmacol 13: S225–228

Ialenti A, Ianaro A, Moncada S, Di Rosa M 1992 Modulation of acute inflammation by endogenous nitric oxide. Eur J Pharmacol 211: 117–182

Johns R A, Peach M J, Linden J, Tichotsky A 1990 N^G-monomethyl L-arginine inhibits endothelium-derived relaxing factor-stimulated cGMP accumulation on cocultures of endothelial and vascular smooth muscle cells by an action specific to the endothelial cell. Circ Res 67: 979–985

Jutila M A, Rott L, Berg E L, Butcher E C 1989 Function and regulation of the neutrophil MEL-14 antigen *in vivo*: comparison with LFA-1 and MAC-1. J Immunol 143: 3318–3324

Kanse S M, Takahashi K, Lam H-C et al 1991 Cytokine stimulated endothelin release from endothelial cells. Life Sciences 48: 1379–1384

Klabunde R E, Ritger R C 1991 N^G-monomethyl-L-arginine (NMA) restores arterial blood pressure but reduces cardiac output in a canine model of endotoxic shock. Biochem Biophys Res Commun 178: 1135–1140

Kubes P, Granger D N 1992 Nitric oxide modulates microvascular permeability. Am J Physiol 262: H611–615

Kubes P, Suzuki M, Granger D 1991 Nitric oxide: an endogenous modulator of leukocyte adhesion. Proc Natl Acad Sci USA 88: 4651–4655

Laurent T, Markert M, Fliedner V V et al 1994 CD11b\CD18 expression, adherence, and chemotaxis of granulocytes in adult respiratory distress syndrome. Am J Respir Crit Care Med 149: 1534–1538

Ley K, Gaehtgens P, Kennie C et al 1991 Lectin-like cell adhesion molecule-1 mediates leukocyte rolling in mesenteric venules in vivo. Blood 77: 2553–2555

Lorente J A, Landin L, Renes E et al 1993 Role of nitric oxide in the haemodynamic changes of sepsis. Crit Care Med 21: 759–767

Lowenstein C J, Snyder S H 1992 Nitric oxide: a novel biological messenger. Cell 70: 705–707

Luscher T F, Vanhoutte P M 1990 The endothelium: modulator of cardiovascular function. Boca Raton, F L: CRC Press Inc, pp. 1–228

Luscher T F, Yang Z, Tschudi M et al 1990 Interaction between endothelin-1 and endothelium-derived relaxing factor in human arteries and veins. Circ Res 66: 1088-1094

Macnaughton P D, Evans T W 1992 Adult respiratory distress syndrome. Lancet 339: 469–472

Maier J A, Hla T, Maciag T 1990 Cyclo-oxygenase is an immediate-early gene induced by interleukin-1 in endothelial cells. J Biol Chem 265: 10805–10808

Marotta P, Di Rosa M 1992 Modulation of the induction of nitric oxide synthase by eicosanoids in the macrophage cell line J774. Br J Pharmacol 107: 640–641

Meakins K L, Marshall J C 1986 The gastrointestinal tract: the 'motor' of MOF. Arch Surg 121: 197–201

Michael J R, Yang J, Farrukh I S, Gurtner G H 1993 Protein-kinase C-mediated pulmonary vasoconstriction in rabbit: role of Ca^{2+}, AA metabolites, and vasodilators. J Appl Physiol 74: 1310–1319

Michie H R, Manogue K R, Spriggs D R et al 1988 Detection of circulating TNF after endotoxin administration. N Engl J Med 318: 1481–1486

Moncada S, Palmer R M J, Higgs E A 1991 Nitric oxide: physiology, pathophysiology and pharmacology. Pharmacology Rev 43: 109–142

Moncada S, Vane J R 1979 Pharmacology and endogenous roles of prostaglandins endoperoxides, thromboxane A_2 and prostacyclin. Pharmacol Rev 30: 293–331

Muller W A, Weigl S A, Deng X, Phillips D M 1993 PECAM-1 is required for transendo-thelial migration of leukocytes. J Exp Med 178: 449–460

Mulligan M S, Hevel J M, Marletta M A, Ward P A 1991 Tissue injury caused by deposition of immune complexes is L-arginine dependent. Proc Natl Acad Sci USA 88: 6338-6342

Myers A K, Robey J W, Price R M 1990 Relationships between tumour necrosis factor, eicosanoids and platelet-activating factor as mediators of endotoxin-induced shock in mice. Br J Pharmacol 99: 499–502

Nguyen T, Brunson D, Crespi C L et al 1992 DNA damage and mutation in human cells exposed to nitric oxide. Proc Natl Acad Sci USA 89: 3030–3034

Ochoa J B, Udekwu AO, Billiar T R et al 1991 Nitrogen oxide levels in patients after trauma and during sepsis. Ann Surg 214: 621–626

Palmer R M J, Ashton D S, Moncada S 1988 Vascular endothelial cells synthesize nitric oxide from L-arginine. Nature 333: 664–666

Peacock A J, Dawes K, Shock A et al 1992 Endothelin-1 and endothelin-3 induce chemotaxis and replication of pulmonary artery fibroblasts. Am J Respir Cell Mol Biol 7: 492–499

Petrak R A, Balk R A, Bone R C 1989 Prostaglandins, cyclo-oxygenase inhibitors and thromboxane synthetase inhibitors in the pathogenesis of multiple systems organ failure. Crit Care Clin 5: 303–314

Petros A, Bennett D, Vallance P 1991 Effect of nitric oxide inhibitors on hypotension in patients with septic shock. Lancet 338: 1557–1558

Petty R G, Pearson J D 1989 Endothelium: the axis of vascular health and disease. J R Coll Phys Lond 23: 92–102

Phillips P, Tsan M-F 1992 Cytoarchitectural aspects of endothelial barrier function in response to oxidants and inflammatory mediators. In: Johnson A, Ferro T J (eds), Lung vascular injury Ch. 4, Marcel Dekker, New York

Pittet J-F, Morel D R, Hemsen A et al 1991 Elevated plasma endothelin-1 concentrations are associated with the severity of illness in patients with sepsis. Ann Surg 213: 261–264

Radomski M W, Palmer R M J, Moncada S 1990 Glucocorticoids inhibit the expression of an inducible, but not the constitutive, nitric oxide synthase in vascular endothelial cells. Proc Natl Acad Sci USA 87: 10043–10047

Rodman D M, McMurty I F, Peach J L, O'Brien R F 1989 Comparative pharmacology of rat and porcine endothelin in rat aorta and pulmonary artery. Eur J Pharmacol 165: 297–300

Rouslahti E 1991 Integrins. J Clin Invest 87: 1–5

Rubanyi G M, Ho E H, Cantor E H et al 1991 Cytoprotective function of nitric oxide: inactivation of superoxide radicals produced by human leukocytes. Biochem Biophys Res Commun 181: 1392–1397

Ryan G B, Majno G 1977 Acute Inflammation. Am J Pathol 86: 183–286

Schultz P J, Raij L 1992 Endogenously synthesized nitric oxide prevents endotoxin-induced glomerular thrombosis. J Clin Invest 90: 1718–1725

Shimakawa H, Flavahan N A, Lorenz R R, Vanhoutte P M 1988 Prostacyclin releases endothelium-derived relaxing factor and potentiates its action in porcine coronary artery. Br J Pharmacol 95: 1197–1203

Smedly J A, Tonnesen M G, Sanhaus R A et al 1986 Neutrophil-mediated injury to endothelial cells. Enhancement by endotoxin and essential role of neutrophil elastase. J Clin Invest 77: 1233–1243

Suffredini A F, Fromm R E, Parker M M et al 1989 The cardiovascular response of normal humans to the administration of endotoxin. N Engl J Med 321: 280–287

Sugiura M, Inagami T, Kon V 1989 Endotoxin stimulates endothelin release in vivo and in vitro as determined by radioimmunoassay. Biochem Biophys Res Commun 161: 1220–1227

Szabo C, Mitchell J, Thiemermann C, Vane J 1993 Nitric oxide-mediated hyporeactivity to noradrenaline precedes the induction of nitric oxide synthase in endotoxin shock. Br J Pharmacol 108: 786–792

Tabor D R, Burchett S K, Jacobs R F 1988 Enhanced production of monokines by canine alveolar macrophages in response to endotoxin-induced shock. Proc Soc Exp Biol Med 187: 408–415

Thiemermann C, Lidbery P S, Thomas G R, Vane J R 1988 Endothelin-1 inhibits ex vivo platelet aggregation in the rabbit. Eur J Pharmacol 158: 182–186

Vallance P, Collier J, Moncada S 1989 Effects of endothelium-derived nitric oxide on peripheral arteriolar tone in man. Lancet ii: 997–1000

Vaporciyan A A, DeLisser H M, Yan H-C et al 1993 Involvement of platelet-endothelial cell adhesion molecule-1 in neutrophil recruitment in vivo. Science 262: 1580–1582.

Vargas H M, Ignarro L J, Chaudhuri G 1990 Physiological release of nitric oxide is dependent on the level of vascular tone. Eur J Pharmacol 190: 393–397

Vincent J L, Bihari D 1992 Sepsis, severe sepsis, or sepsis syndrome: a need for clarification. Int Care Med 18: 255–257

Voerman H J, Stehouwer C D A, van Kamp G J et al 1992 Plasma endothelin levels are increased in septic shock. Crit Care Med 20: 1097–1101

Waage A, Halstensen A, Epsevik T 1987 Association between TNF in serum and fatal outcome in patients with meningococcal disease. Lancet i: 355–357

Weiland J E, Davis W B, Holter J F et al 1986 Lung neutrophils in ARDS. Am Rev Respir Dis 133: 218–225

Wilkund N P, Persson M G, Gustafson L E et al 1990 Modulatory role of nitric oxide in pulmonary circulation in vivo. Eur J Pharmacol 185: 123–124

Winn R, Harlan J, Nadir B et al 1983 Thromboxane A_2 mediates lung vasoconstriction but not permeability after endotoxin. J Clin Invest 72: 911–918

Wise W C, Cook J A, Eller T, Halushka P V 1980 Ibuprofen improves survival from endotoxic shock in the rat. J Pharmacol Exp Ther 215: 160–164

Wolf F W, Marks R M, Sarma V et al 1992 Characterisation of a novel tumour necrosis factor alpha-induced endothelial response gene. J Biol Chem 267: 1317–1326

Wright C E, Rees D D, Moncada S 1992 Protective and pathological role of nitric oxide in endotoxin shock. Cardiovasc Res 26: 48–57

Yanagisawa M, Kurihara H, Kimura S et al 1988 A novel potent vasoconstrictor peptide produced by vascular endothelial cells. Nature 332: 411–415

Yang Z, Buhler F R, Diederich D, Luscher T F 1989 Different effects of endothelin-1 on cyclic AMP- and GMP-mediated vascular relaxation in human arteries and veins: comparison with norepinephrine. J Cardiovasc Pharmacol 13 (suppl 5): 129–131

5. Oxygen transport

Michelle Hayes David Watson

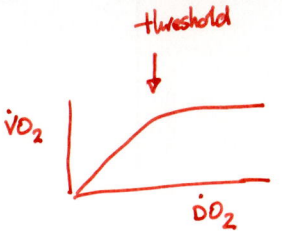

INTRODUCTION

One of the central mechanisms underlying damage to vital organs in criti- *? delivery* cal illness is tissue hypoxia (Sibbald et al 1990). When oxygen delivery (DO_2) is reduced below a critical threshold, oxygen consumption (VO_2) falls because increasing tissue oxygen extraction can no longer compensate for further reductions in DO_2; if DO_2 remains inadequate, increasing meta- *? flow-dependent* bolic derangements eventually lead to cell death and multiple organ fail- ure. In anaesthetised patients undergoing coronary artery bypass grafting in whom blood flow was progressively reduced, the critical level of DO_2 was found to be 330 ml/min/m^2 (Shibutani et al 1983) but the extent to *? extraction ?* which this threshold is altered in critically ill patients has yet to be esta- blished. However, a recent study has suggested that it is lower than that previously reported in normal humans and, perhaps surprisingly, is not altered by the presence of sepsis (Ronco et al 1993a). In the critically ill, tissue hypoxia may be precipitated not only by an inadequate DO_2 but may also be due to an inability of the tissues to extract or utilize the delivered oxygen, in which case cellular oxygenation may be impaired despite nor- mal or increased DO_2 with the development of raised circulating lactate levels.

SUPPLY DEPENDENCY AS AN INDICATOR OF TISSUE HYPOXIA

Total body VO_2 is a measure of global aerobic metabolism and it has been suggested that an inability to consume oxygen is the best early predictor of organ failure (Moore et al 1992). VO_2, is, however, dependent on meta- bolic demands, which can vary widely in critically ill patients and there has therefore been considerable interest in using the relationship between DO_2 and VO_2 as a means of evaluating the adequacy of tissue oxygenation. A number of studies have demonstrated that in apparently stable critically ill patients VO_2 increases when DO_2 is augmented and falls in response to reductions in DO_2, an observation which has been termed 'supply depend- ency' (Powers et al 1973, Danek et al 1980, Kaufman et al 1984, Kariman

SUPPLY DEPENDENCY IN CRITICAL ILLNESS

proportion O_2 extraction fixed ; VO_2 ↓ ; lactaemia → ? oxygen debt ?

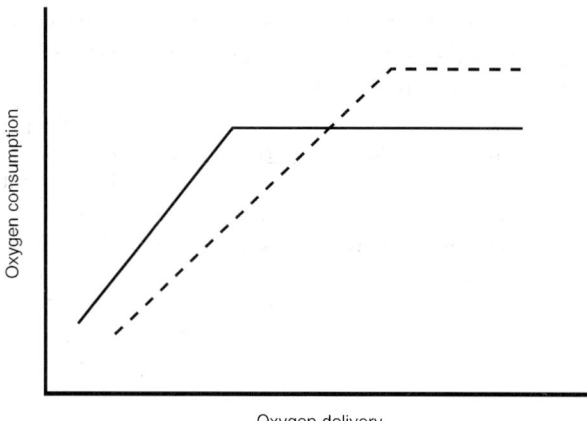

Fig. 5.1 Oxygen delivery (DO_2)/consumption (VO_2) relationships. Solid line: Normal DO_2/VO_2 relationship. Dotted line: DO_2 dependent VO_2 (supply dependency). The slope of the line is displaced to the right as a result of impaired oxygen extraction.

& Burns 1985, Astiz et al 1987, Bihari et al 1987, Mohsenifar et al 1987, Wolf et al 1987, Dorinsky et al 1988). This contrasts with normal physiology, in which VO_2 remains constant at rest once a critical DO_2 has been exceeded (Fig. 5.1). Characteristically, supply dependency is associated with a diminished ability of the tissues to alter oxygen extraction in response to a change in DO_2 (as a result the slope of the 'supply-dependent' relationship is displaced to the right), increased oxygen demand and raised lactate levels (Cain & Curtis 1991). The demonstration of supply dependency has been regarded as indirect evidence of occult tissue oxygen debt (Bihari et al 1987) and some (Gutierrez & Pohil 1986, Bihari et al 1987) but not all (Palazzo and Suter 1991) studies have suggested that supply dependency is associated with a high mortality.

Supply dependency was initially described in patients with ARDS (Powers et al 1973) and subsequently confirmed in patients with sepsis (Kaufman et al 1984, Astiz et al 1987, Bihari et al 1987, Wolf et al 1987), but more surprisingly has also been demonstrated in hypovolaemic shock (Kaufman et al 1984), congestive cardiac failure (Mohsenifar et al 1987) and chronic obstructive lung disease (Brent et al 1984).

RELATIONSHIP BETWEEN RAISED LACTATE LEVELS, SUPPLY DEPENDENCY, TISSUE HYPOXIA AND OUTCOME

The most common cause of hyperlactaemia is thought to be hypoperfusion and cellular hypoxia. However, systemic lactate levels represent a balance between lactate production, washout from the tissues and clearance, and

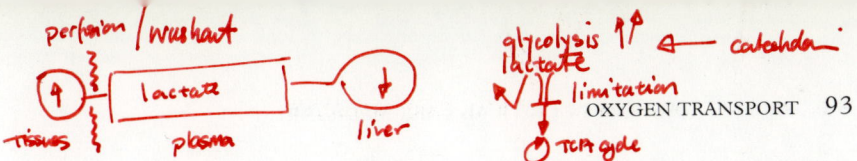
[handwritten annotations at top: "perfusion / washout", "lactate", "plasma", "liver", "glycolysis ↑↑ ← catecholam", "lactate", "✓ limitation", "TCA cycle"]

since lactate is cleared from the circulation predominantly by the liver, impaired hepatic function commonly contributes to hyperlactaemia. It is also important to appreciate that drugs and chemicals can elevate lactate levels by interfering with gluconeogenesis and that catecholamines may induce hyperlactaemia by stimulating glycolysis in excess of the ability of pyruvate to enter the tricarboxylic acid cycle (Green 1961). Inactivation of pyruvate dehydrogenase by endotoxin has also been postulated as a cause of raised lactate levels in patients with sepsis and ARDS; this inactivation could result in a backup of glycolysis leading to a proportional increase in lactate and pyruvate levels (Cain & Curtis 1991). Finally, it has been suggested that washout of lactate following reperfusion may cause an increase in lactate levels at a time when tissue hypoxia is resolving, although such increases are likely to be shortlived. *[handwritten: "endotoxin (inhib⁰ of TCA cycle)"]*

The observation that 70% of patients with lactate levels of greater than 2 mmol/l are not acidotic (Gutierrez et al 1989), has also raised questions about its value as a definitive marker of anaerobic glycolysis. Nevertheless in many studies, patients with hyperlactaemia have been found to exhibit supply dependency (Haupt et al 1985, Gilbert et al 1986, Kruse et al 1990, Vincent et al 1990), in keeping with the suggestion that both are markers of tissue hypoxia. Controversially, this observation has not been reproduced in some recent studies (Ronco et al 1991) and in one supply dependency was demonstrated in patients with normal lactates but not in those in whom blood lactate levels were elevated (Steffes et al 1991). *[handwritten: "supply dependence as c. lactaemia?"]*

Despite these apparent limitations, lactate levels have been shown repeatedly to correlate with outcome in critically ill patients (Peretz et al 1965, Schweizer & Howland 1968, Weil and Afifi 1979, Henning et al 1982, Vincent et al 1983, Cowan et al 1984, Tuchschmidt et al 1989, Bakker et al 1991), although serial determinations are a more useful indication of prognosis and response to therapy than isolated measurements (Vincent et al 1983, Cowan et al 1984, Hayes et al 1993). Furthermore, it has been suggested that blood lactate levels may be superior to oxygen transport variables in predicting outcome in human septic shock (Bakker et al 1991). *[handwritten: "outcome?"]*

DETERMINATION OF DO$_2$, VO$_2$ AND SUPPLY DEPENDENCY

For a number of reasons studies investigating DO$_2$/VO$_2$ relationships should be interpreted with caution. First, VO$_2$ has usually been determined by the reverse Fick method, partly because of the simplicity of the calculation but also because of the inaccuracies which can arise when VO$_2$ is measured directly from an analysis of inspired and expired gas, especially when patients are ventilated with high oxygen concentrations and when airway pressures are increased. Unfortunately, VO$_2$ determined by the reverse Fick method shares measured variables (haemoglobin, cardiac output and arterial oxygen saturation) with calculated DO$_2$ and this may lead to an appar-

[handwritten at bottom: "Direct analysis of VO₂ technically difficult, esp. at high FiO₂ and increased pressure."]

[handwritten: "Reversed Fick method?"]

[handwritten: "RISK OF 'MATHEMATICAL COUPLING'!!"]

[handwritten equations: $VO_2 = CO \times Hb \times 2.34 \times (SaO_2 - SvO_2)$]

[handwritten: $DO_2 = CO \times Hb \times 2.34 \times SaO_2$]

ent relationship between the two due to the phenomenon of 'mathematical coupling' (Archie 1981, Stratton et al 1987). Some studies have found no evidence of supply dependency when VO_2 and DO_2 were determined independently (Vermeij et al 1990, Ronco et al 1991, 1993b) suggesting that this phenomenon may explain the dependent relationship found in many of the studies in which the reverse Fick method has been used.

Secondly, demand-driven increases in DO_2 can be misinterpreted as evidence of 'supply dependency'. Metabolic rate varies spontaneously in critically ill patients (Villar et al 1990), and may also increase in response to stimulation, such as during physiotherapy. Acute changes in body temperature, shivering, pain, anxiety, resisting the ventilator, change of body position, airway suctioning and other routine intensive care procedures are common causes of sudden significant changes in VO_2 in the critically ill (Weissman et al 1984, 1991); even movement of a limb during blood sampling may be associated with an increase in VO_2 of as much as 10–15% (Weissman et al 1991). These changes in VO_2 would be expected to be associated with an appropriate increase in DO_2 and such 'physiological coupling' can mimic supply dependency.

Finally, the apparent dependence of VO_2 on DO_2 may no longer be seen when the effects of sedation are taken into account (Boyd et al 1992) and in septic shock the response to increased DO_2 may vary from time to time in the same patient (Palazzo & Suter 1991).

MANOEUVRES TO DEMONSTRATE SUPPLY DEPENDENCY

An 'oxygen flux test', in which the response of VO_2 to abrupt alterations in oxygen transport is measured, can be used to reveal the presence of supply dependency. DO_2 can be manipulated by fluid loading (Haupt et al 1985, Gilbert et al 1986), blood transfusion (Gilbert et al 1986), changing the level of positive end-expiratory pressure (PEEP) (Powers et al 1973) and by administering inotropes (Shoemaker et al 1986, Vincent et al 1990) or vasodilators (Palazzo et al 1991). It is clearly important that the chosen technique does not increase VO_2 independently of changes in DO_2. This applies particularly to the use of catecholamines such as noradrenaline, adrenaline and dopamine which can directly increase oxidative metabolism leading to marked increases in VO_2, thereby obscuring the true DO_2/VO_2 relationship (Ensinger et al 1993). Increases in VO_2 have also been observed following incremental doses of dobutamine in normal volunteers (Bhatt et al 1992), although other studies in animals (Lewis et al 1989) and humans (Ronco et al 1993b) have concluded that this drug does not primarily influence tissue VO_2. The use of phentolamine has been advocated as an alternative to catecholamines since it can augment DO_2 without increasing VO_2 in healthy individuals (Palazzo et al 1991). There is nevertheless some controversy as to whether vasodilatation is the most appropriate means of achieving increases in DO_2 in the critically ill as some compounds (particularly sodium nitroprusside) may exacerbate flow maldistribution and worsen tissue hypoxia, despite increasing cardiac output and DO_2.

Although blood transfusion can augment DO_2 by increasing oxygen carrying capacity, its effects on VO_2 are inconsistent and it has a variable effect on blood lactate levels (Dietrich et al 1990, Lucking et al 1990, Steffes et al 1991). This has been attributed to the use of stored blood which, despite significantly increasing haemoglobin concentration, may be associated with only limited improvements in tissue oxygenation. It has also been observed that transfusion of old blood adversely influences surrogate markers of tissue oxygenation such as intramucosal pH, raising the possibility that microvascular occlusion by poorly deformable red cells impedes oxygen transport (Marik & Sibbald 1993).

RELATIONSHIP BETWEEN OXYGEN TRANSPORT AND OUTCOME

Cardiac reserve

Survival following surgery is dependent on an adequate cardiac reserve (Boyd et al 1959, Clowes & del Guericio 1960, Clowes et al 1966) and is associated with early increases in cardiac index (CI), DO_2 and VO_2 (Shoemaker et al 1983, Bland et al 1985a, Hankeln et al 1987, Russell et al 1990). By contrast, non-survivors maintain normal or near-normal cardiac function and levels of DO_2 and VO_2 which are significantly lower than those of survivors (Shoemaker et al 1983, Bland et al 1985a). In adult patients with the acute respiratory distress syndrome (ARDS) (Hankeln et al 1987, Cryer et al 1989, Russell et al 1990), sepsis (Abraham et al 1984) or following liver transplantation (Nasraway et al 1995), there is a close relationship between the level of DO_2 and the subsequent development of multiple organ dysfunction syndrome (MODS) and/or a poor outcome. Similarly, failure to increase VO_2 in response to treatment has also been shown to be associated with an increased incidence of MODS (Moore et al 1992). Of particular interest is the observation that in patients who developed MODS, administration of prostacyclin was associated with an increase in DO_2 and VO_2 (determined by the reverse Fick method), suggesting that the rise in DO_2 had revealed a tissue oxygen debt. By contrast, in those patients who subsequently survived, VO_2 was unchanged following prostacyclin administration despite an increase in DO_2 suggesting that in these cases tissue oxygen demands were already being satisfied (Bihari et al 1987). A further study involving postoperative patients has demonstrated that patients who develop MODS have greater oxygen debts than those who do not (Shoemaker et al 1982).

ARDS.
sepsis
liver Tx } *risk of MODS ass. c̄ lower DO_2 — reandable c̄ PGI_2 (oxygen debt?)*

THE USE OF 'SURVIVOR VALUES' OF OXYGEN DELIVERY AND CONSUMPTION AS GOALS FOR TREATMENT

There are sound theoretical arguments to support the concept that outcome from critical illness could be improved by attempting to replicate the haemodynamic and oxygen transport patterns of survivors. Such treatment might prevent or reverse tissue hypoxia by compensating for the increased oxygen demands imposed by critical illness, as well as for the maldistribution of blood flow which occurs both regionally and within the microcirculation and could also correct the oxygen debt which might have developed following initial hypoperfusion.

Parameters affecting survival: increased O_2 demand, maldistribution of blood flow, oxygen debt : can they be modified : clinically useful ways?

The influence of treatment aimed at augmenting DO_2 and VO_2 on outcome

Surgical patients   *$CI > 4.5$; $DO_2 > 600 ml/min/m^2$; $VO_2 > 170 ml/min/m^2$*

The temporal sequence of haemodynamic and oxygen transport patterns in surviving and non-surviving general surgical patients was described in 1985 (Bland et al 1985a) and from this database a physiological algorithm was developed which successfully predicted outcome prospectively (Bland et al 1985b). Therapeutic goals were developed from this algorithm and from the median maximum values of survivors (Shoemaker et al 1973, Shoemaker et al 1983, Bland et al 1985a). It was suggested that prevention, or early correction of the oxygen debt estimated from oxygen transport variables would reduce the incidence of organ failure (and therefore death) and that treatment should be directed at increasing CI, DO_2 and VO_2 to the median maximum values observed in survivors (i.e. > 4.5 l/min/ m^2, > 600 ml/min/m^2, > 170 ml/min/m^2 respectively) (Shoemaker et al 1988a). The hypothesis that in high-risk surgical patients early, aggressive, prophylactic therapy designed to achieve these goals would improve outcome was tested prospectively using a protocol involving fluid replacement and inotropes in two series of high-risk patients (Shoemaker et al 1988b). In the first, there were 168 operations on 151 control patients, 57 (38%) of whom died and 108 operations on 101 protocol patients 21 (21%) of whom died (Shoemaker et al 1982). In the second series, patients were prospectively randomized before surgery to standard care or to treatment aimed at achieving the previously defined target values for cardiac output and oxygen transport (Shoemaker et al 1988b). Mortality was 33% in controls and only 4% in those randomized to the treatment protocol (Shoemaker et al 1988b). Additionally, the average number of days spent on mechanical ventilation was reduced from 9 to 2, ICU days were reduced from 16 to 10 and hospital days from 25 to 19. Finally, the cost per survivor was 50% less for the protocol group who had only one-third the number of complications of controls (Shoemaker et al 1988b). Although

Elective high-risk surgery : preoperatively increasing DO_2 beneficial (major effect achieved by FLUID LOADING)

these results are impressive, it is important to note that the protocols received twice as much fluid as the controls (Shoemaker et al 1988b), suggesting that volume replacement may have been inadequate in the control
group, and that two-thirds of the protocol patients managed to achieve the
therapeutic goals with fluids alone, suggesting that these patients had good
physiological reserve. The protocol group also contained fewer patients with
septic shock (Shoemaker et al 1988b). Unfortunately, APACHE II scores
were not recorded making comparisons between the patients in this study
and with those recruited to other studies difficult.

In a more recent investigation involving high-risk surgical patients, treatment with dopexamine aimed at achieving $DO_2 > 600$ ml/min/m^2 instituted
mostly preoperatively or in the early postoperative period reduced 28-day
mortality by 75% (Boyd et al 1993). In this study an increase in VO_2 was
not targetted, DO_2 in the controls was very low, the elevation of DO_2 in the
treatment group was only transient and modest and VO_2 was unchanged.
The impressive reduction in mortality may therefore have been due to factors unrelated to alterations in oxygen transport such as the use of
dopexamine hydrochloride, an agent which has been shown to significantly
increase hepatosplanchnic blood flow (Leier 1988), perhaps combined with
more aggressive volume replacement in the protocol group. Alternatively,
preoperative optimization of protocol patients to normal haemodynamic
values, a manoeuvre which has previously been shown to reduce mortality
(Schultz et al 1985, Berlauk et al 1991) may have been responsible for the
improvement in outcome. *Probably benefit in elective surgery.*

Trauma

In trauma patients treatment aimed at achieving elevated values for CI,
DO_2 and VO_2 was associated with a trend towards improved survival in the
protocol group, although when analysed on the basis of intention to treat
this difference was not statistically significant (Fleming et al 1992). However, when the analysis was restricted to those who achieved target values
within 24 h, a larger proportion of protocol patients survived, perhaps
suggesting that the early ability to attain higher levels of oxygen transport
is associated with better outcome.

More recently Shoemaker's group have repeated a prospective randomized
trial of survivor values for cardiac index and oxygen transport as resuscitation end-points in severe trauma (Bishop et al 1995). The 50 protocol
patients had a significantly lower mortality and fewer organ failures than
did the 75 control patients for whom the resuscitation goals were normal
vital signs, urine output and central venous pressure. Importantly, however, the protocol patients received significantly more colloid solution from
12 to 72 h after admission. They were also given significantly more blood
and had a higher total fluid intake during the second day after admission.

Benefit less clearly established in trauma
(FLUID LOADING beneficial)

Septic shock

The evidence that such treatment can benefit patients with septic shock is conflicting. In one study it was shown that target values for CI, DO_2 and VO_2 could always be attained using a combination of fluid loading, dobutamine and noradrenaline, although in some cases only when very high doses of dobutamine (up to 200 µg/kg/min) were used (Edwards et al 1989). Unfortunately, this study was uncontrolled and suggestions that the management plan reduced mortality relied on retrospective comparisons with previous results from the same institution and with mortality rates reported in other studies (Parker et al 1987, Ruiz et al 1979, Groeneveld 1986). In a prospective, randomized study of the effects of increasing CI and DO_2 in septic shock there was no difference in outcome between the two groups when analysed by intention to treat, although there appeared to be a trend towards a lower mortality in the protocol group (Tuchschmidt et al 1992). When all patients from both groups were analysed together mortality was closely related to post-resuscitation oxygen delivery and when patients in the optimal treatment group with a CI > 4.5 $l/min/m^2$ were retrospectively compared with patients in the normal treatment group whose CI remained below 4.5 $l/min/m^2$, there was a significant difference in mortality. Although the authors claimed that these results supported the concept that targeting high levels of CI improves outcome from septic shock, many believe that their findings can only be interpreted as confirming that survival is associated with the ability to attain higher levels of CI and DO_2.

BENEFIT NOT SHOWN IN SEPTIC SHOCK

Table 5.1   Descriptive information

	Controls (n = 50)	Protocols (n = 50)	SA (n = 9)
Age	63.5 (21–88)	62 (21–84)	46 (19–80)
APACHE II (lst 24 h)	18 (7–34)	18 (6–35)	11 (6–18)
APACHE III (1st 24 h)	58 (32–117)	63 (26–127)	39 (18–56)
Organ failure score (Knaus – 1st 24 h)	1 (0–3)	1 (0–4)	1 (0–2)
Colloid administered from t0–t1	1 (0–9)	1 (0–6)	1 (1–3.5)
Blood administered from t0–t1 (units)	1 (0–26)	0 (0–14)	0 (0–4)
ARDS	15	16	2
Septic shock	23	24	1
Days in unit	10 (1–64)	10 (1–48)	10 (1–29)
Days ventilated	8 (0–54)	8 (0–41)	2 (0–26)
Number of patients ventilated	44	46	7
Days in hospital	23.5 (1–244)	19 (1–187)	20 (11–102)
In-unit mortality (%)	30	50*	0
Hospital mortality (%)	34	54*	0
Predicted risk of death	34 (3–91)	34 (3–85)	6 (3–32)

Data as median (range)   * $P < 0.05$ Controls vs Protocols

Heterogeneous groups of critically ill patients

Not only were the results of these studies inconclusive, but aggressive attempts to augment DO_2 and VO_2 may be associated with a number of potential dangers. In the most seriously ill patients, for example, it often proves difficult or impossible to achieve target values (especially VO_2) despite the use of large doses of inotropes and vasoactive agents; in such patients the prognosis is very poor (Hayes et al 1993) and the administration of high-dose adrenergic agents might precipitate complications such as tachyarrhythmias and myocardial ischaemia, as well as exacerbating maldistribution of flow.

In an attempt to resolve some of these controversies a prospective, randomized, controlled study was performed in a heterogeneous group of 109 critically ill patients in order to evaluate the effects of treatment aimed at increasing CI, DO_2 and VO_2 to previously recommended levels, initiated on admission to the intensive care unit (Hayes et al 1994). Importantly, patients were randomized only if target values (CI >4.5 l/min/m², DO_2 >600 ml/min/m² and VO_2 >170 ml/min/m²) were not achieved with fluid resuscitation alone. In the protocol group, incremental doses of dobutamine (up to 200 µg/kg/min) were administered until all three goals were achieved simultaneously, unless tachyarrhythmias or evidence of myocardial ischaemia developed. In controls, dobutamine was administered only if the CI < 2.8 l/min/m². In both groups, noradrenaline was infused to maintain mean arterial pressure (MAP) at 80 mmHg. 109 patients were studied, 50 patients were randomized to each group since 9 patients achieved target values with fluids alone. Patients were well matched (Table 5.1), and there were no differences in MAP, VO_2 or lactate between the two groups despite significantly higher (P <0.05) levels of CI and DO_2 in the protocol patients. In-hospital mortality was significantly higher (P =0.04) in the protocol group (54%, predicted risk of death (PRD) 34%) than in the control group (34%, PRD 34%). All patients who achieved the haemodynamic and oxygen transport goals with fluid alone survived to leave hospital (PRD 6%) (Table 5.1).

Despite the use of high doses of dobutamine in an attempt to increase VO_2, only four patients in the protocol group, compared to two in the control group died of sudden cardiac events. The majority of excess deaths in the protocol group occurred late and were due to MODS. It is conceivable that the large doses of dobutamine administered to some of the patients in this group may have exacerbated flow maldistribution thereby reducing perfusion of vital organs, such as the gut, and contributing to the greater incidence of multiple organ failure.

Although in this study VO_2 increased significantly after resuscitation, the increase was of similar magnitude in both groups, a finding which is consistent with previous observations in patients with septic shock (Tuchschmidt et al 1992) and in a mixed group of critically ill patients (Yu et al 1993). In neither of these studies was there any difference in VO_2

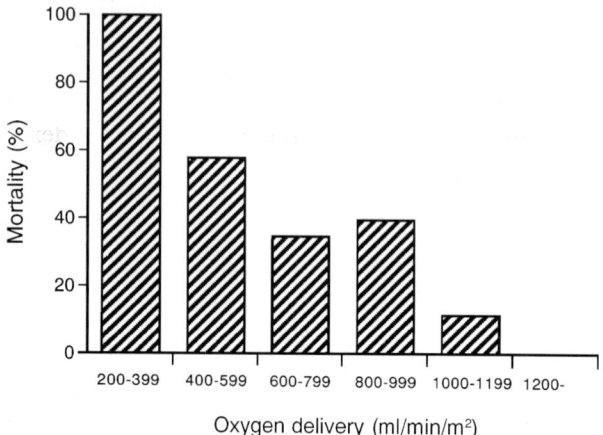

Fig. 5.2 Relationship between mortality rate and oxygen delivery in critical illness — as DO$_2$ increases mortality rate falls.

between those in the conventional and optimally treated groups, and in one (Tuchschmidt et al 1992) there was no difference in lactate, nor was there any statistical difference in outcome until the groups were retrospectively redefined. If 'optimal treatment' was responsible for the trend to improved outcome, and this was related to reversal of an oxygen debt, one would have expected VO$_2$ to be higher and lactate levels to be lower in the protocol group.

In a recent prospective, randomized, controlled trial (Gattinoni et al 1995) treatment aimed at increasing the cardiac index to supranormal levels or at maintaining normal values of mixed venous oxygen saturation in the early stages of critical illness was compared with conventional management. The principle finding of this trial was that neither form of 'goal-orientated haemodynamic therapy' improved morbidity or mortality. Significantly this negative result was perhaps at least partly a consequence of being unable to consistently attain the targets of treatments, since only 45% of the cardiac index group and 67% of the oxygen saturation group actually reached and sustained their therapeutic goals during the five-day treatment period. This compared with the 94% of patients in the control group who achieved and maintained their target of a normal cardiac index. Similarly in the studies of Hayes et al (1994), Yu et al (1993) and Tuchschmidt et al (1992) 70%, 34% and 27% of protocol patients respectively failed to achieve target values. In all these studies, in which patients were randomized after admission to the intensive therapy unit the use of 'survivor values' as treatment goals failed to influence outcome when analysed according to intention to treat and one suggested that such a strategy utilizing high-dose dobutamine might actually be detrimental (Hayes et al 1994). Although Gattinoni and his co-workers did not observe any trend towards higher mortality in the protocol groups those who failed to achieve target values were older, sicker, and had more frequent recourse to fluid administration, with higher doses of dobutamine superimposed on inotropic doses of dopamine. Electrocardiographic alterations suggestive of myocardial ischaemia led to abandonment of the protocol in significantly more patients randomly allocated to the supranormal cardiac index group (9 of 253 patients).   *GOAL- oriented THERAPY INEFFECTIVE IN CRITICAL ILLNESS*

TARGETS FOR THERAPY OR MARKERS OF PHYSIOLOGICAL RESERVE?

In one study involving a heterogeneous group of critically ill patients (Hayes et al 1994), an inverse relationship between DO_2 and mortality emerged when all patients, including the nine who were not randomized, were grouped together (Fig. 5.2). In this study all but 2 of the 33 patients from all groups who achieved the target values for CI, DO_2 and VO_2 survived, suggesting that the ability to achieve higher values of DO_2 and VO_2 in response to resuscitation may be indicative of greater physiological reserve, a less severe illness and consequently a better prognosis. A recent study in patients with the sepsis syndrome also demonstrated that survivors responded to a short-term infusion of dobutamine with a significantly greater increase in DO_2 and VO_2 than non-survivors (Vallet et al 1993). 'Goal-directed therapy' may therefore serve only to identify those patients who have the ability to attain survivor values if and when they need to. It is, however, important to note that 15 of the 33 'achievers' in the study of Hayes et al were in the protocol group, and that 14 of those achieved the target values for CI, DO_2 and VO_2 with 25 µg/kg/min or less of dobutamine. This group had a lower mortality than predicted (13% with a PRD of 25%) and it is possible that they may have been benefited by dobutamine administration.   *? Ability to achieve ci/DO2/VO2 targets a mark of physiological reserve and (lesser) severity of illness?*

DETERMINANTS OF OUTCOME

Timing of therapy

When all the randomized controlled trials of 'goal-directed therapy' are analysed on the basis of intention to treat only three (Shoemaker et al 1988b, Boyd et al 1993, Bishop et al 1995) have clearly demonstrated a significant improvement in outcome. Two others suggest a favourable trend (Fleming et al 1992, Tuchschmidt et al 1992) and three have shown no improvement (Yu et al 1993, Hayes et al 1994, Gattinoni et al 1995). It is noteworthy that the three studies showing a significant reduction in mortality were performed on high-risk surgical or multiply-injured patients and treatment (mainly expansion of the circulating volume) was instituted preoperatively or early postoperatively. It seems likely that the attenuated response of non-survivors to treatment seen in some studies may be at least in part related to delays in instituting treatment. Whereas early in shock peripheral

EARLY expansion of circulating volume in high-risk surgical and trauma patients beneficial

defects in oxygen utilization may be overcome by increases in DO_2, if resuscitation is delayed progressive and irreversible damage to the cellular metabolic apparatus may prove refractory to subsequent treatment.

Cardiac reserve

In one of the studies involving heterogeneous groups of critically ill patients the haemodynamic and oxygen transport responses of survivors and non-survivors were qualitatively similar, regardless of whether patients were allocated to receive treatment aimed at achieving survivor values or to a control group (Hayes et al 1994). In both groups those who survived responded with greater increases in CI, left ventricular stroke work index (LVSWI), mean arterial pressure (MAP) and DO_2 and had lower lactate levels than those who died. Moreover in non-survivors from the protocol group even very high doses of dobutamine failed to significantly increase CI, LVSWI and DO_2, suggesting that these patients were suffering from severe myocardial depression, unresponsive to the inotropic action of this agent. These observations are consistent with Gattinoni's findings, as well as with studies involving postoperative patients in which cardiac reserves were greater in survivors than non-survivors (Timmins et al 1992, Shoemaker et al 1973, Bland et al 1985a) and demonstrate that survival is associated with the ability to increase myocardial performance and hence achieve a level of DO_2 sufficient to sustain a hypermetabolic state.

Survival ass. ε ability to recruit myocardial reserve.

Oxygen extraction capabilities

Administration of small doses of endotoxin to normal human volunteers produces a significant increase not only in DO_2 but also VO_2 (Suffredini et al 1992) and patients with uncomplicated sepsis have a greater capacity to extract oxygen and consequently a higher VO_2, despite a lower CI and DO_2 than more severely ill patients with sepsis syndrome (Kreymann et al 1993). Clearly hypermetabolism is an important component of a successful host response, particularly in sepsis. This view is supported by the observation that following caecal ligation and puncture, surviving rats remained hypermetabolic, whilst preterminal animals became hypometabolic. Regardless of their diets, surviving animals demonstrated a mean increase of 15% in resting energy expenditure from presepsis levels, whilst the resting energy expenditure of preterminal animals decreased by 22% (Fried et al 1986).

It is perhaps not surprising, therefore, that impaired oxygen utilization, as reflected by significantly falling oxygen extraction, has been clearly associated with non-survival (Hayes et al 1993), an observation which is consistent with the finding that low oxygen extraction is related to death in paediatric septic shock (Pollack et al 1985). This impairment of oxygen uptake may be due to vasolidation-induced maldistribution of flow

Hypermetabolic host response in critical illness; inability to increase metabolic rate ux- ε poor prognosis.

low $\dot{V}O_2$ ass. c̄ poor outcome
failve to recruit $\dot{V}O_2$ ~ defective aerobic metabolic / impaired peripl'd
O_2 utilizath.

OXYGEN TRANSPORT 103

(Groeneveld et al 1986, Samsel et al 1988) and/or defective cellular oxygen utilization. Although in the study of Hayes et al (1993) CI and DO_2 increased in survivors and non-survivors from both control and protocol groups, in non-survivors this was offset by a fall in oxygen extraction which prevented, or limited any rise in VO_2. By contrast, survivors were characterized by a greater increase in DO_2, a lesser reduction in oxygen extraction and consequently a significant increase in VO_2 (Figs 5.3 and 5.4). At the time of maximal resuscitation (tmax) both control and protocol survivors had significantly higher VO_2's than non-survivors. Importantly, VO_2 was higher in control survivors than protocol non-survivors at tmax, a finding consistent with previous work demonstrating that low VO_2 is associated with a poor outcome (Wilson et al 1972), whereas increased VO_2 is characteristic of survivors (Hankeln et al 1987, Kreymann et al 1993). Similarly trauma patients who failed to increase VO_2 to survivor levels had persisting hyperlactaemia which was predictive of MODS (Moore et al 1992), and the authors suggested that this was related to defective aerobic metabolism. Furthermore, in a proportion of surgical patients with sepsis and raised blood lactate levels, VO_2 did not rise when DO_2 was increased by blood transfusion, an observation which was attributed to impaired peripheral oxygen utilization unresponsive to improvements in DO_2. This

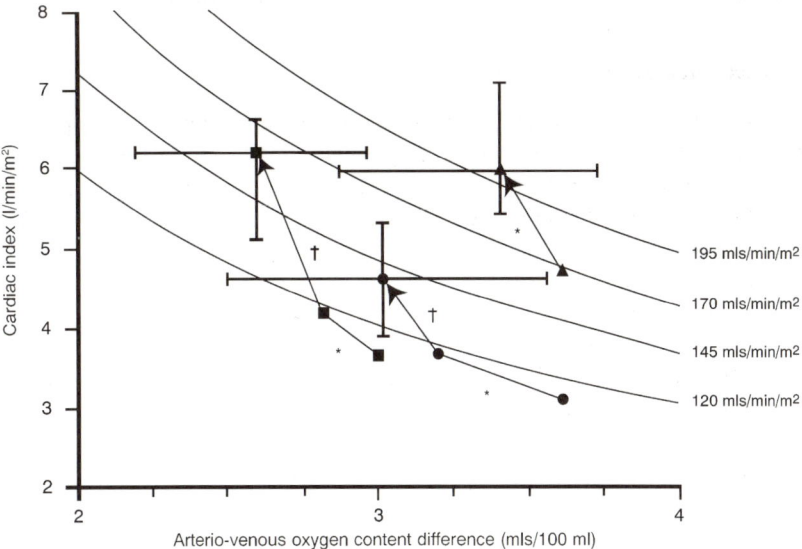

Fig. 5.3 Changes in cardiac index, arterio-venous oxygen content difference and VO_2 in response to fluids and maximal resuscitation in survivors. Data as medians with the interquartile ranges drawn at maximal resuscitation. Closed circles: control survivors. Closed squares: protocol survivors. Closed triangles: spontaneous achievers. Star: t0–t1, Cross: t1–tmax.

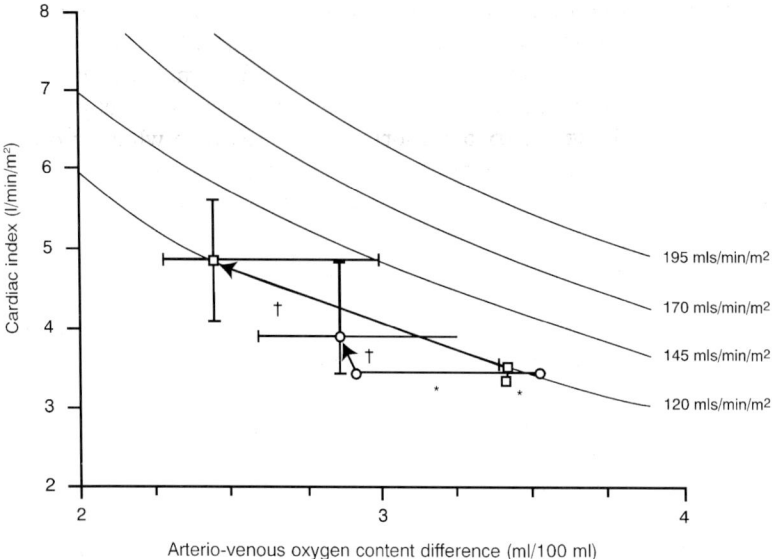

Fig. 5.4   Changes in cardiac index, arterio-venous oxygen content difference and VO₂ in response to fluid and maximal resuscitation in non-survivors. Data as medians with the interquartile ranges drawn at maximal resuscitation. Open circles: control non-survivors. Open squares: protocol non-survivors. Star: t0–t1, Cross: t1–tmax.

defect in oxygen utilization was associated with a poor outcome (Steffes et al 1991).

CONCLUSION

In conclusion, although persistent tissue hypoxia is clearly associated with the onset of multiple organ failure and a poor outcome, studies to date suggest that it may be the ability to achieve higher levels of DO_2 and VO_2, rather than the use of a specific treatment regimen in an attempt to achieve 'survivor values', which is associated with survival. Early institution of therapy, especially expansion of the circulating volume, and appropriate monitoring before patients have developed irreversible defects in oxygen extraction and severe myocardial depression is of paramount importance. Preoperative or early institution of resuscitative therapy in the shocked patient, in high-risk patients requiring operative care and the multiply injured should be routine clinical practice. Studies analysed according to intention to treat have failed to demonstrate that management protocols targeted to survivor values, when instituted following admission to intensive care, improve outcome. In many seriously ill patients, such as those with respiratory failure, septic shock or postoperative complications, a delay after the initial insult is often unavoidable; for such categories of patients aggressive, unselected therapy other than adequate fluid resuscitation, restoration of blood pressure and maintenance of a normal cardiac output cannot be recommended (Hinds & Watson 1995). It remains to be seen whether newer inotropic agents can have a more favourable effect on oxygen consumption. It will also be important to investigate whether other novel agents such as N-acetylcysteine or NG-methyl-L-arginine, which may improve oxygen extraction, have a beneficial effect on outcome.

KEY POINTS FOR CLINICAL PRACTICE

- Early institution of therapy before patients have developed irreversible defects in oxygen extraction and severe myocardial depression is of paramount importance.
- Preoperative resuscitation is likely to improve outcome.
- Adequate volume replacement is essential in all cases.
- Maintain a mean arterial pressure of at leat 80 mmHg with reference to premorbid levels.
- Haemodynamic support should attempt to maintain SvO_2 and correct hyperlactataemia, whilst avoiding complications such as tachycardia or myocardial ischaemia.
- In selected cases with continued evidence of impaired tissue oxygenation attempt to increase DO_2 and VO_2 to median survivor values with moderate doses of inotropes. Aggressive use of inotropes to achieve survivor values can no longer be recommended.
- In those who fail to achieve median survivor levels, aim for normal haemodynamics and DO_2.
- In the future new treatments which improve extraction capabilities may prove more useful.

REFERENCES

Abraham E, Bland R D, Cobo J C, Shoemaker W C 1984 Sequential cardiorespiratory patterns associated with outcome in septic shock. Chest 85: 75–80
Archie J P 1981 Mathematic coupling of data. Ann Surg 193: 296–303
Astiz M, Rackow E C, Falk J L et al 1987 Oxygen delivery and consumption in patients with hyperdynamic septic shock. Crit Care Med 15: 26–28
Bakker J, Coffernils M, Leon M et al 1991 Blood lactate levels are superior to oxygen derived variables in predicting outcome in human septic shock. Chest 99: 956–962
Berlauk J F, Abrams, J H, Gilmour I J et al 1991 Preoperative optimisation of cardiovascular haemodynamics improves outcome in peripheral vascular surgery. Ann Surg 214: 289–299
Bhatt S B, Hutchinson R C, Tomlinson B et al 1992 Effect of dobutamine on supply and uptake on healthy volunteers. Br J Anaesth 69: 298–303
Bihari D, Smithies M, Gimson A et al 1987 The effects of vasodilatation with prostacyclin on oxygen delivery and uptake in critically ill patients. N Engl J Med 317: 397–403
Bishop M H, Shoemaker W C, Appel P L et al 1995 Prospective randomized trial of survivor values of cardiac index, oxygen delivery and oxygen consumption as resuscitation end points in severe trauma. J Trauma, Injury, Infection and Critical Care 38: 780–787

Bland R D, Shoemaker W C 1985 Probability of survival as a prognostic and severity illness score in critically ill surgical patients. Crit Care Med 13: 91–95

Bland R D, Shoemaker W C, Abraham E et al 1985 Haemodynamic and oxygen transport patterns in surviving and non surviving postoperative patients. Crit Care Med 13: 85–90

Boyd O, Grounds R M, Bennett E D 1993 A randomised clinical trial of the effect of deliberate perioperative increase of oxygen delivery on mortality in high-risk surgical patients. JAMA 270: 2699–2707

Boyd O, Grounds M, Bennett E D 1992 The dependency of oxygen consumption on oxygen delivery in critically ill postoperative patients is mimicked by variations in sedation. Chest 101: 1619–1624

Boyd A, Tremblay R, Spencer F C, Bahnson H T 1959 Estimation of cardiac output soon after intrathoracic surgery with cardiopulmonary bypass. Ann Surg 150: 613–626

Brent B N, Matthay R, Mahler D A et al 1984 Relationship between oxygen uptake and oxygen transport in stable patients with chronic obstructive pulmonary disease. Am Rev Respir Dis 129: 682–686

Cain S M, Curtis S E 1991 Experimental models of pathologic oxygen supply dependency. Crit Care Med 19: 603–612

Clowes G H Jr, Del Guericio L R 1960 Circulatory response to trauma of surgical operations. Metabolism 9: 67–81

Clowes G, Vucinci M, Wiedner M G 1966 Circulatory and metabolic alterations associated with survival or death in peritonitis. Ann Surg 163: 866–885

Cowan B N, Burns H J G, Boyle P et al 1984 The relative prognostic value of lactate and haemodynamic measurements in early shock. Anaesthesia 39: 750–755

Cryer H G, Richardson J D, Longmuir-Cook S, Brown M 1989 Oxygen delivery in patients with adult respiratory distress syndrome who undergo surgery. Arch Surg 124: 1378–1385

Danek S J, Lynch J, Weg J, Dantzker D 1980 The dependence of oxygen uptake on oxygen delivery in the adult respiratory distress syndrome. Am Rev Respir Dis 122: 387–295

Dietrich K A, Conrad S A, Herbert C A et al 1990 Cardiovascular and metabolic response to red blood cell transfusion in critically ill, volume-resuscitated, nonsurgical patients. Crit Care Med 18: 940–944

Dorinsky P, Costello J, Gadek J 1988 Relationships of oxygen uptake and oxygen delivery in respiratory failure not due to the adult respiratory distress syndrome. Chest 93: 1013–1019

Edwards J D, Brown C G S, Nightingale P et al 1989 Use of survivors cardiorespiratory values as therapeutic goals in septic shock. Crit Care Med 17: 1098–1103

Ensinger H, Weichel T, Lindner K H et al 1993 Effects of norepinephrine, epinephrine and dopamine infusions on oxygen consumption in volunteers. Crit Care Med 21: 1502–1508

Fleming A, Bishop M, Shoemaker W et al 1992 Prospective trial of supranormal values as goals of resuscitation in severe trauma. Arch Surg 127: 1175–1181

Fried R C, Bailey P M, Mullen J L et al 1986 Alterations in exogenous substrate metabolism in sepsis. Arch Surg 21: 173–178

Gattinoni L, Brazzi L, Pelosi P et al 1995 A trial of goal-oriented hemodynamic therapy in critically ill patients. N Engl J Med 333: 1025–1032

Gilbert E M, Haupt M T, Mandanas R Y et al 1986 The effect of fluid loading, blood transfusion and catecholamine infusion on oxygen delivery and consumption in patients with sepsis. Am Rev Resp Med 134: 873–878

Green N M 1961 Effect of epinephrine on lactate, pyruvate and excess lactate production in normal human subjects. J Lab Clin Med 58: 682–693

Groenveld A B J, Bronsveld W, Thijs L G 1986 Haemodynamic determinants of mortality in human septic shock. Surgery 99: 140–152

Gutierrez G, Lund N, Bryan-Brown C W 1989 Cellular oxygenation during multiple organ failure. Crit Care Clin 5: 271–287

Gutierrez G, Pohil R J 1986 Oxygen consumption is linearly related to oxygen supply in critically ill patients. J Crit Care 1: 45–53

Hankeln K B, Senker R, Schwarten J U et al 1987 Evaluation of prognostic indices based on haemodynamic and oxygen transport variables in shock patients with adult respiratory distress syndrome. Crit Care Med 15: 1–7

Haupt M T, Gilbert E M, Carlson R W 1985 Fluid loading increases oxygen consumption in septic patients with lactic acidosis. Am Rev Resp Med 131: 912–916

Hayes M A, Yau E H S, Timmins A C et al 1993 Response of critically ill patients to treatment aimed at achieving supranormal oxygen delivery and consumption: relationship to outcome. Chest 103: 886–895

Hayes M A, Timmins A C, Yau E H S et al 1994 Elevation of systemic oxygen delivery in the treatment of critically ill patients. N Engl J Med 330: 1717–1722

Henning R J, Weil M H, Weiner F 1982 Blood lactate as a prognostic indicator of survival in patients with acute myocardial infarction. Circulatory Shock 9: 307–331

Hinds C J, Watson J D 1995 Manipulating hemodynamics and oxygen transport in critically ill patients. N Eng J Med 333: 1074–1075

Kariman B S, Burns S 1985 Regulation of tissue oxygen extraction is distributed in the adult respiratory distress syndrome. Am Rev Respir Dis 132: 109–114

Kaufman B S, Rackow E C, Falk J L 1984 The relationship between oxygen delivery and consumption during fluid resuscitation of hypovolaemic and septic shock. Chest 85: 336–340

Kreymann G, Grosser S, Buggisch P et al 1993 Oxygen consumption and resting metabolic rate in sepsis, sepsis syndrome and septic shock. Crit Care Med 21: 1012–1019

Kruse J A, Haupt M T, Puri V K et al 1990 Lactate levels as predictors of the relationship between oxygen delivery and consumption in ARDS. Chest 98: 959–962

Leier C V 1988 Regional blood flow responses to vasodilators and inotropes in congestive heart failure. Am J Cardiol 62: 86E–96E

Lewis T, Samsel R W, Sanders W M et al 1989 The effect of adrenergic agents on oxygen delivery and consumption (abstract). Am Rev Respir Dis 139: A311

Lucking J E, Williams T M, Chaten F C et al 1990 Dependence of oxygen consumption on oxygen delivery in children with hyperdynamic septic shock and low oxygen extraction. Crit Care Med 18: 1316–1319

Marik P, Sibbald W 1993 Effect of store-blood transfusion on oxygen delivery in patients with sepsis. JAMA 269: 3024–3029

Mohsenifar Z, Amin D, Jasper A C et al 1987 Dependence of oxygen consumption on oxygen delivery in patients with chronic congestive heart failure. Chest 92: 447–450

Moore F A, Haenel J B, Moore E E et al 1992 Incommensurate oxygen consumption in response to maximal oxygen availability predicts post injury multiple organ failure. J Trauma 33: 58–67

Nasraway S, Klein R, Spencer T et al 1995 Haemodynamic correlates of outcome in patients undergoing orthoptic liver transplantation: evidence for early postoperative myocardial depression. Chest 107: 218–224

Palazzo M G, Morel D R, Lopez J 1991 Effect of phenotolamine on the relationship between oxygen consumption and delivery in sheep. Eur J Appl Physiol 63: 223–227

Palazzo M G, Suter P M 1991 Delivery dependent oxygen consumption in patients with septic shock: daily variations, relationship with outcome and the sick euthyroid syndrome. Int Care Med 17: 325–332

Parker M M, Shelhamer J H, Natanson C et al 1987 Serial cardiovascular variables in survivors and non-survivors of human septic shock: heart rate as an early predictor of prognosis. Crit Care Med 15: 923–929

Peretz D I, Scott H M, Duff J et al 1965 The significance of lacticacidaemia in the shock syndrome. Ann N Y Acad Sci 119: 1133–1141

Pollack M P, Fields A I, Ruttiman U E 1985 Distribution of cardiopulmonary variables in paediatric survivors and non survivors of septic shock. Crit Care Med 13: 454–459

Powers S R, Mannal R, Neclerio M et al 1973 Physiologic consequences of positive end expiratory pressure (PEEP) ventilation. Ann Surg 178: 265–272

Ronco J J, Phang P T, Wiggs B et al 1991 Oxygen consumption is independent of changes in oxygen delivery in severe adult respiratory distress syndrome. Am Rev Respir Dis 143: 1267–1273

Ronco J J, Fenwick J C, Tweedale M G et al 1993a Identification of the critical oxygen delivery for anaerobic metabolism in critically ill septic and nonseptic humans. JAMA 270: 1724–1730

Ronco J J, Fenwick J C, Wiggs B R et al 1993b Oxygen consumption is independent of increases in oxygen delivery by dobutamine in septic patients who have normal or increased plasma lactate. Am Rev Respir Dis 147: 25–31

Ruiz C E, Weil M H, Carlson R W 1979 Treatment of circulatory shock with dopamine studies on survival. JAMA 242: 165–168

Russell J A, Ronco J L, Lockhat D et al 1990 Oxygen delivery and consumption and ventricular preload are greater in survivors than in non surviros of the adult respiratory distress syndrome. Am Rev Respir Dis 141: 659–665

Samsel R W, Nelson D P, Sanders W M et al 1988 Effect of endotoxin on systemic and skeletal muscle oxygen extraction. J Appl Physiol 65: 1377–1382

Schultz R J, Whitfied G F, Lamura J J et al 1985 The role of physiologic monitoring in patients with fractures of the hip. J Trauma 25: 309–316

Schweizer O, Howland W S 1968 Prognostic significance of high lactate levels. Anesth Analg 47: 383–388

Shibutani K, Komatsu T, Kubal K et al 1983 Critical level of oxygen delivery in anaesthetised man. Crit Care Med 11: 640–643

Shoemaker W C, Montgomery E S, Kaplan E et al 1973 Physiologic patterns in surviving and nonsurviving shock patients. Arch Surg 106: 630–636

Shoemaker W C, Appel P L, Bland R D 1983 Use of physiologic monitoring to predict outcome and to assist in clinical decisions in critically ill postoperative patients. Am J Surg 146: 4350

Shoemaker W C, Appel P L, Waxman K, Schwartz S and Chang P 1982 Clinical trial of survivors' cardiorespiratory patterns as therapeutic goals in critically ill postoperative patients. Crit Care Med 10: 398–403

Shoemaker W C, Appel P L, Kram H B 1986 Haemodynamic and oxygen transport effects of dobutamine in critically ill surgical patients. Crit Care Med 14: 1032–1037

Shoemaker W C, Appel P L, Kram H B 1988a Tissue oxygen debt as a determinant of lethal and non lethal postoperative organ failure. Crit Care Med 16: 1117–1120

Shoemaker W C, Appel P L, Kram H B et al 1988b Prospective trial of supranormal values of survivors as therapeutic goals in high risk surgical patients. Chest 94: 1176–1186

Shoemaker W C, Kram H B, Appel P L, et al 1990 The efficacy of central venous and pulmonary artery catheters and therapy based upon them in reducing morbidity and mortality. Arch Surg 125: 1332–1338

Sibbald W J, Bersten A, Rutledge F S 1990 The role of tissue hypoxia in multiple organ failure. In: K Reinhart and K Eyrich (eds) Clinical aspects of oxygen transport and tissue oxygenation. Springer, Berlin, pp 112–114

Steffes C P, Bender J S, Levison M A 1991 Blood transfusion and oxygen consumption in sepsis. Crit Care Med 19: 512–517

Stratton H H, Feustel P J, Newell J C 1987 Regression of calculated variables in the presence of shared measurement error. J Appl Physiol 62: 2083–2093

Suffredini A, Shelhamer J, Neumann R D et al 1992 Pulmonary and oxygen transport effects of intravenously administered endotoxin in normal humans. Am Rev Respir Dis 145: 1398–1403

Timmins A, Hayes M, Yau E H S et al 1992 The relationship between cardiac reserve and survival in critically ill patients receiving treatment aimed at achieving supranormal oxygen delivery and consumption. Postgrad Med J 68(Suppl 2): S34–S40

Tuchschmidt J, Fried J, Swinney R et al 1989 Early haemodynamic correlates of survival in patients with septic shock. Crit Care Med 17: 719–723

Tuchschmidt J, Fried J, Astiz M et al 1992 Elevation of cardiac output and oxygen delivery improves outcome in septic shock. Chest 102: 216–220

Vallet B, Chopin C, Curtis S E et al 1993 Prognostic value of the dobutamine test in patients with sepsis syndrome and normal lactate values: a prospective multicentre study. Crit Care Med 21: 1868–1875

Vermeij C J, Feenstra B W A, Bruining H A 1990 Oxygen delivery and oxygen uptake in post-operative and septic patients. Chest 98: 415–420

Villar J, Slutsky A, Hew E et al 1990 Oxygen transport and oxygen consumption in critically ill patients. Chest 98: 687–692

Vincent J L, Dufaye P H Berre J et al 1983 Serial lactate determinations during circulatory shock. Crit Care Med 11: 449–451

Vincent J L, Roman A, De Backer D et al 1990 Oxygen uptake/supply dependency: Effects of short term dobutamine infusion. Am Rev Respir Med 142: 2–7

Weil M H, Afifi A A 1970 Experimental and clinical studies on lactate and pyruvate as indicators of the severity of acute circulatory failure (shock). Circulation 41: 989–1001

Weissman C, Kemper M 1991 The oxygen uptake–oxygen delivery relationship during ICU interventions. Chest 99: 430–435

Weissman C, Kemper M, Damask M C et al 1984 Effect of routine intensive care interactions on metabolic rate. Chet 86: 815–818

Wilson R F, Christenson C, LeBlanc L P 1972 Oxygen consumption in critically ill patients. Ann Surg 176: 801–804

Wolf Y, Cotev S, Perel A et al 1987 Dependance of oxygen consumption on cardiac output in sepsis. Crit Care Med 15: 198–203

Yu M, Levy M M, Smith P et al 1993 Effect of maximising oxygen delivery on morbidity and mortality rates in critically ill patients: a prospective, randomised, controlled study. Crit Care Med 21: 830–838

Gram -ve infect. → endotox/LPS → Mφ/monocytes → cytokines

Individual variation –

— 3-deoxy-D-manno-octulosonic acid link (KDO)

Lipid A   oligosaccharide   o-chain
                            serotypic variability

conserved

disaccharide (diglucosane) + } u. 6 fatty acids — chiefly responsible for toxic actions but activity enhanced by presence of KDO

Endotoxin receptors: — scavenger receptor (Mφ) – endocytosis + detoxification
— 73kD endotox rec — macrophage activation (also appear to Staph. peptidoglycan + pertussis toxin)
— CD14   55kD glycoprotein   monocytes, Mφ + activated granulocytes.
↓
(IL-1 / IL-6 / IL-8 / TNF) ↑
Endotoxin binding enhanced by lipopolysaccharide binding protein in serum

Receptor activation → ↑ tyrosine kinase activity – phosphorylation of   Mitogen Activated Protein Kinase (TNF role?)   65kD cytosolic protein (IL-1 role?)

→ NF-κB endotoxin-inducible nuclear transcription factor (cytokine + acute-phase gene activation.

6. Endotoxin responsiveness

Karoline F. Bruin   Marijke von der Möhlen
Sander J. H. van Deventer

INTRODUCTION

Animal and clinical studies have identified endotoxin, the lipopolysaccharide component of the outer membrane of Gram-negative bacteria, as the main trigger of septic shock in Gram-negative infection. Immunocompetent cells such as monocytes and macrophages are the main cellular targets of endotoxin, and many of the symptoms associated with septic shock are mediated by endotoxin-induced cytokines that are synthesized and secreted by these cells. Although endotoxin triggers septic shock, it is well known that individuals may differ substantially in their susceptibility to its biological effects. Many factors that modulate the effects of endotoxin on the host have been identified, including the binding of endotoxin to serum proteins, endotoxin signal transduction and the transcription, translation and release of various cytokines. In the first section of this chapter, we review the molecular structure and its importance for the biological activity of endotoxin, cellular receptors for endotoxin and the endotoxin signal transduction pathway. Next, cytokine induction by endotoxin, and the gene structure and regulation of tumour necrosis factor (TNF), an important mediator of the biological effects of endotoxin, is discussed. The influence of serum constituents and genetic factors on endotoxin sensitivity is then reviewed. Finally, the induction of sensitization and tolerance to the biological effects of endotoxin in several in vivo models of endotoxicity is outlined.

THE STRUCTURE OF ENDOTOXIN AND ITS RELATIONSHIP TO BIOLOGICAL ACTIVITY

Endotoxin is a lipopolysaccharide molecule which is a structural component of the outer membrane of Gram-negative bacteria. It consists of a species-specific O-chain, a core oligosaccharide and a lipid A moiety. The core oligosaccharide and lipid A are relatively well conserved amongst common pathogenic Gram-negative bacteria, whereas the extensive structural variability of the O-chain accounts for the antigenic differences that form the basis of serotyping. Lipid A consists of a disaccharide backbone (usually a diglucosamine) which is covalently linked to the core oligosaccharide by the unusual sugar 3-deoxy-D-manno-octulosonic acid (KDO).

Experiments with synthetic lipid A analogues have demonstrated that the number, structure and position of the fatty acids (usually six) attached to the disaccharide lipid A backbone determine its biological activity in various test systems, such as pyrogenicity in rabbits, the dermal Shwartzman reaction and the Limulus assay (Rietschel et al 1990). These experiments also confirmed that lipid A is responsible for most, if not all, of the biological properties of endotoxin, and indicated that maximal endotoxic activity requires a disaccharide carrying two phosphate groups and six fatty acid chains in any asymmetrical distribution pattern (Rietschel et al 1990). Monophosphorylation of the disaccharide or alterations in the number of fatty acid chains attached to it (i.e. four, five or seven side chains) reduced endotoxic activity, whereas monosaccharide backbones or disaccharides with less than two fatty acid side chains are completely inactive (Rietschel et al 1990) Thus, partial detoxification of endotoxin can be achieved by removal of fatty acid side chains from lipid A. In accordance with these findings, acyloxyacyl hydrolysis of endotoxin by a neutrophil enzyme has been shown to reduce toxicity of endotoxin while preserving its immunostimulatory properties (Munford & Hall 1986). It should be noted, however, that in some systems the complete endotoxin molecule is somewhat more active than lipid A alone, apparently due to the presence of KDO in the core oligosaccharide, and that some of the actions of endotoxin require at least one KDO molecule to be attached to lipid A (Rietschel et al 1990). Presumably the attachment of KDO to lipid A results in a conformational change of lipid A that provides optimal biological activity.

ENDOTOXIN RECEPTORS

Although several membrane-associated structures that can interact with endotoxin or lipid A have been identified, their distinct roles in the endotoxin signal transduction pathway remain to be identified. The CD11/CD18 family of glycoproteins, for example, can bind endotoxin (Wright et al 1989a), but binding does not result in activation of monocytes or macrophages (Couturier et al 1992) and phagocytes express other lipid A binding sites (Golenbock et al 1990).

The scavenger receptor

One of the lipid A binding sites has been characterized as the scavenger receptor (Kodama et al 1990, Rohrer et al 1990), a macrophage receptor that binds a large variety of known ligands (Maor et al 1991). Binding of the lipid A analogue lipid IV_A to scavenger receptors is followed by internalization of the ligand-receptor complex, and subsequent degradation of the molecule (Hampton et al 1991). Thus, the scavenger receptor may play a role in the detoxification of endotoxin. However, interaction of endotoxin with the scavenger receptor does not result in activation of macrophages as reflected by the absence of TNF production.

The 73 kD endotoxin receptor

A membrane-associated endotoxin-binding protein of 73 kD originally identified on murine splenocytes is now known to have an analogue which is expressed by human monocytes (Lei & Morrison 1989a, b, Lei et al 1991). A monoclonal antibody generated against this receptor activates macrophages, as indicated by induction of cell-mediated cytotoxicity (Bright et al 1990, Chen et al 1990, Green et al 1992). Interestingly, this receptor not only recognizes endotoxin, but also peptidoglycans from *Staphylococcus aureus* (Dziarski 1991) as well as pertussis toxin (Clark 1990, Lei & Morrison 1992, 1993a, b, van't Wout et al 1992) suggesting the possibility of a 'final common pathway' for monocyte activation by Gram-negative and Gram-positive microorganisms.

CD14

The endotoxin receptor that has been most extensively characterized is CD14. CD14 is a 55 kD cell membrane-associated glycoprotein originally classified as a differentiation antigen on cells of the myelomonocytic lineage. It is present on monocytes, macrophages and activated granulocytes, as well as on some mature tumour cell lines, but not on cells in earlier stages of differentiation or on immature tumour cell lines such as U937, HL60 or K562 (Griffin et al 1981, Todd et al 1981, Maliszewski et al 1985, Goyert et al 1986). The gene for CD14 has been cloned and mapped to the long arm of chromosome 5, to a region encoding several growth factors and receptors such as interleukin-3 (IL-3), granulocyte-macrophage colony-stimulating factor (GM-CSF), the platelet-derived growth factor (PDGF), the β_2-adrenergic receptor and endothelial cell growth factor (ECGF) (Goyert et al 1987). This localization already prompted speculation regarding a role for CD14 as a receptor in the early 1980s, although a ligand for CD14 was not identified until 1990, when it became clear that activation of macrophages by endotoxin could be partially blocked by specific anti-CD14 antibodies (Wright et al 1990). It has since become clear that the release of IL-1, IL-6, IL-8 and TNF by human monocytes upon activation by endotoxin is mediated by CD14.

The binding of endotoxin to human monocytes is greatly enhanced by, but not completely dependent on, the presence of lipopolysaccharide binding protein (LBP) in serum, as will be discussed in detail below (Wright et al 1990, Couturier et al 1991, Mathison et al 1992, Dentener et al 1993). However, in order to further understand the properties of CD14 as an endotoxin receptor, its structure will be discussed first. From the predicted amino acid sequence of CD14 it became clear that, although a character-istic leader peptide was present, the protein contained no membrane span-ning hydrophobic domain (Haziot et al 1988). CD14 is anchored to the cell membrane by a glycophosphatidylinositol (GPI) anchor (Simmons et al 1989), which seemed to exclude a function as a cell-signalling protein. However, it has been recently postulated that even though GPI-anchored proteins have neither a transmembrane nor a cytoplasmic region, they may be involved in signal transduction (for a review, see Robinson 1991). The GPI-anchoring of CD14 has two consequences. First, it allows rapid cleav-age from the cell membrane by GPI-specific phospholipases C or D (PI-PLC and -D). Shedding of CD14 from activated monocytes has been observed in vitro (Bazil & Strominger 1991), and may occur in vivo as well, since soluble forms of CD14 have been detected both in urine and in plasma (Bazil et al 1986, Haziot et al 1988). Secondly, GPI-anchoring results in a high lateral mobility of CD14 within the cell membrane, which may also be important for its function as an endotoxin receptor. Binding of specific monoclonal antibodies to CD14 results in clustering of CD14 (Jonas et al 1989), and specific immobilization of CD14 by adherence of macrophages to anti-CD14-coated plastic wells results in inhibition of activation of these cells by endotoxin (Wright et al 1990).

As has been mentioned above, the CD14-mediated activation of monocytes and macrophages is partly dependent on the presence of LBP. Macrophage responsiveness to endotoxin, lipid A, or lipid A partial struc-tures, as measured by TNF production in vitro, was a thousand-fold higher in the presence of normal serum than in the presence of LBP-depleted serum (Mathison et al 1992). In addition, the potentiating effect of nor-mal serum could be reversed by preincubation of monocytes with an anti-CD14 monoclonal antibody (My4) or by enzymatic removal of CD14 from the cell surface by PI-PLC (Wright et al 1990, Heumann et al 1992). A similar effect was observed when monocytes from patients with paroxys-mal nocturnal haemoglobinuria (PNH), that lack GPI-anchored proteins including CD14, were stimulated with endotoxin. These CD14-negative cells were able to react to endotoxin, but were approximately a hundred-fold less sensitive to endotoxin when compared to normal cells. Thus, CD14 cleavage may be a mechanism of preventing cell activation by endotoxin. However, CD14 deficiency does not cause complete endotoxin-unrespon-siveness and it would appear that an additional, CD14-independent, path-way of endotoxin signal transduction exists. Alternatively, CD14 may interact with other (low affinity) endotoxin receptors to upregulate the efficiency of signal transduction (Fig. 6.1).

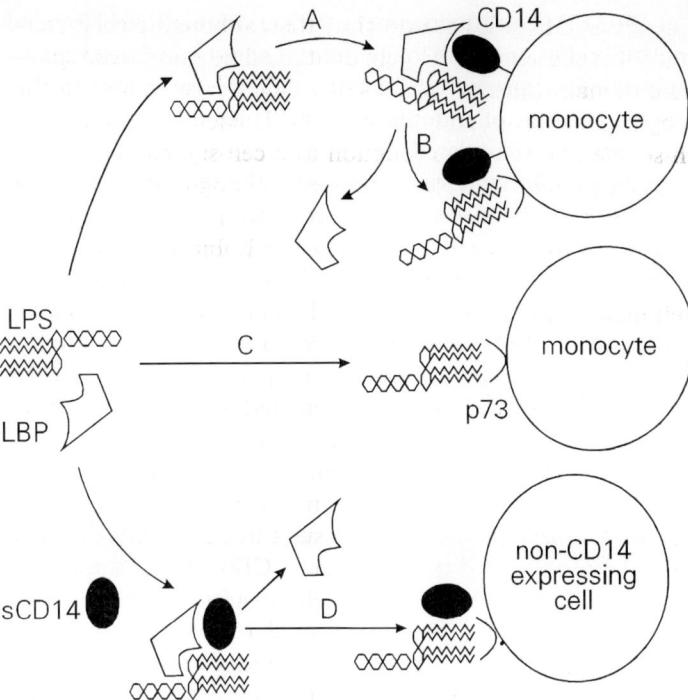

Fig. 6.1   The endotoxin signal transduction pathway. Endotoxin forms complexes with LBP present in plasma. LBP may serve to facilitate binding of endotoxin to CD14 present on monocytes and macrophages (A), leading to cell activation. Alternatively, endotoxin bound to CD14 may result in signal transduction through a second (low-affinity) endotoxin receptor, possibly p73(B). This low affinity endotoxin receptor may be activated directly by endotoxin if high doses of endotoxin are present (C). Endotoxin complexed to LBP may also bind soluble CD14; the resulting endotoxin-soluble CD14 complex may subsequently activate cells that do not express CD14 on their cell surface, possibly through a low affinity endotoxin receptor (D).

POST RECEPTOR SIGNAL TRANSDUCTION

Protein phosphorylation

An early event in endotoxin-induced macrophage activation is the phosphorylation of tyrosine residues on several proteins (Weinstein et al 1991, 1993). Blocking tyrosine kinase activity has been shown to block endotoxin-induced TNF release (Weinstein et al 1993), as well as endo-toxin-induced tumoricidal activity (Dong et al 1993) and the release of eicosanoids (Weinstein et al 1991). CD14 is known to interact with pro-tein kinases (Stefanova et al 1991), and protein tyrosine phosphorylation was shown to be CD14-dependent at low concentrations of endotoxin

(Weinstein et al 1993). At endotoxin concentrations higher than 10 ng/ml, CD14-blocking antibodies could no longer inhibit endotoxin-induced TNF tyrosine phosphorylation, providing further evidence for a low affinity, CD14-independent pathway of endotoxin signal transduction. At least two of the proteins that are phosphorylated are mitogen-activated protein (MAP) kinase isozymes, and phosphorylation leads to increased enzyme activity (Weinstein et al 1992). MAP kinases have been implicated in the regulation of a wide range of cellular processes including mitogenesis (Cobb et al 1991, Thomas 1992) and activation of MAP kinases by endotoxin may be a critical step in the induction of the biological effects of endotoxin.

Another protein that is phosphorylated after endotoxin stimulation of macrophages is an abundant cytosolic 65 kD protein (Shinomiya et al 1991). Phosphorylation of this protein is, however, on serine rather than tyrosine residues. P65 phosphorylation can be inhibited by protein kinase C (PKC) inhibitors, which results in an inhibition of the endotoxin-induced TNF and IL-1 release (Nakano et al 1993). Phosphorylation of P65 can also be blocked by treatment with a calmodulin antagonist. Interestingly, this treatment blocked IL-1 but not TNF mRNA accumulation and release of the protein (Shinomiya & Nakano 1987, Kovacs et al 1988). Thus, the induction of TNF and IL-1 synthesis by endotoxin is regulated differentially (Zuckerman et al 1991b). Finally, phosphorylation of P65 did not occur in macrophages from endotoxin-resistant C3H/HeJ mice nor in endotoxin-tolerant macrophages (Shinomiya et al 1991).

NF-κB

NF-κB is an endotoxin-inducible nuclear transcription factor that was first identified in endotoxin-stimulated B cells (Sen & Baltimore 1986, Libermann & Baltimore 1991). However, the signalling pathway controlling activation of NF-κB is incompletely understood. NF-κB is present in the cytosol bound to an inhibitory polypeptide called IκB (Baeuerle & Baltimore 1988a, b). Activation of NF-κB occurs upon phosphorylation of this subunit, which results in the dissociation of NF-κB and its migration into the nucleus (Ghosh & Baltimore 1991). Interestingly, non-phosphorylated IκB can not only bind NF-κB in the cytosol, but also dissociates NF-κB from κB enhancer sequences present in DNA (Zabel & Baeuerle 1990). NF-κB binds to DNA as a dimer, consisting of either homo- or heterodimers of p50 and p65 NF-κB polypeptides, with differential effects on activation of transcription (Baeuerle 1991, Müller et al 1993). NF-κB is involved in activation of the transcription of many genes involved in defensive functions, such as cytokines and acute phase proteins (reviewed in Müller et al 1991). NF-κB-mediated transcriptional activation can thus play a role in the coordinate gene expression required in immune responses.

Arachidonic acid metabolites

Some endotoxin-induced biological effects, such as phagocytosis and synthesis of IL-1 require the action of lipoxygenases (Schade 1986). It was found that endotoxin-stimulated macrophages contained more 13-hydroxyoctadecadienoic acid (13-HODD), a 15-lipoxygenase product derived from linoleic acid, than unstimulated controls (Schade et al 1987). When D-galactosamine sensitized mice were treated with several lipoxygenase inhibitors, TNF production after endotoxin administration was reduced (Schade et al 1989). This effect was also found in cultured macrophages. Later, it was shown that lipoxygenase inhibitors could prevent endotoxin-induced leukopenia and death in vivo, but not leukopenia induced by TNF (Schade et al 1991). When several site-specific lipoxygenase inhibitors were tested in vivo and in vitro, it was found that 15-lipoxygenase inhibitors were ineffective and that the inability to interfere with the biological effect of endotoxin correlated well with interference in 13-HODD synthesis. Thus, 15-lipoxygenase products seem to play a critical role in endotoxin signal transduction. However, when we tested a specific 15-lipoxygenase inhibitor in vitro, the endotoxin-induced TNF release was not inhibited (unpublished results).

ENDOTOXIN-INDUCED CYTOKINE RELEASE

Monocyte and macrophage activation by endotoxin results in the release of cytokines, such as TNF, IL-1, IL-6 and IL-8, and many of the biological effects of endotoxin are mediated by these cytokines. In experimental endotoxaemia in humans, the appearance of TNF in the circulation coincides with the onset of clinical symptoms of endotoxaemia, and the peak levels of TNF that are induced correlate with the severity of these symptoms. Furthermore, injection of recombinant TNF into healthy volunteers reproduces many of the clinical and laboratory manifestations of Gram-negative septic shock. These data indicate that the release of TNF is a pivotal step for induction of the biological effects of endotoxin. However, human monocytes markedly differ in their capacity to produce TNF following stimulation by endotoxin. Hence, the variability in the biological effects of endotoxin observed after intravenous administration may be related to inter-individual differences in the induction and release of TNF. We therefore briefly review TNF, its gene structure, TNF gene polymorphism and the relation of TNF gene polymorphism with TNF secretory capacity, the regulation of the induction of TNF synthesis and release, and finally, TNF receptors.

TNF levels correlated with time-course and severity of clinic endotoxaemia

The structure of TNF   3 × 17kD = OOO 51kD

Circulating, biologically-active human TNF is a 51 kD protein composed of three identical, non-covalently bound 17 kD subunits (Jones et al 1989), synthesized as 26 kD precursors of 233 amino acids. The 17 kD mature form of 157 amino acids is processed by cleavage of a signal peptide (Pennica et al 1984). TNF can also be expressed in a membrane-associated form (Kriegler et al 1988).

The TNF gene

The gene encoding TNF-α was cloned in 1984 (Pennica et al 1984), and was mapped to the short arm of chromosome 6 (Nedwin et al 1985), within the region encoding the human major histocompatibility (MHC) class III gene products (Spies et al 1986). It is situated 200 kb centromeric of the genes encoding HLA-B (HLA class I) and 350 kb telomeric of the HLA class III complement/steroid gene cluster (Fig. 6.2) (Carroll et al 1987). The TNF-α gene is flanked by the genes encoding lymphotoxin-α (or TNF-β)(5′) and lymphotoxin-β(3′) (Nedwin et al 1985, Nedespasor et al 1986, Browning et al 1993). The TNF-α and LT-α genes are arranged in a similar manner and consist of four exons and three introns (Nedwin et al 1985). Maximal homology (56%) between TNF-α and LT-α is found in the last exon of the genes, which encodes 89% and 80% of the secreted forms of TNF-α and LT-α respectively.

TNF gene polymorphism   TNF_a locus highly conserved.

The positioning of the TNF locus within the region encoding the human MHC has prompted questions regarding the linkage of TNF gene polymorphism with HLA-haplotypes, in particular those that are associated with autoimmune disorders. Somewhat disappointly, however, the TNF locus proved to be highly conserved in the population and the conventional approach of identifying restriction fragment length polymorphisms (RFLP) identified only two RFLPs in the human TNF locus. An EcoRI RFLP that appeared to be linked to a subgroup of HLA-B40-positive individuals was found in the TNF-β gene (Partanen & Koskimies 1988) A possible relation of this RFLP with TNF inducibility has not been investigated. In 1989, an NcoI RFLP was discovered in the TNF-α gene (Fugger et al 1989), but was later mapped to the first intron of the TNF-β gene (Messer et al 1991). After NcoI treatment, two restriction fragments, named TNFB*1 and TNFB*2 (of 5.3 and 10.5 kb respectively), were detectable. The frequency of the TNFB*2 allele was decreased significantly in patients with primary biliary cirrhosis (Fugger et al 1989). The TNFB*1 allele was associated with an increased production of TNF-β (Messer et al 1991), and was strongly associated with HLA-DR3, HLA-B8 and HLA-A1 haplotypes (Fugger et al 1989).

A different strategy for identifying gene polymorphism is the detection of simple sequence length polymorphisms (SSLP), or 'microsatellites', that exist throughout the human genome (Litt & Luty 1989, Tautz 1989, Weber & May 1989). Several microsatellites, named TNFa, TNFb, TNFc, TNFd and TNFe, have been identified in the vicinity of the human TNF locus (Nedospasov et al 1992, Udalova et al 1993). Extensive polymorphism exists within these microsatellites, and the relationship of different alleles with HLA-haplotypes has been thoroughly investigated (Jongeneel et al 1991). Combination of HLA class I and II, TNFB*1 and *2, and TNFa haplotypes resulted in the formation of four 'extended haplotypes' that correlated with TNF-α secretory capacity. Interestingly, one of these haplotypes (HLA-DQw8, HLA-DR3(Dw4), HLA-C4, TNFB*2, TNFa2, HLA-B15) occurred more frequently in patients with insulin-dependent diabetes mellitus (IDDM)) (Pociot et al 1993).

Finally, a biallelic polymorphism in the human TNF-α promoter region detecting a point mutation was described recently (Wilson et al 1992). The uncommon allele of this polymorphism was found to be strongly associated with the HLA-A1, B8 and DR3 antigens (Wilson et al 1993). It is not yet clear whether this polymorphism is related to the capacity to secrete TNF-α.

The regulation of transcription, translation and release of TNF

The synthesis and release of TNF is under tight control, and is regulated at the levels of transcription (Collart et al 1986, 1987, Sariban et al 1988, Horiguchi et al 1989, Jongeneel et al 1989, Taffet et al 1989, Collart et al 1990), TNF-α mRNA half-life (Beutler et al 1986, Sariban et al 1988, Jongeneel et al 1989, Taffet et al 1989), translational efficiency (Han et al 1990) and probably also the release of soluble TNF.

Initial studies focused on the regulation of the TNF promoter in the 5'-flanking region of the TNF gene. The 5'-untranslated region (UTR) of the TNF gene was analysed for DNA-protein interactions by electrophoretic mobility shift assays (EMSAs) using restriction fragments of the 5'-UTR and nuclear extracts from resting and endotoxin-stimulated macrophages. Functional analysis of the TNF promoter region was performed by transfection experiments with constructs, containing truncated 5' flanking regions of the TNF gene coupled to a chloramphenicol transferase (CAT) reporter gene (Jongeneel 1992). Finally, sequence analysis of the 5' flanking region of the murine TNF-α gene revealed five κB enhancer sequences, which may be important for inducible promoter activity (Lenardo & Baltimore 1989), as well as an MHC class II Y-box, a binding site for nuclear factor (NF)-Y, which is thought to be involved in baseline rather than inducible promoter activity (Fig. 6.2) (Jongeneel 1992). These experiments indicate an important role for NF-κB as a regulator of TNF gene transcription. NF-κB is an endotoxin-inducible transcription factor that consists of a 50/67 kD protein heterodimer (Sen & Baltimore 1986, Collart et al 1990, Pomeranz et al 1990, Shakov et al 1990). Functional analysis of the murine TNF promoter showed that the five κB sites present in the murine TNF promoter can all bind NF-κB, although with different affinities (Collart et al 1990, Jongeneel 1992). At least two of the κB sites (κB1 and κB2) can also bind another transcription factor (Jongeneel 1992), nuclear factor granulocyte/monocyte-a (NF-GMa) (Shannon et al 1988, 1990, Schreck 1990), although it is not yet clear whether binding of this factor usually results in increased TNF gene transcription. Even though much of the evidence presented above points to NF-κB as a principal regulator of TNF gene transcription, other transcription factors, such as NF-Y, may also play a role. However, in experiments using constructs containing combinations of the potential transcription factor binding sequences in the TNF promoter coupled to an enhancerless reporter promoter, it was shown that only the combinations of two specific κB sites (κB2 and κB3) had endotoxin-inducible enhancer activity, whereas the κB1, κB4 and the NF-Y binding sites showed no enhancer activity, even in combination with κB3 (Shakov et al 1990, Jongeneel 1992).

In addition to the tight regulation of TNF transcription, TNF expression is also regulated at the level of translation. TNF mRNA has a very short half-life, due to its rapid degradation. The vulnerability of TNF mRNA is related to the presence of an AU-rich sequence (UUAUUUAU) in the 3'-UTR of the TNF mRNA molecule (Caput et al 1986). Interestingly, this AU-motif is conserved in the 3'-UTR of several other cytokine and proto-oncogene mRNAs, and may represent an RNAse attack site (Shaw & Kamen 1986, Wilson & Treisman 1988). Furthermore, these AU-rich sequences were shown to decrease translational efficiency (Kruys et al 1986, 1989, Han et al 1990). Recently, it was reported that the 3'-UTR of the TNF gene may contain repressor sequences silencing the TNF gene in cells that do not normally express TNF (Han et al 1991, Kruys et al 1992). In these experiments, constructs containing 5'- and 3'-UTR sequences coupled to a CAT reporter gene were transfected into non-hematopoietic cells. In cells containing the 3'-UTR CAT expression was silenced, whereas in cells without the 3'-UTR CAT expression was present even in the absence of NF-κB sites in the 5'-UTR.

In conclusion, NF-κB and possibly NF-GMa play an important role in the regulation of TNF gene transcription. TNF mRNA abundance and translational efficiency is regulated by an AU-rich motif in the 3'-UTR. Finally, regulation of TNF expression can be modulated by dominant repressor sequences in the 3'-UTR.

very short ½-life of TNF-mRNA (AV-rich sequence ?-RNASe attack site?)

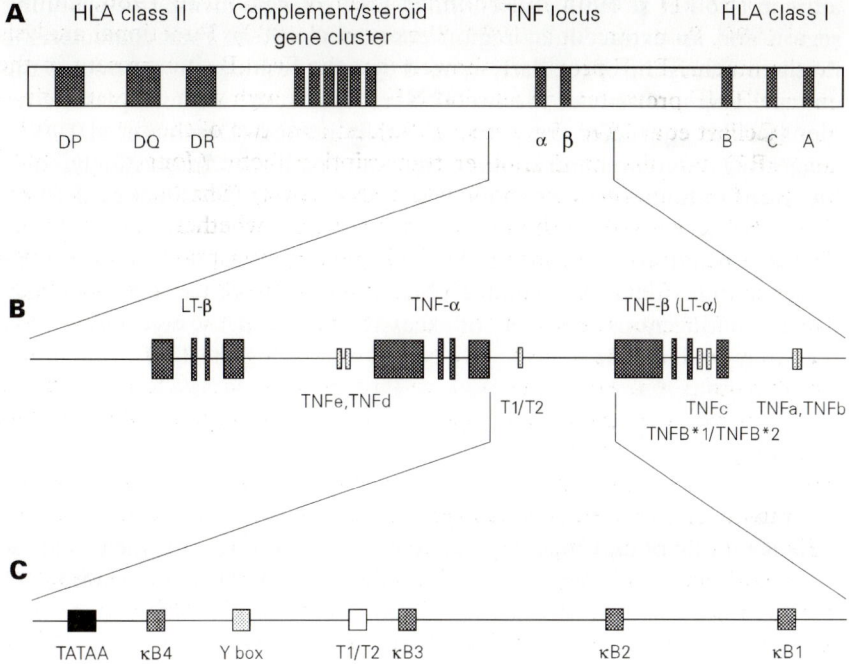

Fig. 6.2 Schematic diagram of the short arm of human chromosome 6. In (A) the position of the TNF locus in the region encoding the human major histocompatibility complex class I and II antigens is illustrated. In (B) the structure of the TNF-α, TNF-β (lymphotoxin (LT)-α) and LT-β is shown. Each of these genes consists of four exons (dark grey bars). In addition, the position of the microsatellites TNFa-e, as well as the TNFB′1/TNFB′2 and T1/T2 polymorphisms are shown (light grey bars). (C) represents the TNF-α promoter region, containing four κB sites and a Y box. Furthermore, the positions of the TNFc microsatellite and the T1/T2 polymorphism are indicated.

The TNF receptors

Two receptors for TNF with molecular weights of 55 and 75 kD respectively, that can bind both TNF-α and lymphotoxin, have been identified, cloned and characterized (Loetscher et al 1990a, b, Schall et al 1990). Comparison of the amino acid sequences of these receptors revealed sequence homology in the extracellular domains (Dembic et al 1990). The TNF receptors belong to a superfamily of receptors, the nerve growth factor (NGF) receptor family (Smith et al 1990, Mallet & Barclay 1991), which also includes NGF (Johnson et al 1992), CD27 (Camerini et al 1991), CD30 (Dürkop et al 1992), CD40 (Stamenkovic et al 1989) and the Fas antigen (Itoh et al 1991), all of which have a single membrane-spanning region and an extracellular region containing two to four characteristic domains consisting of regularly-spaced cysteine residues. In contrast to the extracellular similarity of the two TNF receptors, the intracytoplasmic regions of the molecules are not structurally related (Dembic et al 1990), suggesting differential intracellular signalling pathways. Interestingly, soluble forms of both TNF receptors exist (Gray et al 1990, Heller et al 1990, Kohno et al 1990, Nophar et al 1990, Porteu & Nathan 1990). These probably result from enzymatic cleavage of the extracellular domain of the receptors. The function of soluble TNF receptors is not yet clear: they may serve as endogenous inhibitors of excessive TNF activity, or, alternatively, they may prolong the half-life of TNF by stabilizing the TNF trimer.

sTNF-R

SERUM FACTORS THAT MODULATE ENDOTOXIN SENSITIVITY

Endotoxin that is liberated from live or disintegrating Gram-negative bacteria is rapidly bound by many molecules present in serum, such as albumin, transferrin and complement components C1 and C3 (Berger & Beger 1987, Tesh et al 1987). Whereas some endotoxin-protein interactions may be aspecific (endotoxin binds avidly to positively charged surfaces), others are highly specific and may play a role in the clearance and detoxification of endotoxin or modulate its biological effects.

Endotox — neg. charged — binds to cations

Endotoxin-lipoprotein interactions

Endotoxin binds to high density lipoprotein (HDL) in serum after modification by a non-lipid serum component (Ulevitch et al 1979). Binding to HDL results in partial detoxification of endotoxin as reflected by a reduced pyrogenicity and an inability to produce neutropenia in rabbits and a reduced lethality of HDL-bound endotoxin in adrenalectomized mice, as well as decreased abilities to activate complement and induce TNF, IL-1 and IL-6 production by monocytes and macrophages (Ulevitch & Johnston 1978, Mathison et al 1988, Cavaillon et al 1990, Baumberger et al 1991). Nevertheless, HDL-bound endotoxin can still produce shock, disseminated intravascular coagulation and death (Ulevitch et al 1981). The alterations in biological activity of endotoxin in vivo that are caused by binding to HDL may be related to different cellular targeting of free versus HDL-bound endotoxin. Whereas free endotoxin is taken up mainly by macrophages, HDL-endotoxin complexes are taken up by tissues that metabolize cholesterol, in particular by the adrenal gland (Mathison & Ulevitch 1979). It has been suggested that uptake of HDL-endotoxin complexes by this organ may function as a detoxification pathway of endotoxin, thus providing a possible explanation for the enhanced toxicity of endotoxin

HDL — bind endotoxin: less potent

observed in adrenalectomized mice (Freudenberg et al 1986). Another likely explanation for this effect, however, is the inability of adrenalectomized animals to produce cortisol.

Interactions of endotoxin with LBP and bactericidal/permeability increasing protein (BPI)

Two endotoxin-binding proteins, LBP and BPI, that specifically interact with the lipid A moiety of endotoxin and modulate its biological effects, have recently been characterized (Marra et al 1990, Schumann et al 1990). LBP is a 60 kD acute phase protein that was first identified by its ability to decrease binding of endotoxin to HDL (Tobias & Ulevitch 1983, Tobias et al 1986). It is present in low concentrations (<100 ng/ml) in normal serum, but in acute phase serum LBP levels increase substantially to 30–50 μg/ml. BPI is present in the primary granules of neutrophilic granulocytes, but a soluble form is detectable in plasma from septic patients (von der Möhlen and van Deventer, unpublished results). The primary structures of LBP and BPI were deduced from the cloned and sequenced genes (Gray et al 1989, Schumann et al 1990). LBP shares 45% amino acid sequence identity with BPI at its NH_2 terminal end. Both these proteins specifically bind endotoxin at their NH_2 terminal and form high affinity complexes with lipid A, the biologically active moiety of endotoxin (Tobias et al 1989, Gazzano-Santoro et al 1992). Recently, the genes encoding LBP and BPI were mapped to the same region of the long arm of human chromosome 20, suggesting that the proteins are members of a family of endotoxin-binding proteins (Tobias et al 1988, Gray et al 1993).

Interestingly, the biological effects of LBP and BPI, are opposed (Dentener et al 1993). As discussed above, binding of LBP to endotoxin results in interaction of the LBP-endotoxin complex with CD14 (Wright et al 1989b, 1990) LBP also binds to Gram-negative bacteria and endotoxin-coated erythrocytes, and promotes adhesion of these particles to macrophages, thus serving as an opsonin (Wright et al 1989b). It is presently unknown how LBP modulates endotoxin sensitivity in vivo. However, increased serum levels of LBP in acutely ill patients would be expected to increase the endotoxin sensitivity of these patients.

BPI was first identified as a bactericidal protein that was present in the primary granules of neutrophils (Weiss et al 1978, Ooi et al 1987). It was later shown that BPI specifically binds endotoxin, and neutralizes several of its biological effects in vitro (Marra et al 1990, Ooi et al 1991). Recombinant BPI has a protective effect in experimental endotoxaemia in several animal models (Marra et al 1992). Since circulating BPI is detectable in serum from septic patients it is tempting to speculate on its role as a naturally-occurring endotoxin antagonist.

Soluble CD14

Normal serum levels of soluble CD14 in humans are rather high (2–6 µg/ ml) and may vary in the course of several disease processes. In polytraumatized patients and in those with severe burns, serum CD14 levels were initially depressed, but subsequently increased and remained elevated for some time thereafter (Krüger et al 1991). The role of soluble CD14 in endotoxicity has been the topic of much debate. First, it may act as a naturally-occurring endotoxin antagonist by binding LBP-endotoxin complexes in the systemic circulation, thereby preventing activation of monocytes or macrophages (Maliszewski 1991). There is some evidence that soluble CD14 can indeed reduce endotoxin-induced monocyte activation in vitro in the presence of serum (Schütt et al 1992). However, even in severe sepsis, the molar excess of soluble CD14 to lipopolysaccharide does not prevent endotoxin-induced biological effects, which suggests that this mechanism is not very important in vivo. Secondly, soluble CD14 may be shed by monocytes as a way of preventing (further) activation of monocytes by endotoxin. On the other hand, soluble CD14 has the exciting property of enabling cells that do not express CD14 on their membranes, such as endothelial cells, to respond to endotoxin-LBP complexes in the systemic circulation (Frey et al 1992, Patrick et al 1992).

GENETICALLY-DETERMINED ENDOTOXIN RESISTANCE: THE C3H/HEJ MOUSE

C3H/HeJ mice are genetically resistant to the lethal actions of endotoxin (Watson et al 1978). This genetic defect, which has been mapped to chromosome 4, results in a phenotypic resistance to endotoxin due to a defective endotoxin response of C3H/HeJ macrophages. The defect acts at multiple levels: not only do macrophages require much higher concentrations of endotoxin for TNF mRNA synthesis to be initiated but even in the presence of high intracellular TNF mRNA levels little protein is translated (Beutler et al 1986).

SENSITIZATION TO THE BIOLOGICAL EFFECTS OF ENDOTOXIN

Many substances that modulate host responses to endotoxin have been identified. Depending on the substance used and the temporal relationship between pretreatment and subsequent challenge, both sensitization and induction of tolerance to the effects of endotoxin have been observed.

D-galactosamine sensitization

One of the most widely studied models involves sensitization to endotoxin by previous administration of D-galactosamine. Treatment with D-galactosamine renders rabbits, rats and mice multiple orders of magnitude

D-galactosamine — sensitizat to TNF
lead

more sensitive to the lethal action of endotoxin (Galanos et al 1979). D-galactosamine is a well-known hepatotoxic agent, which induces biochemical alterations in the hepatocyte including depletion of UTP and accumulation of UDP. These lead to an impaired synthesis of RNA and other cellular macromolecules. Reversal of the early biochemical changes induced by D-galactosamine by administration of uridine leads to reversal of endotoxin-sensitization. Sensitization by D-galactosamine requires endotoxin-responsive macrophages, since endotoxin-resistant C3H/HeJ mice become susceptible to sensitization only after transfer of macrophages from endotoxin-sensitive C3H/HeN mice (Freudenberg et al 1986). However, D-galactosamine enhances susceptibility of both endotoxin-sensitive (C3H/HeN) and endotoxin-resistant (C3H/HeJ) mice to a challenge with killed Gram-negative as well as Gram-positive bacteria (Freudenberg & Galanos 1991) and lethality could be prevented by administering anti-TNF antiserum. In addition, it was demonstrated that sensitization to endotoxin by D-galactosamine is related to an increased susceptibility to TNF released by macrophages. Sensitization to TNF parallelled sensitization to endotoxin and was also present in endotoxin-resistant C3H/HeJ mice (Lehmann et al 1987). The biochemistry of endotoxin sensitization by D-galactosamine administration is not clear, but the biochemical changes leading to impairment or cessation of RNA synthesis are a prerequisite for this effect. Interestingly, it has been found that other, less specific, inhibitors of RNA synthesis, such as lead acetate, actinomycin D (ActD), α-amanitin and cycloheximide also sensitize animals to endotoxin (Berry & Smythe 1964, Seyberth et al 1972). For example, combined administration of endotoxin and lead acetate renders rats about 100 000 times more sensitive to the lethal action of endotoxin (Seyle et al 1966). Lead treatment resulted in a higher peak serum TNF concentration as well as a higher total production of TNF (Honchel et al 1991). The effects of some endotoxin sensitizers on endotoxin-induced synthesis of tumour necrosis factor by monocytes in vitro has been studied, but the reported data are inconclusive with respect to the mechanism of action: TNF release was inhibited by cycloheximide, but not by actinomycin D or α-amanitin (Voitenok et al 1989).

Bacterial infections

Inoculation of mice with sublethal doses of certain bacterial strains, such as *Coxiella burnetti*, *Salmonella typhimurium*, *Klebsiella pneumoniae*, *Escherichia coli*, *Bordetella pertussis*, *Propionibacterium acnes*, *Myco-bacterium bovis Bacille Calmette-Guérin* (BCG) and *Corynebacterium parvum*, induces hypersensitivity to a subsequent endotoxin challenge (Schramek et al 1984, Matsuura & Galanos 1990, Vogel et al 1990). Remarkably, this sensitization also occurs in endotoxin-resistant C3H/HeJ mice. As in the D-galactosamine sensitization model, increased sensitivity to endotoxin induced by bacterial infection is accompanied by an increased sensitivity to the toxic actions of TNF (Matsuura & Galanos 1990). In some models,

Bacterial sensitizat to endotox — inc. BCG
+ asymptomatic Gm in intact. INF-γ !

hypersensitivity to endotoxin may persist for up to 60 days after inoculation. These studies suggest that asymptomatic (Gram-negative) bacterial
infections may profoundly influence host responses to endotoxin. The
mechanism of sensitization to endotoxin in the course of infection is not
yet clear. Induction of interferon γ production by T lymphocytes may play
a role (Vogel et al 1990), since it was shown to augment TNF biosynthesis
in response to endotoxin by macrophages, even in endotoxin-resistant
C3H/HeJ mice (Beutler et al 1986).

INDUCTION OF TOLERANCE TO THE BIOLOGICAL EFFECTS
OF ENDOTOXIN

Low-dose endotoxin pretreatment

It is known that administration of very low doses of endotoxin can induce
tolerance to a subsequent lethal endotoxin challenge in both humans and
animals (Johnston & Greisman 1985). Binding-studies using ^{3}H-labelled
endotoxin showed a decreased binding of endotoxin to monocytes after
induction of tolerance by endotoxin pretreatment, probably due to a decrease in the number of binding sites for endotoxin available on the
monocyte cell surface (Larsen & Sullivan 1984). In the endotoxin-tolerant
state, the toxicity of exogenous TNF is also reduced. One explanation for
this effect may be internalization (or shedding) of TNF receptors on
monocytes caused by stimulation with endotoxin (Ding et al 1989). Experimental injection of endotoxin results in transient TNF and IL-1 peaks
in serum. The induction of IL-1 depends partly on the previously released
TNF as was demonstrated by a significant decrease in circulating IL-1 levels
after pretreatment with an anti-TNF monoclonal antibody (Zuckerman
et al 1991). A second injection of endotoxin no longer resulted in TNF
release, but the IL-1 response remained. Thus, IL-1 induction by endotoxin is at least partly regulated by a separate mechanism (see also p. 127),
and the IL-1 that is induced in tolerant mice may have different cellular
sources. Abrogation of TNF release after induction of tolerance to endotoxin in macrophages appears to be due to a decrease in endotoxin-induced
TNF mRNA without an effect on mRNA stability (Mathison et al 1990,
Evans & Zuckerman 1991, Takasuka et al 1991). However, there is one
report in which neither TNF mRNA levels nor cellular levels of the 26 kD
TNF precursor were reduced in refractory macrophages when compared
to those in macrophages actively secreting TNF (Zuckerman et al 1989).

Monophosphoryl lipid A (MPLA) and other lipid A derivatives

Since the identification of the lipid A moiety of endotoxin as the trigger of
its toxic effects, the toxicity of various chemically-modified forms of this
lipid were investigated. A study that compared the in vivo toxicity of

endotoxin, diphosphoryl lipid A and monophosphoryl lipid A (MPLA) surprisingly showed that endotoxin and diphosphoryl lipid A were toxic, whereas MPLA was not, despite the fact that similar amounts of TNF were induced (Kiener et al 1988). By contrast, investigation of TNF production in whole blood ex vivo after stimulation with endotoxin, lipid A, MPLA and two other lipid A derivatives (lipid IV_A and lipid X) revealed that these structures exhibit a decreasing capacity to stimulate synthesis and release of TNF (Kovach et al 1990). Purified lipid X was later shown to have no immunostimulatory activity; previous reports of immunostimulatory capacity were shown to be due to contamination of the lipid X preparation used (Lam et al 1991). Simultaneous incubation of lipid IV_A with endotoxin or lipid A inhibited the release of TNF in whole blood. Furthermore, it inhibited the induction of TNF mRNA in endotoxin-stimulated mononuclear cells (Kovach et al 1990).

Lipid X and 3-aza-lipid X (a diamino analogue) can also inhibit some of the actions of endotoxin. Endotoxin-induced priming of neutrophils is inhibited by lipid X in a manner suggesting competition for cellular binding sites (Danner et al 1987). 3-aza-lipid X is a partial agonist of endotoxin when administered in high doses. Inhibition of neutrophil priming is strongest when lipid X is added before endotoxin. Administration of lipid X in vivo to counteract the actions of endotoxin may therefore be most useful as a preventive measure in patients with a high risk of developing Gram negative infections.

? inhibition of endotoxin acting by lipidX ? competition for cellular binding sites

Low dose TNF and IL-1 pretreatment

Administration of sublethal doses of recombinant TNF to rats resulted in tolerance to the toxic effects of this cytokine as well as to the effects of a lethal dose of endotoxin (Fraker et al 1988). Thus, these substances can induce reciprocal tolerance. In rats, treatment with recombinant TNF before induction of Gram-negative septicemia by cecal ligation and puncture, also protected against the lethality of this condition (Alexander et al 1991). One of the biochemical differences between treated and control groups is an enhanced hepatic induction of manganese superoxide dismutase in TNF-treated rats just before clinical differences between the groups are first observed. In addition, it was demonstrated in vitro that one of the early effects of administration of TNF in combination with protein synthesis inhibitors is phosphorylation of a small heat-shock protein, HSP27 (Koning et al 1991). After pretreatment of cells with TNF (without protein synthesis inhibitors), challenge with TNF and protein synthesis inhibitors no longer resulted in phosphorylation of HSP27. This may reflect that in hyporesponsiveness, a step early in TNF signal transduction is impaired.

Administration of a sublethal dose of IL-1 24 hours before challenge with a lethal dose of several Gram-negative bacteria could prevent death in a murine model (Van der Meer et al 1990). Some protection was also found in infections with Gram-positive bacteria and in cerebral malaria. If IL-1 was administered intraperitoneally 2 hours before a lethal challenge with recombinant TNF, protection against the lethal actions of this cytokine ensued (Sheppard et al 1991). This protection persisted for 8 days after the IL-1 treatment. The mechanism whereby IL-1 exerts its protective effects is as yet unclear.

pre-treatment c̄ (low-dose) TNF + IL-1 protective
? impaired cytokine signal transduction ?

CONCLUSION

Critically ill patients may develop septicemia triggered by small amounts of endotoxin (plasma levels usually do not exceed 100 ng/l). In addition, despite obvious differences in clinical outcome, cytokine levels in septic patients usually do not exceed those observed in volunteers that are challenged with a low dose of endotoxin. These findings point towards sepsis being a state of susceptibility to the biological effects of endotoxin or cytokines. In this review we have discussed many factors that determine host sensitivity to the toxic effects of bacterial lipopolysaccharides. Causes for this increase in susceptibility can be found at multiple levels including binding of endotoxin to plasma proteins, presentation of endotoxin to immunocompetent cells, endotoxin signal transduction, and the transcription, release, receptor binding and signal transduction of the various induced cytokines. In addition, genetic factors that in humans seem to be located on chromosome 6, may determine the amount of TNF that is produced by monocytes in vitro, as well as by volunteers in vivo, after a standard endotoxin challenge. A more detailed knowledge of the mechanisms that lead to endotoxin tolerance or susceptibility will increase our knowledge of the pathogenesis of Gram-negative sepsis, and may lead to novel therapeutic interventions.

Sepsis - increased sensitivity to endotoxin or cytokines

KEY POINTS FOR CLINICAL PRACTICE

- Endotoxin is a major bacterial factor in the pathogenesis of gram-negative sepsis
- The structure of endotoxin and its receptors on immune competent cells have been partially elucidated
- The biological activity of endotoxin depends on interaction with endotoxin-binding proteins in plasma
- Extensive differences in endotoxin sensitivity exist between individuals
- Bacterial infections and endotoxin itself can dramatically influence the sensitivity to endotoxin
- The effects of endotoxin are mediated by proinflammatory cytokines

Binding proteins
feedback
Cytokines

REFERENCES

Alexander H R, Sheppard B C, Jensen J C et al 1991 Treatment with recombinant human tumor necrosis factor-alpha protects rats against the lethality, hypotension, and hypothermia of Gram-negative sepsis. J Clin Invest 88: 34–39

Baeuerle P A 1991 The inducible transcription factor NF-κB: regulation by distinct protein subunits. Biochem Biophys Acta 1072: 63–80

Baeuerle P A, Baltimore D 1988a Activation of DNA-binding activity in an apparently cytoplasmic precursor of the NF-κB transcription factor. Cell 53: 211–217

Baeuerle P A, Baltimore D 1988b IκB: a specific inhibitor of the NF-κB transcription factor. Science 242: 540–546

Baumberger C, Ulevitch R J, Dayer J-M 1991 Modulation of endotoxic activity of lipopolysaccharide by high-density lipoprotein. Pathobiology 59: 378–383

Bazil V, Strominger J L 1991 Shedding of CD14 as a mechanism of downmodulation of CD14 on stimulated human monocytes. J Immunol 147: 1567–1574

Bazil V, Horejsi V, Baudys M et al 1986 Biochemical characterization of a soluble form of the 53-kDa monocyte surface antigen. Eur J Immunol 16: 1583–1589

Berger D, Beger H G 1987 Quantification of the endotoxin binding capacity of human transferrin. In: Levin J, Ten Cate J W, Büller H R, van Deventer S J H, Sturk A (eds) Bacterial endotoxins: Pathophysiological effects, clinical significance, and pharmacological control. Alan R Liss, New York, pp 115–124

Berry L J, Smythe D S 1964 Effects of bacterial endotoxins on metabolism VII. Enzyme induction and cortisone protection. J Exp Med 120: 721–732

Beutler B, Krochin N, Milsark I W, Luedke C, Cerami A 1990 Control of cachectin (tumor necrosis factor) synthesis: mechanisms of endotoxin resistance. Science 232: 977–980

Beutler B, Tkacenko V, Milsark I, Krochnin N, Cerami A 1986 The effect of A interferon on cachectin expression by mononuclear phagocytes reversal of the lps^d (endotoxin resistance) phenotype. J Exp Med 164: 1791–1796

Bright S W, Chen T Y, Flebbe L M, Lei M G, Morrison D C 1990 Generation and characterization of hamster-mouse hybridomas secreting monoclonal antibodies with specificity for lipopolysaccharide receptor. J Immunol 145: 1–7

Browning J L, Ngam-ek A, Lawton P et al 1993 Lymphotoxin β, a novel member of the TNF family that forms a heteromeric complex with lymphotoxin on the cell surface. Cell 72: 847–856

Camerini D, Walz G, Loenen W A M, Borst J, Seed B 1991 The T cell activation antigen CD27 is a member of the NGF/TNF receptor family. J Immunol 147: 3165–3169

Caput D, Beutler B, Hartog K, Thayer R, Brown-Shimer S, Cerami A 1986 Identification of a common nucleotide sequence in the 3'-untranslated region of mRNA molecules specifying inflammatory mediators. Proc Natl Acad Sci USA 83: 1670–1674

Carroll M C, Katzman P, Alicot E M et al 1987 Linkage map of the human histocompatibility complex including the tumor necrosis factor genes. Proc Natl Acad Sci USA 84: 8535–8539

Cavaillon J M, Fitting C, Haeffner-Cavaillon N, Kirsch S J, Warren H S 1990 Cytokine response by monocytes and macrophages to free and lipoprotein-bound lipopolysaccharide. Infect Immun 58: 2375–2382

Chen T Y, Bright S W, Pace J L, Russell S W, Morrison D C 1990 Induction of macrophage-mediated tumor cytotoxicity by a hamster monoclonal antibody with specificity for lipopolysaccharide receptor. J Immunol 145: 8–12

Clark C G, Armstrong G D 1980 Lymphocyte receptors for pertussis toxin. Infect Immun 58: 3840–3846

Cobb M H, Boulton T G, Robbins D J 1991 Extracellular signal-related kinase: ERKs in progress. Cell Regul 2: 965–978

Collart M A, Belin D, Vassali J D, de Kossodo S, Vassali P 1986 γ-Interferon enhances macrophage transcription of tumor necrosis factor/cachectin, interleukin-1, and urokinase genes, which are controlled by short-lived repressors. J Exp Med 164: 2113–2118

Collart M A, Belin D, Vassali J D, Vassali P 1987 Modulations of functional activity in differential macrophages are accompanied by early and transient increase or decrease of C-fos gene transcription. J Immunol 139: 949–955

Collart M A, Bauerle P, Vassali P 1990 Regulation of tumor necrosis factor α transcription in macrophages: involvement of four κB-like motifs and of constitutive and inducible forms of NF-κB. Mol Cell Biol 10: 1498–1506

Couturier C, Haeffner-Cavaillon N, Caroff M, Kazatchkine M D 1991 Binding sites for endotoxins (lipopolysaccharides) on human monocytes. J Immunol 147: 1899–1904

Couturier C, Jahns G, Kazatchkine M D, Haeffner-Cavaillon N 1992 Membrane molecules which trigger the production of interleukin-1 and tumor necrosis factor by lipopolysaccharide-stimulated human monocytes. Eur J Immunol 22: 1461–1466

Danner R L, Joiner K A, Parillo J E 1987 Inhibitionof endotoxin-induced priming of human neutrophils by lipid X and 3-aza-lipid X. J Clin Invest 80: 605–612

Dentener M A, Bazil V, Von Asmuth E J U, Ceska M, Buurman W A 1993 Involvement of CD14 in lipopolysaccharide-induced tumor necrosis factor-α, IL-6 and IL-8 release by human monocytes and alveolar macrophages. J Immunol 150: 2885–2891

Ding A H, Sanchez E, Srimal S, Nathan C F 1989 Macrophages rapidly internalize their tumor necrosis factors receptors in response to bacterial lipopolysaccharide. J Biol Chem 264: 3924–3929

Dembic Z, Loetscher H, Gubler U et al 1990 Two human TNF receptors have similar extracellular, but distinct intracellular, domain sequences. Cytokine 2: 231–237

Dentener M A, Von Asmuth E J U, Francot G J M, Marra M N, Buurman W A 1993 Antagonistic effects of lipopolysaccharide binding protein and bactericidal/permeability-increasing protein on lipopolysaccharide-induced cytokine release by mononuclear phagocytes. J Immuno 151: 4258–4265

Dong Z, O'Brian C A, Fidler L J 1993 Activation of tumoricidal properties in macrophages by lipopolysaccharide requires protein tyrosine kinase activity. J Leukocyte Biol 53: 53–60

Dürkop H, Latza U, Hummel M, Eitelbach F, Seed B, Stein H 1992 Molecular cloning and expression of a new member of the nerve growth factor receptor family that is characteristic for Hodgkin's disease. Cell 68: 421–427

Dziarski R 1991 Peptidoglycan and lipopolysaccharide bind to the same binding site on lymphocytes. J Biol Chem 266: 4719–4728

Evans G F, Zuckerman S H 1991 Glucocorticoid-dependent and -independent mechanisms involved in lipopolysaccharide tolerance. Eur J Immunol 21: 1973–1979

Fraker D L, Stovroff M C, Merino M J, Norton J A 1988 Tolerance to tumor necrosis factor in rats and the relationship to endotoxin tolerance and toxicity. J Exp Med 168: 95–105

Freudenberg M A, Galanos C 1991 Tumor necrosis factor alpha mediates lethal activity of killed Gram-negative and Gram-positive bacteria in D-galactosamine- treated mice. Infect Immun 59: 2110–2115

Freudenberg M A, Keppler D, Galanos C 1986 Requirement for lipopolysaccharide-responsive macrophages in galactosamine-induced sensitization to endotoxin. Infect Immun 51: 891–895

Frey E A, Miller D S, Gullstein Jahr T et al 1992 Soluble CD14 participates in the response of cells to lipopolysaccharide. J Exp Med 176: 1665–1671

Fugger L, Morling N, Ryder L P et al 1989 Ncol restriction fragment length polymorphism (RFLP) of the human tumour necrosis factor (TNF-α) region in primary biliary cirrhosis and in healthy Danes. Scand J Immunol 30: 185–189

Galanos C, Freudenberg M A, Reutter W 1979 Galactosamine-induced sensitization to the lethal effects of endotoxin. Proc Natl Acad Sci USA 76: 5939–5943

Gazzano-Santoro H, Parent J B, Grinna L et al 1992 High-affinity binding of the bactericidal/permeability-increasing protein and a recombinant amino-terminal fragment to the lipid A region of lipopolysaccharide. Infect Immun 60: 4754–4761

Ghosh S, Baltimore D 1991 Activation in vitro of NF-κB by phosphorylation of its inhibitor IκB. Nature 344: 678–682

Golenbock D T, Hampton R Y, Raetz C R H, Wright S D 1990 Human phagocytes have multiple lipid A-binding sites. Infect Immun 58: 4069–4075

Goyert S M, Ferrero E M, Seremetis S V, Winchester R J, Silver J, Mattison A C 1986 Biochemistry and expression of myelomonocytic antigens. J Immunol 137: 3909–3914

Goyert S M, Ferrero E, Rettig W J, Yenamandra A Y, Obata F, Le Beau M M 1987 The CD14 monocyte differentiation antigen maps to a region encoding growth factors and receptors. Science 239: 497–500

Gray P W, Flaggs G, Leong S R, Gumina R J 1989 Cloning of the cDNA of a human neutrophil bactericidal protein. J Biol Chem 264: 9505–9509

Gray P W, Barrett K, Chantry D, Turner M, Feldman M 1990 Cloning of the human tumor necrosis factor (TNF) receptor cDNA and expression of recombinant soluble TNF-binding protein. Proc Natl Acad Sci USA 87: 7380–7384

Gray P W, Corcorran A E, Eddy R L, Byers M G, Shows T B 1993 The genes for lipopolysaccharide binding protein (LBP) and the bactericidal/permeability-increasing protein (BPI) are encoded in the same region of human chromosome 20. Genomics 15: 188–190

Green S J, Chen T Y, Crawford R M, Nacy C A, Morrison D C, Meltzer M S 1992 Cytotoxic activity and productin of toxic nitrogen oxides by macrophages treated with IFNγ and monoclonal antibodies against the 73 kDa lipopolysaccharide receptor. J Immunol 149: 2069–2075

Griffin J D, Ritz J, Nadler L M, Schlossman S F 1981 Expression of myeloid differentiation antigens on normal and malignant myeloid cells. J Clin Invest 68: 932–941

Hampton R Y, Golenbock D T, Penman M, Krieger M, Raetz C R H 1991 Recognition and plasma clearance of endotoxin by scavenger receptors. Nature 352: 342–344

Han J, Brown T, Beutler B 1990 Endotoxin-responsive sequences control cachectin/ tumor necrosis factor biosynthesis at the translational level. J Exp Med 171: 465–475

Han J, Huez G, Beutler B 1991 Interactive effects of the tumor necrosis factor promoter and 3'-untranslated regions. J Immunol 146: 1843–1848

Haziot A, Chen S, Ferrero E M, Low M C, Silber R, Goyert S M 1988 The monocyte differentiation antigen, CD14, is anchored to the cell membrane by phosphatidylinositol phosphate. J Immunol 141: 547–552

Heller R A, Song K, Onasch M A, Fischer W H, Chang D, Ringold G M 1990 Complementary DNA cloning of a receptor for tumor necrosis factor and demonstration of a shed form of the receptor. Proc Natl Acad Sci USA 87: 6151–6155

Heumann D, Gallay P, Barras C et al 1992 Control of lipopolysaccharide (LPS) binding and LPS–induced tumor necrosis factor secretion in human peripheral blood monocytes. J Immunol 148: 3505–3512

Honchel R, Marsano L, Cohen D, Shedlofsky S, McClain C J 1991 Lead enhances lipopolysaccharide and tumor necrosis factor liver injury. J Lab Clin Med 117: 202–208

Horiguchi J, Spriggs D, Imumura K, Stone R, Luebbers R, Kufe D 1989 Role of arachidonic acid metabolism in transcriptional induction of tumor necrosis factor gene expression by phorbol ester. Mol Cell Biol 9: 252–258

Itoh N, Yonehara, Mitzushima S I et al 1991 The polypeptide encoded by the cDNA for human cell surface antigen Fas can mediate apoptosis. Cell 66: 233–243

Johnson D, Lanahan A, Buck C R et al 1992 Expression of the NGF receptor. Cell 68: 421–427

Jonas L, Schütt C, Neels P, Walzel H, Siegl E 1989 Electron microscopic visualization of receptor internalization induced by a monoclonal antibody recognizing the monocyte specific glycoprotein CD14. Acta Histochem 85: 167–173

Johnston C A, Greisman S E 1985 Mechanisms of endotoxin tolerance. In: Hinshaw L B (ed) Handbook of endotoxin vol. 2: Pathophysiology of endotoxin. Elsevier Amsterdam, pp 359–401

Jones E Y, Stuart D I, Walker N P C 1989 Structure of tumor necrosis factor. Nature 338: 225–228

Jongeneel C V 1992 The TNF and lymphotoxin promoters. In: Beutler B (ed) Tumor necrosis factors. The molecules and their emerging role in medicine. Raven Press, New York, pp 539–559

Jongeneel C V, Shakhov A N, Nedospasov S A, Cerottini J C 1989 Molecular control of tissue-specific expression at the mouse TNF locus. Eur J Immunol 19: 549–552

Jongeneel C V, Briant L, Udalova I A, Sevin A, Nedospasov S A, Cambon-Thomsen A 1991 Extensive genetic polymorphism in the human tumor necrosis factor region and relation to extended HLA haplotypes. Proc Natl Acad Sci USA 88: 9717–9721

Kiener P A, Marek F, Rodgers G, Lin P F, Warr G, Desiderio J 1988 Induction of tumor necrosis factor, IFN-γ, and acute lethality in mice by toxic and non-toxic forms of lipid A. J Immunol 141: 870–874

Kodama T, Freeman M, Rohrer L, Zabrecky J, Matsudaira P, Krieger M 1990 Type I macrophage scavenger receptor contains α-helical and collagen-like coiled coils. Nature 343: 531–535

Kohno T, Brewer M T, Baker S L et al 1990 A second tumor necrosis factor receptor gene product can shed a naturally occurring tumor necrosis factor inhibitor. Proc Natl Acad Sci USA 87: 8331–8335

Konig M, Wallach D, Resch K, Holtmann H 1991 Induction of hyporesponsiveness to an early post-binding effect of tumor necrosis factor by tumor necrosis factor itself and interleukin 1. Eur J Immunol 21: 1741–1745

Kovach N L, Yee E, Munford R S, Raetz C R H, Harlan J M 1990 Lipid IV_A inhibits synthesis and release of tumor necrosis factor induced by lipopolysaccharide in human whole blood ex vivo. J Exp Med 172: 77–84

Kovacs F J, Radzioch D, Young H A, Varesio L 1988 Differential inhibition of IL-1 and TNF-α mRNA expression by agents which block second messenger pathways in murine macrophages. J Immunol 141: 3101–3105

Kriegler M, Perez C, De F K, Albert I, Lu S D 1988 A novel form of TNF/cachectin is a cell surface cytotoxic transmembrane protein: ramifications for the complex physiology of TNF. Cell 53: 45–53

Krüger C, Schütt C, Obertacke U et al 1991 Serum CD14 levels in polytraumatized and severely burnt patients. Clin Exp Immunol 85: 297–301

Kruys V I, Wathelet M G, Huez G A 1988 Identification of a translation inhibitory element (TIE) in the 3' untranslated region of the human interferon-β mRNA. Gene 72: 191–200

Kruys V, Marinx O, Shaw G, Deschamps J, Huez G 1989 Translational blockade imposed by cytokine-derived AU-rich sequences. Science 245: 852–855

Kruys V, Kemmer K, Shakhov A, Jongeneel V, Beutler B 1992 Constitutive activity of the tumor necrosis factor promoter is canceled by the 3'-untranslated region in non-macrophage cell lines; a transdominant factor overcomes this suppressive effect. Proc Natl Acad Sci USA 89: 673–677

Lam C, Hildebrandt J, Schutze E et al 1991 Immunostimulatory, but not anti-endotoxin, activity of lipid X is due to small amounts of contaming N,O-acylated disaccharide-1-phosphate: in vitro and in vivo re-valuation of the biological activity of synthetic lipid X. Infect Immun 59: 2351–2358

Larsen N E, Sullivan R 1984 Interaction between endotoxin and human monocytes: Characteristics of the binding of ^{3}H-labeled lipopolysaccharide and ^{51}Cr-labeled lipid A before and after the induction of endotoxin tolerance. Proc Natl Acad Sci USA 81: 3491–3495

Lehmann V, Freudenberg M A, Galanos C 1987 Lethal toxicity of lipopolysaccharide and tumor necrosis factor in normal and D-galactosamine-treated mice. J Exp Med 165: 657–663

Lei M G, Morrison D C 1989a Specific endotoxic lipopolysaccharide-binding proteins on murine splenocytes. I. Detection of lipopolysaccharide-binding sites on splenocytes and splenocyte subpopulations. J Immunol 141: 996–1005

Lei M G, Morrison D C 1989b Specific endotoxic lipopolysaccharide binding proteins on murine splenocytes. II. Membrane localization and binding characteristics. J Immunol 141: 1006–1011

Lei M G, Morrison D C 1992 Interrelationships of LPS, pertussis toxin and the p73 LPS receptor on lymphoreticular cells. In: Levin J, Alving C R, Munford R S, Stütz PL (eds) Endotoxin research series vol. 2, Bacterial endotoxin: recognition and effector mechanisms. Elsevier, Amsterdam, pp 143–150

Lei M G, Morrison D C 1993a Lipopolysaccharide interaction with S2 subunit of pertussis toxin. J Biol Chem 268: 1488–1493

Lei M G, Morrison D C 1993b Evidence that lipopolysaccharide and pertussis toxin bind to different domains on the same p73 receptor on murine splenocytes. Infect Immun 61: 1359–1364

Lei M G, Stimpson A, Morrison D C 1991 Specific endotoxic lipopolysacchride-binding receptors on murine splenocytes. III. Binding specificity and characterization. J Immunol 147: 1925–1932

Lenardo M J, Baltimore D 1989 NF-κB: a pleiotropic mediator of inducible and tissue-specific gene control. Cell 58: 227–229

Libermann T A, Baltimore D 1991 Transcriptional regulation of immunoglobulin gene expression. In: Cohen P, Foulkes J G (eds) Molecular aspects of cellular regulation vol. 6. Hormonal control regulation of gene transcription. Elsevier, Amsterdam, pp 399–422

Litt M, Luty J A 1989 A hypervariable microsatellite revealed by in vitro amplification of a dinucleotide repeat within the cardiac muscle actin gene. Am J Hum Genet 44: 397–401

Loetscher H, Pan Y C E, Lahm H W et al 1990a Molecular cloning and expression of the human 55 kd tumor necrosis factor receptor. Cell 61: 351–359

Loetscher H, Schlaeger E J, Lahm H W, Pan Y C, Lesslauer W, Brockhams M 1990b Purification and partial amino acid sequence analysis of two distinct tumor necrosis factor receptors from HL60 cells. J Biol Chem 265: 20131–20138

Maliszewski C R 1991 CD14 and the immune response to lipopolysaccharide. Science 252: 1321–1322

Maliszewski C R, Ball E D, Graziano R F, Fanger M W 1985 Isolation and characterization of My 23, a myeloid cell-derived antigen reactive with the monoclonal antibody AML-2-23, J Immunol 135: 1929–1936

Mallet S, Barclay A N 1991 A new superfamily of cell surface proteins related to the nerve growth factor receptor. Immunol Today 12: 220–223

Maor I, Brook G J, Aviram M 1991 Platelet secreted lipoprotein-like particle is taken up by the macrophage scavenger receptor and enhances cellular cholesterol accumulation. Atherosclerosis 88: 163–174

Marra M N, Wilde C G, Griffith J E, Snable J L, Scott R W 1990 Bactericidal/permeability-increasing protein has endotoxin-neutralizing activity. J Immunol 144: 662–666

Marra M N, Wilde C G, Collins M S, Snable J L, Thornton M B, Scott R W 1992 The role of bactericidal/permeability-increasing protein as a natural inhibitor of bacterial endotoxin. J Immunol 148: 532–537

Mathison J C, Ulevitch R J 1979 The clearance, tissue distribution, and cellular localization of intravenously injected lipopolysaccharide in rabbits. J Immunol 123: 2133–2143

Mathison J C, Wolfson N, Ulevitch R J 1988 Participation of tumor necrosis factor in the mediation of Gram-negative bacterial lipopolysaccharide-induced injury in rabbits. J Clin Invest 81: 1925–1937

Mathison J C, Virca G D, Wolfson E, Tobias P S, Glaser T K, Ulevitch R J 1990 Adaptation to bacterial lipopolysaccharide controls lipopolysaccharide-induced tumor necrosis factor production in rabbit macrophages. J Clin Invest 85: 1108–1118

Mathison J C, Tobias P S, Wolfson E, Ulevitch R J 1992 Plasma lipopolysaccharide binding protein. A key component in macrophage recognition of Gram-negative LPS. J Immunol 149: 200–206

Matsuura M, Galanos C 1990 Induction of hypersensitivity to endotoxin and tumor necrosis factor by sublethal infection with Salmonella typhimurium. Infect Immun 58: 935–937

Messer G, Spengler U, Jung M C et al 1991 Polymorphic structure: of the tumor necrosis factor (TNF) locus: an NcoI polymorphism in the first intron of the human TNF-beta gene correlates with a variant amino acid in position 26 and a reduced level of TNF-beta production. J Exp Med 173: 209–219

Müller J M, Ziegler-Heitbrock H W L, Baeuerle P A 1993 Nuclear factor kappa B, a mediator of lipopolysaccharide effects. Immunobiology 187: 233–256

Munford R S, Hall C L 1986 Detoxification of bacterial lipopolysaccharides (endotoxins) by a human neutrophil enzyme. Science 234: 203–205

Nakano M, Saito S, Nakano Y, Yamasu H, Matsuura M, Shinomiya H 1993 Intracellular protein phosphorylation in murine peritoneal macrophages in resposne to bacterial lipopolysaccharide (LPS): effects of kinase-inhibitors and LPS-induced tolerance. Immunobiol 187: 272–282

Nedospasov S A, Shakhov A, Turetskaya R et al 1986 Tandem arrangement of genes coding for tumor necrosis factor (TNF-α) and lymphotoxin (TNF-β) in the human genome. Cold Spring Harbor Symp Quant Biol LI: 611

Nedospasov S A, Udalova I A, Kuprash D Y, Turetskaya R L 1992 DNA sequence polymorphism at the human tumor necrosis factor (TNF) locus. Numerous TNF/lymphotoxin alleles tagged by two closely linked microsatellites in the upstream region of the lymphotoxin (TNF-β) gene. J Immunol 147: 1053–1059

Nedwin G E, Naylor S L, Sakaguchi A Y et al 1985 Human lymphotoxin and tumor necrosis factor genes: structure, homology and chromosomal localization. Nucl Acids Res 13: 6361–6373

Nophar Y, Kemper O, Brakebusch C et al 1990 Soluble forms of tumor necrosis factor receptors (TNF-Rs). The cDNA for the type I TNF-R, cloned using amino acid sequence data for its soluble form, encodes both a cell surface and a soluble form of the receptor. EMBO J 9: 3269–3278

Ooi C E, Weiss J, Elsbach P, Frangione B, Mannion B 1987 A 25-kDa NH$_2$-terminal fragment carries all the antibacterial activities of the human neutrophil 60-kDa bactericidal/permeability-increasing protein. J Biol Chem 262: 14891–14894

Ooi C E, Weiss J, Doerfler M E, Elsbach P 1991 Endotoxin-neutralizing properties of the 25 kD N-terminal fragment and a newly isolated 30 kD C-terminal fragment of the

55–60 kD bactericidal/permeability-increasing protein of human neutrophils. J Exp Med 174: 649–655

Partanen J, Koskimies S 1988 Low degree of DNA polymorphism in the HLA-linked lymphotoxin (tumour necrosis factor β) gene. Scand J Immunol 28: 313–316

Patrick D, Bettes J, Frey E A, Prameya R, Doroviv-Zis K, Finlay B B 1992 Hemophilus influenzae lipopolysaccharide disrupts confluent monolayers of bovine brain endothelial cells via a serum-dependent cytotoxic pathway. J Infect Dis 165: 865–872

Pennica D, Nedwin G E, Hayflick J S et al 1984 Human tumor necrosis factor: precursor structure, expression and homology to lymphotoxin. Nature 312: 724–729

Pociot F, Briant L, Jongeneel C V et al 1993 Association of tumor necrosis factor (TNF) and class II major histocompatibility complex alleles with the secretion of TNF-α and TNF-β by human mononuclear cells: a possible link to insulin-dependent diabetes mellitus. Eur J Immunol 23: 224–231

Pomeranz R J, Feinberg M B, Trono D, Baltimore D 1990 Lipopolysaccharide is a potent monocyte/macrophage–specific stimulator of human immunodeficiency virus type I expression. J Exp Med 172: 253–261

Porteu F, Nathan C 1990 Shedding of tumor necrosis factor receptors by activated human neutrophils. J Exp Med 172: 599–607

Rietschel E T, Brade L, Schade U et al 1990. Chemical structure and biological activities of lipopolysaccharides. In: Calandra T, Baumgartner J, Carlet J (eds) Endotoxin: From pathophysiology to therapeutic approaches. Flammarion, Paris, pp 6–18

Robinson P J 1991 Phosphatidylinositol membrane anchors and T cell activation. Immunology Today 12: 35–41

Rohrer L, Freeman M, Kodama T, Penman M, Krieger M 1990 Coiled-coil fibrous domains mediate ligand binding by macrophage scavenger receptor type II. Nature 343: 570–572

Sariban E, Imamura K, Luebbers R, Kufe D 1988 Transcriptional and posttranscriptional regulation of tumor necrosis factor expression in human monocytes. J Clin Invest 81: 1506–1510

Schade U F 1986 Involvement of lipoxygenases in the activation of mouse macrophages by endotoxin. Biochem Biophys Res Comm 138: 842–849

Schade U F, Burmeister I, Engel R 1987 Increased 13-hydroxyoctadecadeinoic acid content in lipopolysaccharide stimulated macrophages. Biochem Biophys Res Commun 147: 695–700

Schade U F, Ernst M, Reinke M, Wolter D T 1989 Lipoxygenase inhibitors suppress formation of tumor necrosis factor in vivo and vitro. Biochem Biophys Res Commun 159: 748–754

Schade U F, Engel R, Jakobs D 1991 Differential protective activities of site specific lipoxygenase inhibitors in endotoxic shock and production of tumor necrosis factor. Int J Immunopharmac 13: 565–571

Schall T J, Lewis M, Koller K J et al 1990 Molecular cloning and expression of a receptor for human tumor necrosis factor. Cell 61: 361–370

Schramek S, Kazar J, Sekeyova Z, Freudenberg M A, Galanos C 1984 Induction of hypersensitivity to endotoxin in mice by Coxiella burnetii. Infect Immun 45: 713–717

Schreck R, Bauerle P A 1990 NF-κB as inducible transcriptional activator of the granulocyte-macrophage colony-stimulating factor gene. Mol Cell Biol 10: 1281–1286

Schumann R R, Leong S R, Flaggs G W et al 1990 Structure and function of lipopolysaccharide binding protein. Science 249: 1429–1431

Schütt C, Schilling T, Grunwald U, Schönfeld W, Krüger C 1992 Endotoxin-neutralizing capacity of soluble CD14. Res Immunl 143: 71–78

Sen R, Baltimore D 1986 Multiple nuclear factors interact with the immunoglobulin enhancer sequence. Cell 46: 705–716

Seyberth H W, Schmidt-Gay K H, Hackenthal E 1972 Toxicity, clearance and distribution of endotoxin in mice as influenced by actinomycin D, cycloheximide, α-amanitin and lead acetate. Toxicon 10: 491–500

Seyle H, Tuchweber B, Bertok L 1966 Effect of lead acetate on the susceptibility of rats to bacterial endotoxins. J Bacteriol 91: 884–890

Shakhov A N, Collart M A, Vassali P et al 1990 κB-type enhancers are involved in lipopolysaccharide-mediated transcriptional activation of the tumor necrosis factor α gene in primary macrophages. J Exp Med 171: 35–47

Shannon M F, Gamble J R, Vadas M A 1988 Nuclear proteins interacting with the promoter region of the human granulocyte/monocyte colony-stimulating factor gene. Proc Natl Acad Sci USA 85: 674–678

Shannon M F, Pell L M, Lenardo M J et al 1990 A novel tumor necrosis factor-responsive transcription factor which recognizes a regulatory element in the hemopoietic growth factor genes. Mol Cell Biol 10: 2950–2959

Shaw G, Kamen R 1986 A conserved A U-rich sequence from the 3' untranslated region of GM-CSF mRNA mediates selective mRNA degradation. Cell 46: 659–667

Sheppard B C, Norton J A 1991 Tumor necrosis factor and interleukin-1 protection against the lethal effects of tumor necrosis factor. Surgery 109: 698–705

Shinomiya H, Nakano M 1987 Calcium ionophore A23187 does not stimulate lipopolysaccharide non-responsive C3H/HeJ peritoneal macrophages to produce IL-1. J Immunol 139: 2730–2736

Shinomiya H, Hirata H, Nakano M 1991 Purification and characterization of a 65 kDa protein phosphorylated in murine macrophages stimulated with bacterial lipopolysaccharide. J Immunol 146: 3617–3625

Simmons D L, Tan S, Tenen D G, Nicholson-Weller A, Seed B 1989 Monocyte antigen CD14 is a phospholipid anchored membrane protein. Blood 73: 284–289

Smith C A, Davis T, Anderson D et al 1990 A receptor for tumor necrosis factor defines an unusual family of cellular and viral proteins. Science 248: 1019–1023

Spies T, Morton C C, Nedospasov S A, Fiers W, Pious D, Strominger L J 1986 Genes for the tumor necrosis factors alpha and beta are linked to the human major histocompatibility complex. Proc Natl Acad Sci USA 83: 8699–8702

Stamenkovic I, Clark E A, Seed B 1989 A B-lymphocyte activation molecule related to the nerve growth factor family and induced by cytokines in carcinomas. EMBO J 8: 1403–1410

Stefanova L, Horejsi V, Ansotegui I J, Knapp W, Stockinger H 1991 GPI-anchored cell surface molecules complexes to protein tyrosine kinases. Science 254: 1016–1019

Taffet S M, Singhel K J, Overholtzer J F, Shurtleff S A 1989 Regulation of tumor necrosis factor expression in a macrophage-like cell line by lipopolysaccharide and cyclic AMP. Cell Immunol 120: 291–300

Takasuka N, Tokunaga T, Akagawa K S 1991 Pre-exposure of macrophages to low doses of lipopolysaccharide inhibits the expression of tumour necrosis factor-α mRNA but not of IL-1β mRNA. J Immunol 146: 3824–3830

Tautz D 1989 Hypervariability of simple sequences as a general source of polymorphic DNA markers. Nucleic Acids Res 17: 6463–6471

Tesh V L, Vukajlovich S W, Morrison D C 1987 Endotoxin interactions with serum proteins: relationship to biological activity. In: Levin J, Ten Cate JW, Büller HR, van Deventer S J H, Sturk A (eds) Bacterial endotoxins: Pathophysiological effects, clinical significance, and pharmacological control. Alan R Liss, New York, pp 47–62

Thomas G 1992 MAP kinase by any other name smells just as a sweet. Cell 68: 3–6

Tobias P S, Ulevitch R J 1983 Control of lipopolysaccharide-high density lipoprotein binding by acute phase protein(s). J Immunol 131: 1913–1916

Tobias P S, Soldau K, Ulevitch R J 1986 Isolation of a lipopolysaccharide-binding acute phase reactant from rabbit serum. J Exp Med 1989 164: 777–793

Tobias P S, Mathison J C, Ulevitch R J 1988 A family of lipopolysaccharide binding proteins involved in responses to gram-negative sepsis. J Biol Chem 263: 13479–13481

Tobias P S, Soldau K, Ulevitch R J 1989 Identification of a lipid A binding site in the acute phase reactant lipopolysaccharide binding protein. J Biol Chem 264: 10867–10871

Todd III R F, Nadler L M, Schlossman S F 1981 Antigens on human monocytes identified by monoclonal antibodies. J Immunol 126: 1435–1442

Udalova I A, Nedospasov S A, Webb G C, Chaplin D D, Turetskaya R L 1993 Highly informative typing of the human TNF locus using six adjacent polymorphic markers. Genomics 16: 180–186

Ulevitch R J, Johnston A R 1978 The modification of biophysical and endotoxic properties of bacterial lipopolysaccharides by serum. J Clin Invest 62: 1313–1324

Ulevitch R J, Johnston A R, Weinstein D B 1979 New function for high density lipoproteins: Their participation in intravascular reactions of bacterial lipopolysaccharides. J Clin Invest 64: 1516–1524

Ulevitch R J, Johnston A R, Weinstein D B 1981 New function for high density lipoproteins. Isolation and characterization of a bacterial lipopolysaccharide-high density lipoprotein complex formed in rabbit plasma. J Clin Invest 67: 827–837

van der Meer J W M, Vogels M T E 1990 Interleukin 1 as a therapeutic agent in serious infections. In: Sturk A, van Deventer S J H, Ten Cate J W, Büller H R, Thys L G, Levin J (eds) Bacterial endotoxins: Cytokine mediators and new therapies for sepsis. Wiley–Liss, New York, pp 197–206

van't Wout J, Burnette W N, Mar V L, Rozdzinski E, Wright S D, Tuomanen E I 1992 Role of carbohydrate recognition domains of pertussis toxin in adherence of *Bordetella pertussis* to human macrophages. Infect Immun 60: 3303–3308

Vogel S N, Moore R N, Sipe J D, Rosenstreich D J 1990 BCG-induced enhancement of endotoxin sensitivity in C3H/HeJ mice I. *In vivo* studies. J Immunol 124: 2004–2009

Voitenok N N, Misuno N I, Panyutich A V, Kolesnikova T S 1989 Induction of tumor necrosis factor synthesis in human monocytes treated by transcriptional inhibitors. Immunol Lett 20: 77–82

Watson J, Kelly K, Largen M, Taylor B A 1978 The genetic mapping of a defective LPS response gene in C3H/HeJ mice. J Immunol 120: 422–424

Weber J L, May P E 1989 Abundant class of human DNA polymorphisms which can be typed using the polymerase chain reaction. Am J Hum Genet 44: 388–396

Weinstein S L, Gold M R, DeFranco A L 1991 Bacterial lipopolysaccharide stimulates protein tyrosine phosphorylation in macrophages. Proc Natl Acad Sci USA 88: 4148–4152

Weinstein S L, Sanghera J S, Lemke K, DeFranco A L, Pelech S L 1992 Bacterial lipopolysaccharide induces protein tyrosine phosphorylation and activation of MAP kinases in macrophages. J Biol Chem 267: 14955–14962

Weinstein S L, June C H, DeFranco A L 1993 Lipopolysaccharide-induced protein tyrosine phosphorylation in human macrophages is mediated by CD14. J Immunol 151: 3829–3838

Weiss J, Elsbach P, Olsson I, Odeberg H 1978 Purification and characterization of a potent bactericidal and membrane active protein from the granules of human polymorphonuclear proteins. J Biol Chem 253: 2664–2672

Wilson A G, di Giovine F S, Blakemore A I, Duff G W 1992 Single base polymorphism in the human tumour necrosis factor alpha (TNF alpha) gene detectable by NcoI restriction of PCR product. Hum Mol Genet 1: 353

Wilson A G, de Vries N, Pociot F, di Giovine F S, van der Putte L B, Duff G W 1993 An allelic polymorphism within the human tumor necrosis factor alpha promoter region is strongly associated with HLA A1, B8, and DR3 alleles. J Exp Med 177: 557–560

Wilson T, Treisman R 1988 Removal of poly(A) and consequent degradation of c-fos mRNA facilitated by 3' AU-rich sequences. Nature 336: 396–399

Wright S D, Levin S M, Jong M T C, Chad Z, Kabbash L G 1989a CR3 (CD11b/CD18) expresses one binding site for Arg-Gly-Asp-containing peptides and a second site for bacterial lipopolysaccharide. J Exp Med 169: 175–183

Wright S D, Tobias P S, Ulevitch R J, Ramos R A 1989b Lipopolysaccharide (LPS) binding protein opsonizes LPS bearing particles for recognition by a novel receptor on macrophages. J Exp Med 170: 1231–1241

Wright S D, RAmos R A, Tobias P S, Ulevitch R J, Mathison J C 1990 CD14, a receptor for complexes of lipopolysaccharide (LPS) and LPS binding protein. Science 249: 1431–1433

Zabel U, Baeuerle P A 1990 Purified human IκB can rapidly dissociate the complex of NF-κB transcription factor with its cognate DNA. Cell 61: 255–265

Zuckerman S H, Evans G F, Snyder Y M, Roeder W D 1989 Endotoxin-macrophage interaction: post-translational regulation of tumor necrosis factor expression. J Immunol 143: 1223–1227

Zuckermann S H, Evans G F, Butler L D 1991a Endotoxin tolerance: Independent regulation of interleukin-1 and tumor necrosis factor expression. Infect Immun 59: 2774–2780

Zuckerman S H, Evans G F, Guthrie L 1991b Transcriptional and posttranscriptional mechanisms involved in the differential expression of LPS-induced IL-1 and TNF mRNA. Immunology 73: 460–465

7. Identification and management of life-threatening asthma

Michael J. Moan   Christopher H. Fanta

Hospital admission ⇒ potentially life-threatening illness

INTRODUCTION

*Baseline spirometry + ABG
Steroids + bronchodilators
Monitor response to Rx*

In recent years the number of hospital admissions for asthma in the United States has approached 500 000/year (Brenner 1985, Summer 1985). Although only a small percentage of these hospitalizations involve the monitoring and care provided in an intensive care unit, most patients with asthmatic exacerbations severe enough to require in-hospital treatment are at some risk of deterioration and should be considered to have potentially life-threatening disease. 25–30% of the approximately 5000 annual deaths due to asthma in the United States occur among hospitalized patients (Sly 1988). Occasional failure on the part of both patients and their physicians to recognize the severity of life-threatening asthmatic attacks has been identified as a potentially remediable cause of associated deaths (Benatar 1986). In one hospital-based study, deaths from asthma were associated with failure to obtain baseline spirometry and blood gas analysis in 50% of cases, underuse of corticosteroids in 93% of cases, underuse of nebulized bronchodilators in 100% of cases, and inadequate monitoring of response to treatment in 100% of cases (Ormerod & Stableforth 1980). Although this study is now more than 15 years old, it does indicate areas of asthma care that require continued emphasis. These include prompt recognition of the severe attack, aggressive therapy with bronchodilators and anti-inflammatory therapy, and close monitoring for critical derangements in oxygenation and ventilation.

In this review we focus on the evaluation and medical treatment of patients with severe exacerbations of asthma; in the following chapter the indications for, and the management of, mechanically-assisted ventilation of asthmatic patients are discussed.

PRECIPITATING FACTORS IN ASTHMA

Asthma can be defined as a clinical syndrome characterized by increased responsiveness of the tracheobronchial tree to a variety of stimuli (American Thoracic Society 1987). Hyperresponsive airways can be made to narrow by exposure to numerous different triggers, some of which are listed

Table 7.1 Potential triggers of asthmatic attacks

Inhaled aeroallergens
Physical factors
  Hyperventilation of cold air
  Inhaled irritants (e.g. smoke)
  Strong odours and fumes
  Direct airway stimulation (bronchoscopy or intubation)
Exercise
(Viral) respiratory infections
Drug sensitivity (aspirin, non-steroidal anti-inflammatory agents,
  non-selective β-blockers)
Undermedication or discontinuation of medication, especially steroids
Emotional stress

in Table 7.1. Some stimuli, such as exercise or hyperventilation of cold air, cause generally short-lived attacks that typically resolve spontaneously over 30-60 minutes. Other precipitants, such as inhalation of allergens in the sensitized patient, may induce both immediate and later asthmatic responses, causing airflow obstruction hours after the initial exposure. In general, the longer the duration of an attack prior to hospitalization, the slower the response to therapy.

Patients seeking emergency care for their asthma most often indicate that a preceding upper respiratory tract infection (presumably of viral origin) triggered their attack (Edelson & Rebuck 1985, Summer 1985), yet in many instances no particular inciting factor can be identified. A bacterial infection (bronchitis or sinusitis) probably precipitates only a small minority of cases.

Once the asthmatic attack has been initiated, the airways respond in a characteristic manner, the two major features being smooth muscle contraction and inflammation (Hogg 1982, American Thoracic Society 1987). The inflammatory response includes mucous gland hypersecretion, mucosal and submucosal edema, inflammatory cell infiltration (especially by eosinophils), dysfunction and desquamation of the epithelial lining cells, and plugging of small airways. The relative contributions of bronchoconstriction, airway inflammation and intraluminal obstruction cannot be determined with any certainty on clinical grounds, although the component persisting after intensive bronchodilator therapy presumably reflects predominantly airway inflammation.

DEFINITION OF LIFE-THREATENING ASTHMA

The cause of death in asthma is most often asphyxiation: extreme airflow obstruction induces severe hypoxia and hypercapnia (with acidaemia), ultimately culminating in respiratory arrest. Asthma that causes significant hypoxaemia (arterial oxygen tension less than 8.0 kPa) and hypercapnia (arterial carbon dioxide tension greater than 6.0 kPa), or that alters the

Signs of life-threatening ulcer – *hypoxaemia*
– *hypercapnia*
– *altered level of consciousness*

LIFE-THREATENING ASTHMA   139

level of consciousness (and thereby interferes with conventional modes of administration of therapy) should be considered to be life-threatening.

Traditionally, life-threatening asthma or status asthmaticus was defined as an attack lasting greater than 24 hours. Many studies, however, have demonstrated that deaths can occur within the first few hours of the onset of symptoms (MacDonald et al 1976a, Arnold et al 1982, Sears et al 1986) and it is therefore unhelpful to rely on the duration of an attack as an indication of its severity. Other criteria, based on physical findings and physiological measurements, are more reliable. Moreover, it must be remembered that airflow obstruction in asthma may be quite labile: any patient with severe asthma may deteriorate rapidly, to the point of a life-threatening attack. In part, this risk of deterioration is the justification for hospitalization of all such patients: close observation and early intervention for respiratory failure may be life-saving. Thus, identification of severe attacks constitutes a crucial first step in this management.

RECOGNITION OF THE SEVERITY OF AN ASTHMATIC ATTACK

Severity?

As asthmatic bronchoconstriction and airway inflammation worsen, the ability of the patient to exhale declines. Measures of maximal expiratory flow, such as the peak expiratory flow rate (PEFR) and one-second forced expiratory volume (FEV_1), are thus the best single determinants of severity. By making repeated measurements, changes in severity and the response to treatment can be followed.

PEFR or FEV_1

In addition, widespread airways obstruction impairs oxygenation and ventilation. Hypoxaemia results from mismatching of ventilation and perfusion. Measures of maximal expiratory flow correlate only weakly with the degree of hypoxaemia in severe asthma; other assessments of oxygenation, such as continuous transcutaneous oxygen saturation measurement by oximetry, are needed to detect and monitor significant hypoxaemia. Although hyperventilation is the rule in mild and moderate attacks, severe airways obstruction may be associated with alveolar hypoventilation and resultant hypercapnia. In one series of measurements among patients suffering respiratory arrest from asthma, the mean arterial $PaCO_2$ was 12.9 ± 4.1 kPa (Molfino et al 1991). At the present time, only arterial blood gas analysis can identify accurately the presence of hypercapnia among adults with asthma.

V/Q mismatch

$PaCO_2$ ↑↑ (prior to?) resp'l arrest

As airflow obstruction worsens, pulmonary hyperinflation and increased resistance to inspiratory airflow intensify the work of breathing. A number of important physical findings in severe asthma, such as activity of the accessory muscles and pulsus paradoxus, are a reflection of this additional workload on the respiratory muscles. It is, however, unclear whether the presence of these physical findings, taken together with the severity of airflow obstruction (as measured by the FEV_1 or the PEFR), provides an independent predictor of potentially fatal asthma.

work of breathing

Patient-reported symptoms are an imperfect guide to the severity of asthmatic attacks. Although at times patients may be better able than their physicians to estimate the degree of their airflow obstruction (Shim & Williams 1980), they frequently underestimate the severity of attacks. Studies of induced airflow obstruction following inhalation of bronchoconstrictor substances such as histamine or methacholine and studies of spontaneous asthma during the recovery phase from acute attacks indicate that patients frequently lack awareness of significant airflow obstruction (Rubinfield & Pain 1976, Burdon et al 1982, McFadden 1986). Thus, a patient's reassurance that he or she is 'OK' does not reliably exclude severe asthma.

Certain physical signs are indicative of severe asthmatic attacks. These include:

1. Tachypnoea. Rebuck et al (1982) demonstrated an association between tachypnoea (respiratory rate of >28 breaths/min) and severity of the asthmatic attack, a finding that has been confirmed by others (Edelson & Rebuck 1985). One can often recognize this finding by broken patterns of speech: some patients with severe attacks are too breathless to speak at all; others have their speech restricted to monosyllables or short groups of words.

2. Alterations in heart rate. Tachycardia is a common manifestation of severe asthma: heart rates greater than 110 beats/min are found in the majority of instances, even in the absence of beta-adrenergic stimulation (Rees et al 1968, Rebuck & Read 1971, Edelson & Rebuck 1985, Rebuck et al 1987). Tachycardia should not be considered a contraindication to therapy with sympathomimetic stimulants; as airflow obstruction improves, heart rate may slow despite intensive therapy with sympathomimetics (Rossing et al 1980).

Conversely, the absence of tachycardia does not preclude a severe asthmatic attack. In a series of asthmatic exacerbations with fatal outcomes, the mean pulse rate was 135 beats/min; however, during two of these fatal attacks the pulse rate was less than 100 beats/min (MacDonald et al 1976b). Likewise Molfino et al (1991) reported a patient with sinus bradycardia complicating hypoxaemia and respiratory acidosis during an episode of near-fatal asthma.

3. Systolic arterial paradox. A small decrease in the systolic blood pressure with inspiration is a normal physiological phenomenon. Exaggerated ('paradoxical') falls in this blood pressure are seen in any condition involving severe airflow obstruction, including severe asthma. During an asthmatic attack this physical finding is a consequence of the exaggerated swings in intrathoracic pressures that are caused by the dramatically increased work of breathing. Rebuck & Read (1971) demonstrated significant pulsus paradoxus (an inspiratory fall in systolic blood pressure of ≥10 mmHg) in nearly two-thirds of patients with an FEV_1 <40% of normal and in all patients with an FEV_1 <20%. Comparable findings have been observed by other authors (Knowles & Clark 1973, Edelson & Rebuck 1985). There are two important limitations to the usefulness of pulsus paradoxus in clini-

cal practice. First, in critically ill and tachypnoeic patients, accurate measurement becomes increasingly difficult and secondly, its absence does not exclude severe or life-threatening asthma.

4. Accessory muscle use. Use of accessory muscles of respiration, in particular the sternocleidomastoid and abdominal muscles, is a marker of severe airflow obstruction in asthma (McFadden et al 1973), although as many as half of the patients with a severe asthmatic attack ($FEV_1 < 1$ l) will not manifest this finding (Kelsen et al 1978).

(accessory muscles)

5. Diaphoresis and refusal to lie supine. The finding of diaphoresis and the inability of a patient to lie in a recumbent position during an asthmatic attack have been shown to correlate with severity of airflow obstruction. In a study of asthmatic patients in an emergency department, the average peak expiratory flow for diaphoretic patients was 73.3 ± 5 l/min, for non-diaphoretic patients unable to lie supine 134 ± 21 l/min, and for non-diaphoretic recumbent patients 225 ± 7.5 l/min. In this study no recumbent patient had a PEFR of less than 150 l/min or a $PaCO_2$ of greater than 5.9 kPa (Brenner et al 1983).

Diaphoresis
Erect posture

6. Silent chest. Diffuse wheezing is the usual finding on chest auscultation during severe asthmatic attacks. The finding of a silent chest on auscultation suggests that gas movement is severely reduced as a result of marked and diffuse airways narrowing and/or decreased ventilatory efforts due to respiratory muscle fatigue (Edelson & Rebuck 1985). It should be considered as a harbinger of impending respiratory failure.

Silent chest

7. Cyanosis. It is widely recognized that cyanosis is an imperfect marker of the presence of significant hypoxaemia: its detection is influenced by several factors unrelated to the arterial oxygen content, including lighting conditions, interobserver variability, and skin pigmentation. Although in one series cyanosis was described in as many as one-third of acutely ill asthmatic patients (Rebuck & Read 1971), for the most part cyanosis is a late and infrequent finding even in severe asthma. Severe airflow obstruction may be present in the absence of significant hypoxaemia, cyanosis may be absent despite significant hypoxaemia (arterial oxygen saturation <90%), and cyanosis may be present but overlooked by the majority of observers even in patients with marked hypoxaemia. The problem of early clinical detection of significant hypoxaemia has been circumvented by the widespread availability of transcutaneous oxygen saturation monitors. These oximeters provide reasonably accurate assessment of arterial oxygen saturation provided that there is adequate peripheral perfusion.

(cyanosis)

8. Altered mental status. In the absence of sedating drugs, a depressed mental state complicating an asthmatic attack generally indicates severe hypercapnia and hypoxaemia and heralds impending respiratory failure. In a series of 39 patients with asthmatic exacerbations and altered mental status reported by Westerman et al (1979), 28 (72%) required mechanically-assisted ventilation for respiratory failure. Asthmatic patients presenting unconscious at the time of hospital admission have a particularly poor

depressed consciousness

prognosis. In one report, 10 of 13 asthmatic patients unconscious on arrival to the hospital died (MacDonald et al 1976b).

In summary, patients with asthma attacks who present with one or more of the physical findings described above have severe disease. Others with severe airflow obstruction may, however, manifest none of these signs. The physical findings in severe asthma are neither sensitive nor specific. Other, more objective and quantifiable measures of severity are necessary; central among these are measurements of expiratory airflow limitation.

OBJECTIVE MEASURES IN ASSESSING ASTHMA SEVERITY

We have defined life-threatening asthma in terms of derangements in gas exchange (hypoxaemia and hypercapnia) caused by severe airflow obstruction. In most non-intubated asthmatic patients, however, the severity of the asthmatic episode can be monitored non-invasively utilizing peak expiratory flow measurements and transcutaneous oximetry. Repeated measurements of expiratory flow are particularly useful for identifying patients at risk for hypercapnic respiratory failure, for tracking responses to treatment, and for detecting wide diurnal swings in lung function (the latter a risk factor for a fatal outcome) (Benatar 1986).

1. Quantitative assessment of airflow obstruction. For most patients in whom the diagnosis of asthma is established, expiratory airflow can be satisfactorily monitored with peak expiratory flow measurements; the complete forced expiratory manoeuvre (spirometry) is generally unnecessary and can sometimes temporarily worsen symptoms of asthma. The Wright peak flow meter is widely regarded as the standard for accuracy. Not until the PEFR decreases to less than 30% of predicted (corresponding to an FEV_1 of approximately 25%), does hypercapnia develop in acute asthma (in the absence of sedating medications that depress the respiratory drive) (Nowak et al 1983). Thus, measurement of a PEFR >30% of predicted obviates the need for direct arterial blood sampling. Similarly, among a series of 86 patients with 102 acute asthmatic attacks studied by Nowak et al (1983), all those with a peak expiratory flow rate >200 l/min (or an FEV_1 > 1 l) had a PaO_2 > 8.0 kPa and $PaCO_2$ < 5.6 kPa.

Serial measurements of PEFR (as often as every 6 hours in critically ill patients) can be used to assess the response to therapy and to detect deterioration. In the emergency department, initial lack of improvement following frequent administration of inhaled bronchodilators is evidence that the patient has severe asthma and is likely to require a prolonged course of treatment. For instance, Fanta et al (1982) found that patients who had an initial FEV_1 of less than 30% of the predicted value and whose FEV_1 did not improve 35% or more to at least 40% of predicted after 60 minutes of intense treatment required either prolonged emergency room treatment or hospital admission.

All tests of maximal expiratory flow are dependent on patient cooperation and maximal effort during testing. Reliable results require thorough coaching of patients in the proper testing techniques; results may otherwise overestimate the severity of obstruction.

2. Blood gas analysis. Mild hypoxaemia is seen in the majority of cases of acute asthma. With increasing severity of airflow obstruction, there is a progressive decrease in the PaO_2 although the correlation between PaO_2 and FEV_1 is relatively weak (McFadden & Lyons 1973). In the absence of hypercapnia, severe hypoxaemia is infrequent unless pulmonary complications such as atelectasis, pneumothorax, or eosinophilic pneumonia supervene.

Transient falls in PaO_2 may be induced by bronchodilator therapy; inhaled as well as intravenous β-agonists cause pulmonary arteriolar dilatation and may worsen ventilation-perfusion mismatching (Popa 1986). With non-selective β-agonists such as isoprenaline, the fall in PaO_2 is on average 1.3 kPa (Knudson & Constantine 1967), but with more selective β_2 agents, such as salbutamol, this effect generally becomes insignificant; the average fall in PaO_2 in one study of acute asthma treated with this agent being only 0.3 kPa (Palmer & Diament 1969).

During mild or moderate asthmatic attacks, the $PaCO_2$ initially decreases. With increasing severity however, the $PaCO_2$ normalizes (to 5.3 kPa) and may subsequently rise further. As noted above, hypercapnia may ensue when the PEFR declines to <30% of predicted (Rebuck & Read 1971, McFadden & Lyons 1973). The utility of blood gas analysis in acute, severe asthma is in the detection of hypercapnia (and respiratory acidosis) in patients who, despite treatment, have persistent respiratory distress with a PEFR <30% of predicted. In this subgroup, the measurement of arterial (or mixed venous) $PaCO_2$ is essential; serial determinations of $PaCO_2$ may be necessary to guide decision making regarding the need for intubation and mechanically-assisted ventilation among patients who appear to worsen despite therapy. However, patients with milder disease can be monitored with continuous transcutaneous oximetry and repeated measures of PEFR.

3. Chest radiography. Chest radiographs occasionally detect unsuspected complications of acute asthmatic attacks, such as pneumonia (infectious or non-infectious), lobar or multilobar atelectasis, or pneumothorax/ pneumomediastinum. Although the frequency of these complications among critically ill asthmatic patients receiving treatment in the intensive care unit is unknown, their prevalence in such patients in the emergency department is only approximately 2%. Most often the chest film is normal or shows only hyperinflation (Findley & Sahn 1981). Therapy should not be delayed while obtaining the chest radiograph. The diagnosis should be made and treatment commenced on clinical grounds and the radiograph obtained at an opportune time (Cook et al 1979).

4. Laboratory data. A number of electrolyte abnormalities occur in acute severe asthma, the most common of which is hypokalaemia (serum potas

sium <3.5 mmol), which is found in up to 17% of patients (Cochrane & Clark 1975, Hetzel et al 1977). Rarely, however, does the serum potassium fall below 3.0 mmol or cause clinically significant sequelae. Not surprisingly, hypokalaemia is seen more commonly in patients receiving high doses of β-adrenergic agonists or systemic corticosteroids. It is logical to correct hypokalaemia with supplemental potassium because of the potential risk of cardiac arrhythmias and even sudden death when cardiac stimulants are administered to patients with hypoxia and hypokalaemia. The clinical importance of this risk remains speculative.

Hypophosphataemia has also been reported; it usually occurs in those receiving β-agonist therapy and as respiratory acidosis is resolving (Laaban et al 1990).

The blood count may be normal or show elevations in the leucocyte count or absolute eosinophil count. Leucocytosis may be caused by subcutaneous adrenaline, systemic corticosteroids, or concomitant infection. Neither the eosinophil count nor the total white blood cell count correlates with the severity of the asthmatic attack (Horn et al 1975).

Occasionally, the creatine phosphokinase (CPK) becomes elevated due to excessive use of ventilatory muscles, including the accessory muscles of respiration; the CPK elevation is predominantly due to the release of MM-isoenzyme (Burki & Diamond 1977).

5. Electrocardiography. The eletrocardiogram frequently shows abnormalities such as sinus tachycardia, P-pulmonale, right axis deviation and non-specific ST–T wave changes. These findings reverse with therapy and should not influence management (Rebuck & Read 1971). Atrial and ventricular premature beats and, occasionally, supraventricular tachycardias may complicate the treatment of asthma with sympathomimetics and methylxanthines (Josephson et al 1980).

6. Sputum analysis. In the severe asthmatic attack, expectorated sputum is frequently tenacious and discoloured and may appear infected on gross examination. Microscopically, however, rather than neutrophils and bacteria, one may find eosinophils, crystallized lysophospholipase released from degenerating eosinophils (Charcot-Leydon crystals), bronchiolar casts (Curschmann's spirals), and clusters of epithelial cells (Creola bodies). Occasionally the branching fungal hyphae of aspergillus can be identified in patients with allergic bronchopulmonary aspergillosis (Hogg 1993). A gram stain and culture of purulent sputum should be performed to exclude bacterial infection.

In conclusion, the most important objective tests in the initial evaluation of severe asthmatic attacks are repeated measurements of expiratory flow (spirometry or peak expiratory flow) and transcutaneous oximetry. These tests suffice to identify those individuals at risk for life-threatening asthma: a PEFR <30% of predicted despite initial bronchodilator therapy or an oxygen saturation <90% should dictate arterial blood gas sampling and care in a monitored unit. Other investigations such as chest radiography, electrocardiography, sputum analysis, and various laboratory tests are indicated to exclude treatable complications of asthma. Initiation of therapy must not be delayed while performing these diagnostic investigations.

DIFFERENTIAL DIAGNOSIS

A variety of cardiopulmonary diseases may present with dyspnoea and wheezing, thereby mimicking asthma (Brenner 1983, MacDonnell & Beaucamp 1993). In the differential diagnosis other diffuse obstructive lung diseases (e.g. bronchiolitis obliterans), upper airway obstruction, cardiovascular diseases such as congestive heart failure and pulmonary embolism, and certain predominantly restrictive lung diseases that may have a prominent airway component, such as sarcoidosis, should be considered (Table 7.2). In general, a detailed history and physical examination suffice to establish the diagnosis of asthma; a chest radiograph helps to exclude parenchymal lung diseases. Occasionally, additional tests such as fibreoptic bronchoscopy or computed tomography are required to make alternative diagnoses, such as tracheobronchitis due to infection (especially viral infections such as herpes simplex) or upper airway obstruction by foreign body, stricture, or tumour.

Table 7.2   Differential diagnosis of acute asthmatic attack

A. Diffuse obstructive airways diseases
Chronic bronchitis and emphysema
Bronchiolitis obliterans
Cystic fibrosis
Bronchiectasis

B. Upper airway obstruction
Tracheal or mainstem bronchial tumour
Foreign body
Laryngeal stricture
Vocal cord dysfunction syndrome

C. Cardiovascular diseases
Pulmonary embolism
Congestive heart failure ('cardiac asthma')

D. Chronic infiltrative lung diseases with airway involvement
Sarcoidosis

E. Acute airway infections
Herpetictracheobronchitis
Bronchopneumonia (especially aspiration pneumonia)

F. Miscellaneous
Protozoal infections (e.g. stongyloides, ascaris)
Carcinoid syndrome
Cocaine inhalation
Allergic angiitis and granulomatosis (Churg-Strauss syndrome)

MANAGEMENT OF ACUTE SEVERE ASTHMA

Strategies for the management of acute severe asthma can be divided into three broad categories: general measures, standard therapies, and unconventional approaches.

General measures

A number of ancillary therapies not specifically aimed at reversing airflow obstruction have been used to treat severe asthma, including the administration of supplemental oxygen, antibiotics, fluid administration ('hydration'), and chest physiotherapy.

Supplemental oxygen

Supplemental oxygen by nasal cannulae at low flow rates (1–6 l/min) is usually sufficient to correct significant hypoxaemia and maintain the transcutaneous or arterial oxygen saturation greater than 90%. If higher inspired oxygen concentrations are needed a face mask should be used, in which case bronchodilator solutions can be nebulized 'in line' with the oxygen tubing.

Antibiotics

The routine use of antibiotics in the treatment of severe asthma is not warranted (Graham et al 1982). Bacterial bronchitis or sinusitis are infrequently the triggering event of acute attacks, and when they do occur, their presence is usually suggested by fever and purulent secretions. As noted above, the gross appearance of sputum may be misleading: a yellow-green appearance may result from the inflammatory components of asthma rather than from polymorphonuclear leucocytes.

By contrast, in the severely ill patient with fever and pulmonary infiltrates, empiric antibiotics for community-acquired pneumonia are generally indicated, although with additional evaluation the pulmonary infiltrates may prove to be due to pulmonary eosinophilia rather than infection. We currently advocate the use of either erythromycin or a 3rd generation cephalosporin such as ceftriaxone or cefotaxime to treat likely pathogens in community-acquired pneumonias, pending the results of sputum cultures.

Hydration

Previous recommendations for management of asthma called for the administration of fluid well in excess of that necessary for homeostasis. The rationale was that fluid administration helped to increase the water content of airway secretions, making them less viscous. There is a dearth of scientific evidence to justify this strategy, however, and a counterargument suggests that vigorous fluid administration may have detrimental effects (Stalcup & Mellins 1977). In the presence of large negative intrathoracic pressures, excessive hydration may increase microvascular hydrostatic pressure and decrease plasma colloid osmotic pressure. These effects in theory promote pulmonary oedema formation, with consequent adverse effects on gas diffusion and lung compliance. We recommend correction of any fluid deficit and thereafter attempt to maintain patients in balance.

Chest physiotherapy

Among patients with severe mucus hypersecretion, especially if segmental or lobar atelectasis has developed, chest physiotherapy such as chest clapping and postural drainage may aid in clearing secretions from airways. In most patients, however, we do not recommend chest physiotherapy because: (1) spontaneous cough suffices to clear secretions; (2) lying horizontal is often difficult for the severely dyspneic patient; and (3) repeated treatments may prove unnecessarily fatiguing for the already compromised patient.

Standard therapies

Most cases of acute severe asthma, including life-threatening attacks managed in the intensive care unit, are successfully treated with standard bronchodilator and anti-inflammatory therapies. For the most part these consist of inhaled β-adrenergic agonists and systemic cortico-steroids. Other bronchodilator options include theophylline and anti-cholinergics. Intravenous magnesium is an experimental bronchodilator therapy that has been tried in patients refractory to standard treatment.

β-agonists

Beta-adrenergic agonists are the most potent and rapidly acting of the available bronchodilators. In vitro studies suggest additional potential benefits such as enhanced mucociliary clearance and inhibition or attenuation of the release of chemical mediators of inflammation from mast cells and eosinophils (Popa 1986). However, their primary effect in acute asthma is undoubtedly the induction of airway smooth muscle relaxation, mediated via β receptors on the surface of smooth muscle cells (Popa 1986).

The use of non-selective adrenergic agonists such as isoprenaline, orciprenaline, and adrenaline has largely been superseded by β_2 selective agonists such as salbutamol, terbutaline, isoetharine, and bitolterol (the latter two drugs are not currently available for use in acute asthma in the United Kingdom). These more specific agents retain the potency of the older agonists but have fewer sympathomimetic side effects (Popa 1986, Crane et al 1989).

Table 7.3 Onsets of action, peak effects and durations of action of various routes of β_2-agonists

Route	Onset of action	Peak effect	Duration of action
Subcut	1–3 min	15–30 min	2 h
Oral	30 min	1–2 h	3–6 h
Inhalation	1–6 min	30–60 min	4–6 h

β-agonists can be administered by a number of routes including subcutaneous, oral or intravenous, as well as by inhalation. The onset of action, time to peak effect, and duration of action of the oral, subcutaneous and inhaled routes are outlined in Table 7.3. The inhaled route of administration is preferred in almost all instances (except perhaps the apnoeic patient who cannot be adequately ventilated by manually-assisted ventilation) because greater or equivalent bronchodilation can be achieved with lower serum levels and therefore fewer adverse systemic side-effects (Lawford et al 1978, Rossing et al 1980, Becker et al 1983, Uden et al 1985, Salmeron et al 1994). Following intravenous administration of the non-selective β-agonist isoprenaline or massive doses of subcutaneous adrenaline, myocardial ischaemia and infarction may be observed even among persons without pre-existent coronary artery disease (Kurland et al 1979, Maguire et al 1986). Even with the administration of inhaled selective β-adrenergic agonists, side-effects are common and include anxiety, restlessness, tremor, headache, palpitations, tachycardia, and a mild fall in blood pressure (Popa 1986). Other side-effects of β-agonist therapy, such as hypokalaemia and transient hypoxia, have been discussed above.

Published recommendations regarding routes of administration of β-agonists, in addition to inhalation, in the setting of life-threatening asthma differ. The British Thoracic Society guidelines advocate the use of intravenous β-agonists (for example, salbutamol 200 μg or terbutaline 250 μg over ten minutes) at an earlier stage in the management of individuals with life-threatening disease (British Thoracic Society 1990). On the other hand, the American National Asthma Education Panel guidelines do not recommend administration of β-agonists other than by inhalation except in the case of the intubated apnoeic patient where effective ventilation cannot be achieved due to extremely high airway resistance (National Asthma Education Panel 1991). Our preference is not to administer intravenous or subcutaneous β-agonists in life-threatening asthma except for the rare circumstances noted above and to proceed to intubation at an earlier stage for those patients with evidence of worsening respiratory failure despite continuous inhaled β-agonists and systemic corticosteroids. This approach received support from a recent study, not yet published at the time that the British Thoracic Society guidelines were written, demonstrating that even in severe asthma associated with hypercapnia, inhaled β-agonists have superior efficacy and fewer side-effects than intravenously administered

Table 7.4 Conventional doses of β-agonists for the various routes of administration

Drug	Inhalation dose	Subcutaneous dose	Intravenous injection (slow i.v. push over) 10 min)	Intravenous infusion rate
Salbutamol	2.5 mg	0.5 mg	0.2 mg	3–20 μg/min
Terbutaline	5 mg	0.25–0.5 mg	0.25 mg	3–20 μg/min
Isoetharine (Not available in UK)	5 mg	Not available	Not available	Not available
Bitolterol (Not available in UK)	1–2 mg	Not available	Not available	Not available

β-agonists (Salmeron et al 1994). The conventional doses, by the various routes of administration, of those β-agonists drugs used in the United Kingdom and the United States, for acute asthma are outlined in Table 7.4. In the United States orciprenaline in a dose of 15 mg by inhalation is also available, however, this less β_2-specific agent is being used with ever decreasing frequency.

The optimal dose and frequency of administration of inhaled β-agonists in acute asthma remain to be fully defined. In chronic, stable asthma one can demonstrate incremental bronchodilation to increasing doses of inhaled β-agonists (Lipworth et al 1989, Barnes & Pride 1983), and at least one study in the pediatric literature has indicated that greater bronchodilation can be achieved during asthmatic exacerbations with higher than conventional doses (Schuh et al 1990). Adverse side-effects are also dose-dependent, however, and we continue to use the standard 2.5 mg dose of salbutamol per nebulizer treatment. While the half-life of inhaled β_2-agonists in stable asthma is 4–6 h, the duration of their effect in acute airflow limitation is uncertain; it may vary with the severity and acuity of the obstruction. Numerous studies have demonstrated the safety of β-agonist treatments administered by nebulizer as frequently as every 20 minutes for at least 4 consecutive treatments (e.g. total salbutamol dose of 10 mg over approximately 90 minutes) (Rossing et al 1980, Rossing et al 1981, Fanta et al 1982). Some practitioners opt for continuous nebulization of β-agonists in critically ill asthmatic patients. Although no overall advantage to continuous nebulization has been demonstrated when the total hourly dose is equivalent (Colacone et al 1990, Lin et al 1993, Rudnitsky et al 1993), two studies have suggested that greater bronchodilation is achieved with continuous nebulization among the subset of patients with severe airways obstruction (Lin et al 1993, Rudnitsky et al 1993). In one study using continuously nebulized salbutamol, the recommended dose was 15 mg/h for 2 hours (Lin et al 1993).

Except in the face of impending respiratory arrest, for the majority of severely ill patients hourly administration of nebulized β-agonists (e.g. salbutamol 2.5 mg) provides adequate bronchodilation after the initial treatment period. Hourly treatments can be maintained safely for 24 h or longer if needed without cumulative adverse side-effects or evidence of tachyphylaxis. As the severity of the airflow obstruction lessens, the frequency of administration can be decreased, guided mostly by patient need for the acute relief of dyspnoea.

Recent clinical trials have demonstrated that β-agonists delivered by metered-dose inhalers (MDI) attached to inhalational aids (spacers) achieve the same bronchodilator effect as much larger doses of the same drug administered by hand-held, continuous flow ('updraft') nebulizers (Morgan et al 1982, Cushley et al 1983, Berenberg & Baigelman 1985, Jasper et al 1987). For instance, in patients presenting to an emergency department for treatment of acute asthmatic attacks, orciprenaline 0.65 mg (one 'puff') by MDI with a reservoir bag inhalational aid (Inspir-ease[®]) given once every two minutes for a total of three inhalations (1.95 mg total dose) had the same bronchodilator effect as orciprenaline solution 15 mg given by continuous flow nebulizer (Jasper et al 1987). Optimized particle size and minimized medication loss to the surrounding atmosphere when using an MDI with a spacer (together with carefully coached inhalational technique) may account for the comparable efficacy of the smaller administered dose. As with nebulized β-agonists, the optimal dose (number of inhalations) and schedule of administration of β-agonists by MDI have not yet been clarified. In our hospitalized patients we continue to utilize continuous-flow nebulizers in critically ill asthmatic patients, reserving MDIs for the resolution phase (e.g. PEFR > 200 l/min). During the resolution phase of the asthmatic attack, a significant consideration in the choice of methods of medication delivery becomes patient education in the manual skills important in outpatient asthma care.

Many patients have already pretreated themselves with oral and/or inhaled β-agonists prior to presentation to the emergency department. Patients often report that their bronchodilator inhaler seemed no longer to be effective, and it might be assumed that they had become unresponsive to further sympathomimetic therapy. However, when Rossing et al (1983) compared two groups presenting to the emergency department with acute exacerbations, one group having taken β_2-agonists within 6 h of presentation and the other not, they discovered no difference in the response to sympathomimetic bronchodilator therapy between the two groups. β-agonist bronchodilators are the agents of first choice even among patients with severe airflow obstruction that persists following β-agonist administration outside hospital.

Anticholinergic agents

Anticholinergic agents antagonize the effect of acetylcholine at the post-synaptic muscarinic (cholinergic) receptors located on airway smooth muscle; in the United States their approved use is for treatment of chronic bronchitis and emphysema. Recognition of hyperactive cholinergic responses among persons with asthma and the potential for effecting airway smooth muscle relaxation by a mechanism distinct from β-receptor stimulation led to trials of anticholinergic agents in asthma (Ziment & Au 1986). An early trial in asthmatic exacerbations compared inhaled atropine given in large doses (3.2 mg of atropine per dose) with inhaled orciprenaline (15 mg per dose) by nebulizer in a crossover design. The bronchodilation effected by atropine was slower in onset and less in maximal effect than that achieved with the β-agonist; and no additional bronchodilation resulted from the sequential addition of atropine to orciprenaline. Atropine is well absorbed across the respiratory tract mucosa and can cause systemic side-effects such as dry mouth, dizziness, blurred vision, tachycardia, and prostatism (Karpel et al 1986).

Newer anticholinergic agents such as ipratropium bromide are quaternary derivatives of atropine with minimal systemic absorption, and unlike atropine they do not interfere with mucociliary clearance. In acute asthma, ipratropium bromide has a slower onset of action and less potent bronchodilation than inhaled β-agonists; its potential role relates to possible additive bronchodilation when used in combination with inhaled β-agonists. Published studies evaluating combined β-agonist and anticholinergic therapy in acute asthma have involved relatively small numbers of subjects and have given conflicting results (Ward et al 1985, Rebuck et al 1987, Higgins et al 1988, O'Driscoll et al 1989). Data from on-going, larger scale investigations comparing the effects of salbutamol (2.5 mg by continuous-flow nebulizer) with salbutamol plus nebulized ipratropium (0.5 mg) should be available soon. Inhaled anticholinergic agents may find a role in the management of severe asthma as an adjunctive therapy to β$_2$-agonists, particularly in a subpopulation of patients who have only limited improvement following initial β-agonist therapy.

Theophylline

Theophylline and its widely used salt, aminophylline (theophylline ethylenediamine), are methylxanthines used in the treatment and prophylaxis of both asthma and chronic obstructive pulmonary disease. Among their documented in vitro and in vivo activities are: (1) direct bronchodilation, (2) augmentation of diaphragmatic function, (3) direct central nervous system stimulation of respiratory drive and (4) diuresis (Miech & Stein 1986). The conventionally ascribed mechanism of action for theophylline, namely increasing intracellular cyclic adenosine monophosphate (cAMP) by inhibition of intracellular phosphodiesterase, has been called into question by the observations that (1) the serum levels needed to achieve this effect exceed those obtained in clinical practice, (2) other more potent phosphodiesterase inhibitors are not equally effective bronchodilators, and (3) theophylline-induced relaxation of contracted smooth muscle in isolated organ preparations does not correlate with significant changes in either cAMP or cyclic guanine monophosphate levels (Miech & Stein 1986). Other potential mechanisms of action, such as prostaglandin antagonism or adenosine receptor antagonism, have been proposed but remain to be proven (Miech & Stein 1986).

The use of intravenous aminophylline or theophylline in the treatment of acute severe asthma remains controversial. For many years intravenous methylxanthines were the mainstay of therapy for status asthmaticus. More recently, however, multiple controlled clinical trials have demonstrated that in acute airflow obstruction due to asthma, theophylline is a relatively weak bronchodilator when used alone (Rossing et al 1980) and has no additive bronchodilator activity when used in combination with inhaled β-agonists (Evans et al 1980, Fanta et al 1982, Siegel et al 1985). Studies conducted in emergency departments as well among patients hospitalized for their asthma have demonstrated that improvement in airflow obstruction is not accelerated by the addition of intravenous aminophylline to a regimen of inhaled β-agonists and systemic cortico-steroids.

Aminophylline has a narrow therapeutic-toxic ratio; therapeutic levels up to 20 μg/ml are recommended, while serious toxicities such as cardiac arrhythmias and seizures may be observed at serum levels as low as 40 μg/ml. Unpleasant side-effects such as nausea, vomiting, headaches, palpitations, and tremulousness are common even when blood levels do not exceed the therapeutic range (Miech & Stein 1986). It has been our practice to continue oral theophylline in patients admitted with this medication as part of their treatment programme, but we do not initiate intravenous aminophylline even in critically ill asthmatic patients. For those patients on chronic oral theophylline therapy, levels need to be checked regularly as metabolism of the drug is altered in disease states and by concomitant therapy. Its clearance is reduced, and hence the risk of toxicity increased, by old age, infections, congestive heart failure, liver disease, and drugs such as erythromycin, cimetidine, quinolones (such as ciprofloxacin), troleandomycin, rifampin, propranolol, carbamezepine, allopurinol and oral contraceptives. Its clearance is increased, and hence its efficacy reduced, by cigarette smoking, high protein diets, and drugs that induce hepatic enzymes such as phenytoin and barbiturates (Bukowsky et al 1984).

IV   MgSO4 1 - 2g / 20⁻

Magnesium therapy

Intravenous magnesium (magnesium sulphate at a dose of approximately 1–2 g infused over 20 min) has been shown to have bronchodilator activity when administered to asthmatic patients with severe airflow obstruction that persists following β-agonist therapy (Skobeloff et al 1989); and in case reports prevention of impending respiratory failure has been ascribed to magnesium therapy (Kuitert & Kletchko 1991). The postulated mechanism of action of magnesium relates to its activity as an inhibitor of the intracellular flux of calcium ions; decreased intracellular calcium leading to bronchial smooth muscle relaxation. The side-effects associated with intravenous magnesium therapy are relatively mild and include transient sensations of facial warmth, flushing, and malaise. Despite these encouraging preliminary reports, a double-blind, placebo-controlled trial conducted in an emergency department failed to find any benefit from the addition of intravenous magnesium to a standard regimen of inhaled bronchodilators and systemic corticosteroids (Green & Rothrock 1992). Additional studies are needed before one can justify the routine use of intravenous magnesium in acute severe asthma can be justified.

Systemic corticosteroids

In those asthmatic patients who have persistent severe airflow obstruction despite intensive bronchodilator therapy, airway narrowing is probably predominantly related to luminal plugging by secretions and thickening of the airway wall due to oedema and inflammatory cellular infiltration. Although the exact mechanism of action by which corticosteroids exert their effects in asthma remains unknown, it is widely believed that the primary target of their effect is this inflammatory component of the asthmatic response. Among their myriad effects, corticosteroids reduce airway eosinophilia, decrease microvascular leakage, and inhibit the synthesis and action of the pro-inflammatory derivatives of arachidonic acid (Spector 1985, Ziment 1986).

Several reviews have identified the underuse of systemic corticosteroids in severe asthma as a contributing factor to fatal outcomes (Speizer et al 1968, MacDonald et al 1976a, b, Roussos 1982). Some (Littenberg & Gluck 1986), but not all (Stein & Cole 1990), placebo-controlled trials have demonstrated that systemic corticosteroids reduce the frequency of hospitalizations for asthma when given to patients with acute exacerbations treated in the emergency department. Systemic corticosteroids decrease the frequency of recurrent attacks among patients discharged home from the emergency department following treatment for their asthma (Chapman

Inflammaty cpad — steroids
— eafue ÷ appnte dec .

et al 1991, Fiel et al 1983, Hoffman & Fiel 1988), and they speed the rate of improvement in lung function among patients hospitalized for asthma (Fanta et al 1983, Haskall et al 1983). Systemic corticosteroids are indicated for virtually every patient admitted to the hospital with severe asthma, although controversy exists regarding the optimal dose and route of administration of systemic corticosteroids in asthma (McFadden 1993). We have routinely used a dose of intravenous methylprednisolone equivalent to approximately 4 mg/kg/day (i.e. methylprednisolone 80 mg by intravenous bolus every 8 h). Some studies have suggested that smaller doses may be equally efficacious (Harrison et al 1986); no trials have demonstrated greater benefit from the use of higher doses. Intravenous hydrocortisone is of proven value in acute asthma (dose = approximately 14 mg/kg/day), but it induces more hypokalaemia and fluid retention than methlprednisolone without demonstrable advantages.

Oral steroids are well absorbed and reach peak serum levels within 15 minutes of administration in the absence of factors that interfere with absorption (e.g. malabsorption syndromes, vomiting, or diarrhoea) (Morrison et al 1977). Comparable benefit has been found when similar oral and intravenous doses have been compared (Ratto et al 1988). In one study that specifically excluded patients with respiratory failure, oral methylprednisolone 90 mg over 24 h proved equally effective to the same oral dose plus 1000 mg of intravenous hydrocortisone (Harrison et al 1986). In the absence of additional published experience, most clinicians have continued to rely on intravenously administered corticosteroids for the initial phase of treatment of life-threatening asthma.

It is important to remember that the onset of action of corticosteroids is delayed for a matter of hours following their administration, and severe airflow obstruction may persist for up to several days despite their use. Intensive bronchodilator therapy must be continued together with systemic corticosteroids while awaiting symptomatic and objective improvement (Ziment 1986).

Large doses of systemic corticosteroids may induce numerous adverse side-effects, including muscular weakness due to proximal myopathy and generalized catabolism. In this situation the potential for diaphragmatic weakness also exists. In asthmatic attacks that fail to resolve fully despite several days of high-dose corticosteroid therapy, dose reduction is generally indicated. After approximately 5–7 days, a reduced dose (for example, prednisone 60 mg/day) may be equally effective with fewer adverse consequences.

To summarize, in the initial management of life-threatening asthma, inhaled β-agonists are the mainstay of bronchodilator therapy. They can be administered as frequently as necessary (up to approximately 5.0–10.0 mg/h for salbutamol) in the absence of serious tachyarrhythmias. Inhaled ipratropium by nebulizer solution may provide additive bronchodilation in some patients; its precise role in combination with inhaled β-agonists continues to be investigated. Bronchodilators alone are inadequate therapy for severe asthma; systemic corticosteroids treat the inflammatory causes of airflow obstruction and significantly speed the resolution of asthmatic attacks. Sample medication orders suitable during the early phase of treatment for most patients hospitalized with severe asthma are: salbutamol 2.5 mg by continuous-flow nebulizer every 4 h and every 1 h p.r.n.; and methylprednisolone 80 mg by intravenous bolus every 8 h. For periods of severe respiratory distress, the dose of inhaled salbutamol can be increased transiently to as much as 7.5–10 mg over 1 h. As the asthmatic attack improves, the daily dose of systemic corticosteroids should be reduced rapidly to ≤60 mg of prednisone or the equivalent and the oral route of administration utilized.

Unconventional approaches

In a small minority of asthmatic patients, severe airflow obstruction will prove refractory to the conventional therapies discussed above. In this situation, a number of dramatic, potentially life-saving, and sometimes dangerous measures have been tried in an attempt to stave off intubation or to relieve severe airflow obstruction in the intubated patient. For the most part, the outcomes for these 'heroic' measures have been reported for small numbers of patients in uncontrolled clinical trials. In the absence of prospective controlled trials, their merit must be judged on their relative efficacies and toxicities. At the present time we consider these to be experimental procedures best reserved for use at centres skilled in their application or as part of a controlled clinical trial.

General anaesthesia

General anaesthetic agents have powerful smooth muscle relaxant activity. Agents such as ether, halothane, and ketamine have been tried in refractory asthma, with some reported dramatic successes (O'Rourke & Crone 1982, Schwartz 1984, Robertson et al 1985, Rosseel et al 1985, L'Hommedieu & Arens 1987). Each of these agents has significant disadvantages to their use such as myocardial depression for halothane, risk of explosion and combustion for ether, and the potential for myocardial ischaemia for ketamine; administration in this setting is best supervised by staff experienced in their use. In our experience we have found that the vast majority of patients will respond to conventional measures and in 15 years' experience at our hospital, we have not had to resort to this therapy.

Helium-oxygen mixture   60 - 80% Heliox.

Inhalation of a gas mixture of reduced density utilizing helium in place of nitrogen improves expiratory flow and reduces the work of breathing. In studies of both intubated (Martin-Barbaz et al 1987, Gluck et al 1990) and non-intubated (Shiue & Gluck 1989, Gluck et al 1990) asthmatic patients with hypercapnic respiratory failure, significant falls in $PaCO_2$ and increases in pH were observed within 20 min of breathing helium-oxygen mixtures ranging from 60 to 80% helium. The mixture can be delivered by a partial rebreathing mask with reservoir bag; a helium tank, gas mixer, and oxygen analyser are needed, along with close monitoring of the inspired oxygen concentration (Shiue & Gluck 1989). Heliox carries little or no risk in itself and is easily administered. We feel that it is reasonable to attempt a short trial of heliox but unless there is an immediate improvement, we would not persist with this type of therapy. If respiratory failure persists we would prefer to intubate on an urgent rather than an emergency basis.

Continuous Positive Airway Pressure (CPAP)

In acute asthma there is a substantial increase in the mechanical workload of the muscles of inspiration (diaphragm, intercostal, and accessory muscles) due to the following factors. Hyperinflation occurs due to gas trapping leading to ventilation at higher lung volumes. At these volumes the diaphragm and the other muscles of inspiration are significantly shorter than normal and work at a mechanical disadvantage, leading to a decrease in the efficiency of their action. As a result the inspiratory muscles are forced to maintain their contraction throughout the entire respiratory cycle. These factors are generally considered to be responsible for the respiratory muscle fatigue which can lead to respiratory failure in severe asthma. The strategy of providing positive airway pressure via either a tight-fitting facemask or a nasal mask for severely ill asthmatic patients appears counterintuitive, since impaired exhalation and pulmonary hyperinflation characterize the underlying condition. The rationale for its use, however, is that CPAP provides part of the inflating pressure required for inspiration thus unloading the inspiratory muscles and thereby reducing the possibility of fatigue.

Martin et al demonstrated that in histamine-induced acute airflow obstruction, CPAP decreases the pressure-time product for the inspiratory muscles, thereby reducing inspiratory muscle work (Martin et al 1982). Subsequent investigations by Shivaram et al (1987) found that patients with acute severe asthma described reductions in their sense of respiratory discomfort with the use of CPAP at levels of 5.3 ± 2.6 cmH_2O. There were also reductions in the ratio of the duration of inspiration to the duration of the total respiratory cycle (T_i/T_{tot}), suggesting a reduction in the workload of the inspiratory muscles. This reduction in inspiratory muscle work could potentially avert the need for mechanical ventilation. CPAP face masks are uncomfortable to wear, interfere with expectoration of airway secretions, predispose to gastric distension due to aerophagia, and pose a significant risk for aspiration in patients with emesis. Successful use of CPAP in life-threatening asthma is likely to depend on careful patient selection, with only the most co-operative subjects being suitable candidates.

Whole lung lavage

Overproduction and accumulation of thick tenacious airway secretions compromise ventilation and gas exchange in severe asthma and may contribute to micro- and macro-atelectasis. Attempts have been made to clear these tenacious secretions by whole lung lavage with some reported success. This technique involves bronchoscopy (often with the rigid bronchoscope, the procedure being performed in the operating room) and the instillation and then aspiration of one litre or more of normal saline from first one lung and then the other (Ramirez-R & Obenour 1971). In some reports the instillate has included N-acetylcysteine as a mucolytic. To maintain adequate gas exchange in patients with respiratory compromise due to asthma, intubation and mechanical ventilation are necessary prior to bronchoscopy and whole lung lavage. A potentially serious risk from this procedure is worsened obstruction due to flooding of the airways as well as from the effects of the mucolytic added to the lavage fluid.

Faced with a dying patient, physicians justifiably resort to unproven and potentially hazardous therapies when all standard measures have failed. For instance, successful use of extracorporeal membrane oxygenation (ECMO) has been described in an asthmatic patient whose oxygenation and ventilation could not be sustained with mechanical ventilation and conventional measures of life support (King et al 1986). However, in the vast majority of instances, in a hospital environment asthma improves over time when treated with bronchodilators and anti-inflammatory steroids and rarely does one have to resort to the measures outlined above. Mechanical ventilation may be necessary to support oxygenation and carbon dioxide elimination while airflow obstruction improves; in most reported series the duration of mechanical ventilation varies from 2.8 to 4.9 days (Luksza et al 1986, Zimmerman et al 1993).

OUTCOME FROM LIFE-THREATENING ASTHMA

Patients who experience a near-fatal asthmatic attack need close medical observation over the ensuing months and years. This point is underlined by a 6-year follow-up study of 145 patients who were mechanically ventilated for near-fatal asthma: the in-hospital mortality in this study was 16.5%, and following hospitalization the mortality rates at 1, 3, and 6 years were 10.1%, 14.4% and 22.6% respectively (Marquette et al 1992).

KEY POINTS FOR CLINICAL PRACTICE

- Most asthmatic deaths result from asphyxiation due to severe diffuse airways obstruction. We define life-threatening asthma as asthmatic exacerbations with airflow obstruction of such severity as to cause serious hypoxaemia (arterial PaO_2 < 8.0 kPa) or hypercapnia (arterial $PaCO_2$ > 6.0 kPa).
- The presence of certain physical findings, such as pulsus paradoxus, use of accessory muscles of respiration, diaphoresis and the refusal to lie supine, indicate the presence of severe airways obstruction. However, these clinical clues lack sensitivity and their absence does not exclude severe asthma.
- Identification of patients at risk for life-threatening asthmatic attacks can be achieved non-invasively with objective measurements of airflow obstruction (spirometry or peak expiratory flow) together with transcutaneous oxygen monitoring (oximetry). Arterial blood gas analysis is needed for patients with persistent severe airflow obstruction (PEFR <30% of predicted) and/or hypoxaemia (oxygen saturation <90%).
- The cornerstones to successful treatment of severe asthmatic attacks are intensive bronchodilator therapy and early administration of systemic anti-inflammatory therapy.
- Inhaled β_2-selective adrenergic agonists are the bronchodilators of choice for severe asthma because of their rapid onset of action, potent broncho-dilation, and few serious adverse side-effects.
- Intravenous administration of β-agonists is no more efficacious than, and is associated with significantly more systemic side-effects than, the inhaled route.
- Inhaled anticholinergic agents such as ipratropium bromide are less potent bronchodilators than inhaled β-agonists for asthmatic airflow obstruction.
- Most trials evaluating intravenous theophylline or aminophylline in combination with inhaled β-agonists have found no additive broncho-dilation compared to inhaled β-agonists alone. Medication side-effects tend to be additive with combination therapy. For these reasons we do not recommend routine use of methylxanthines in the treatment of severe asthmatic attacks.
- Airway inflammation in severe asthma is treated with systemic corticosteroids. The optimal dose and route of administration are controversial. We routinely administer intravenous methylprednisolone 80 mg by bolus infusion every 8 hours during the initial phase of treatment of severe asthma, although it is likely that the oral route of administration is equally effective and lower doses may achieve the same outcome.

Strategy f medical ventilation?
Pressure - controlled; long E- time; permise hypercapnia;
CPAP?
Luskae etal Thorax 1986

- Experimental and somewhat unconventional measures, such as lung lavage, administration of general anaesthetic agents, use of continuous positive airway pressure, and inhalation of a helium–oxygen gas mixture, have been utilized for refractory asthmatic attacks when respiratory failure or death seem imminent. We find that conventional therapies plus intubation and mechanical ventilation for respiratory failure are preferable outside of clinical trials or treatment centres skilled in these techniques.
- Patients who have had a life-threatening asthmatic attack need close medical follow-up because of their high risk for a fatal recurrence.

REFERENCES

American Thoracic Society 1987 Chronic bronchitis, asthma and pulmonary emphysema. Am Rev Respir Dis 136: 224–225

Arnold A G, Lane D J, Zapata E 1982 The speed of onset and the severity of acute asthma. Br J Dis Chest 76: 157–163

Barnes P J, Pride N B 1983 Dose-response curves to inhaled beta-adrenoceptor agonists in normal and asthmatic subjects. Br J Clin Pharmacol 15: 677–682

Becker A B, Nelson N A, Simons F E R 1983 Inhaled salbutamol (albuterol) vs injected epinephrine in the treatment of acute asthma in children. J Pediatr 102: 465–469

Benatar S R 1986 Fatal asthma. N Engl J Med 314: 423–429

Berenberg M, Baigelman W 1985 Comparison of metered dose inhaler attached to an aerochamber with an updraft nebulizer for the administration of metaproterenol in hospitalized patients. J Asthma 22: 87–92

Brenner B E 1983 Bronchial asthma in adults: Presentation to the emergency department. Am J Emerg Med 1: 50–70

Brenner B E 1985 The acute asthmatic in the emergency room: The decision to admit or discharge. Am J Emerg Med 3: 74–77

Brenner B E, Abraham E, Simon R R 1983 Position and diaphoresis in acute asthma. Am J Med 74: 1005–1009

British Thoracic Society 1990 Guidelines for management of asthma in adults: II — Acute severe asthma. Br Med J 301: 797–800

Bukowsky M, Nakatsu K, Munt P W 1984 Theophylline reassessed. Ann Intern Med 101: 63–73

Burdon J G W, Juniper E F, Kilian K J et al 1982 The perception of breathlessness in asthma. Am Rev Respir Dis 126: 825–828

Burki N K, Diamond L 1977 Serum creatine phosphokinase activity in asthma. Am Rev Respir Dis 116: 327–331

Chapman K R, Verbeek P R, White J G et al 1991 Effect of a short course of prednisone in the prevention of early relapse after the emergency room treatment of acute asthma. N Engl J Med 324: 788–794

Cochrane G M, Clark T J H 1975 A survey of asthma mortality in patients between ages 35 and 64 in Greater London Hospitals in 1971. Thorax 30: 300–305

Colacone A, Wolkove N, Stern E et al 1990 Continuous nebulization of albuterol (salbutamol) in acute asthma. Chest 97: 693–697

Cook N J, Crompton G K, Grant I W B 1979 Observations on the management of acute bronchial asthma. Br J Dis Chest 73: 157–163

Crane J, Burgess C, Beasley R 1989 Cardiovascular and hypokalemic effects of inhaled salbutamol, fenoterol and isoprenaline. Thorax 44: 136–140

→ See Ch 8.

Zimmerman et al   Crit. Care Med. 1993

Cushley M J, Lewis R A, Tattersfield A E 1983 Comparison of three techniques of inhalation on the airway response to terbutaline. Thorax 38: 908–913

Edelson J D, Rebuck A S 1985 The clinical assessment of severe asthma. Arch Intern Med 145: 321–323

Evans W V, Monie R D H, Crimmins J et al 1980 Aminophylline, salbutamol and combined intravenous infusions in acute severe asthma. Br J Dis Chest 74: 385–389

Fanta C H, Rossing T H, McFadden E R 1982 Emergency room treatment of asthma: relationships among therapeutic options, severity of obstruction and time course of response. Am J Med 72: 416–422

Fanta C H, Rossing T H, McFadden E R 1983 Glucocorticoids in acute asthma: A critical controlled trial. Am J Med 74: 845–851

Fiel S B, Swartz M A, Glanz K et al 1983 Efficacy of short term corticosteroid therapy in outpatient treatment of acute bronchial asthma. Am J Med 75: 259–262

Findley L J, Sahn S A 1981 The value of the chest roentgenograms in acute asthma in adults. Chest 80: 535–536

Gluck E H, Onorato D J, Castriotta R 1990 Helium-oxygen mixtures in intubated patients with status asthmaticus and respiratory acidosis. Chest 98: 693–698

Graham V A L, Milton A F, Knowles G K et al 1982 Routine antibiotics in hospital management of acute asthma. Lancet 1: 418–420

Green S M, Rothrock S G 1992 Intravenous magnesium for acute asthma: Failure to decrease emergency treatment duration or need for hospitalization. Ann Emerg Med 21: 260–265

Harrison B D, Stokes T C, Hart G J et al 1986 Need for intravenous hydrocortisone in addition to oral prednisone in patients admitted to hospital with severe asthma without ventilatory failure. Lancet 1: 181–184

Haskall R J, Wong B M, Hansen J E 1983 A double-blind, randomized clinical trial of methylprednisolone in status asthmaticus. Arch Intern Med 143: 1324–1327

Hetzel M R, Clark T J H Branthwaite M A 1977 Asthma: analysis of sudden deaths and ventilatory arrests in hospital. Br Med J 1: 808–811

Higgins R M, Stradling J R, Lane D J 1988 Should ipratropium bromide be added to beta-agonists in the treatment of acute severe asthma? Chest 94: 718–722

Hoffman I B, Fiel S B 1988 Oral vs repository corticosteroid therapy in acute asthma. Chest 93: 11–13

Hogg J C 1982 The pathophysiology of asthma. Chest 82 (Suppl): 8S–12S

Hogg J C 1993 The pathology of asthma. J Allergy Clin Immunol 92: 1–5

Horn B R, Robin E D, Theodore J et al 1975 Total eosinophil counts in the management of bronchial asthma. N Engl J Med 292: 1152–1155

Jasper A C, Mohsenifar Z, Kahan S et al 1987 Cost-benefit comparison of aerosol bronchodilator delivery methods in hospitalized patients. Chest 91: 614–618

Josephson G W, Kennedy H L, MacKenzie E J et al 1980 Cardiac dysrhythmias during the treatment of acute asthma: a comparison of two treatment regimens by a double blind protocol. Chest 78: 429–435

Karpel J P, Appel D, Briedbart D et al 1986 A comparison of atropine sulfate and metaproterenol sulfate in the emergency treatment of asthma. Am Rev Respir Dis 133: 727–729

Kelsen S G, Kelsen D P, Fleeger B F et al 1978 Emergency room assessment and treatment of patients with acute asthma. Am J Med 64: 622–628

King D, Smales C, Arnold A G et al 1986 Extracorporeal membrane oxygenation as emergency treatment for life-threatening acute severe asthma. Postgrad Med J 62: 855–857

Knowles G K, Clark T J H 1973 Pulsus paradoxus as a valuable sign indicating severity of asthma. Lancet 2: 1356–1359

Knudson R J, Constantine H P 1967 An effect of isoproterenol on ventilation-perfusion in asthmatic versus normal subjects. J Appl Physiol 22: 402–406

Kuitert L M, Kletchko S L 1991 Intravenous magnesium sulfate in acute, life-threatening asthma. Ann Emerg Med 20: 1243–1245

Kurland G, Williams J, Lewiston N J 1979 Fatal myocardial toxicity during continuous infusion intravenous isoproterenol therapy of asthma. J Allergy Clin Immunol 63: 407–411

L'Hommedieu C S, Arens J J 1987 The use of ketamine for the emergency intubation of patients with status asthmaticus. Ann Emerg Med 16: 568–571

Laaban J P, Waked M, Laromiguiere M et al 1990 Hypophosphatemia complicating management of acute severe asthma. Ann Intern Med 112: 68–69

Lawford P, Jones B J M, Milledge J S 1978 Comparison of intravenous and nebulized salbutamol in initial treatment of severe asthma. Br Med J 1: 84

Lin R Y, Sauter D, Newman T et al 1993 Continuous versus intermittent albuterol nebulization in the treatment of acute asthma. Ann Emerg Med 22: 1847–1853

Lipworth B J, Struthers A D, McDevitt D G 1989 Tachyphylaxis to systemic but not to airway responses during prolonged therapy with high dose inhaled salbutamol in asthmatics. Am Rev Respir Dis 140: 586–592

Littenberg B, Gluck E H 1986 A controlled trial of methylprednisolone in the emergency treatment of acute asthma. N Engl J Med 314: 150–152

Luksza A R, Smith P, Coakley J et al 1986 Acute severe asthma treated by mechanical ventilation: 10 years' experience from a district general hospital. Thorax 41: 459–463

MacDonald J B, Seaton A, Williams D A 1976a Asthma deaths in Cardiff 1963–1974: 90 deaths outside hospital. Br Med J 1: 1493–1495

MacDonald J B, MacDonald E T, Seaton A et al 1976b Asthma deaths in Cardiff 1963–1974: 53 deaths in hospital. Br Med J 2: 721–723

MacDonnell K F, Beaucamp H D 1993 Differential diagnosis. In: Weiss E B, Stein M (eds) Bronchial asthma: mechanisms and therapeutics. Little, Brown, Boston, pp. 459–484

Maguire J, Geha R S, Umetsu D T 1986 Myocardial specific creatine phosphokinase isoenzyme elevation in children with asthma treated with intravenous isoproterenol. J Allergy Clin Immunol 78: 631–636

Marquette C H, Saulnier F, Leroy O et al 1992 Long-term prognosis of near-fatal asthma. Am Rev Respir Dis 146: 76–81

Martin J G, Shore S, Engel L A 1982 Effect of continuous positive airway pressure on the respiratory mechanics and pattern of breathing in induced asthma. Am Rev Respir Dis 126: 812–817

Martin-Barbaz F, Barnoud D, Carpentier F et al 1987 Utilisation de mélanges hélium-oxygène au cours de l'état de mal asthmatique. Rev Pneumol Clin 43: 186–189

McFadden E R, Lyons H A 1973 Arterial blood gas tensions in asthma. N Engl J Med 278: 1027–1032

McFadden E R, Kiser R, De Groot W J 1973 Acute bronchial asthma: Relations between clinical and physiologic manifestations. N Engl J Med 1973: 221–225

McFadden E R 1986 Clinical physiologic correlates in asthma. J Allergy Clin Immunol 77: 1–5

Mcfadden E R 1993 Dosages of corticosteroids in asthma. Am Rev Respir Dis 147: 1306–1310

Miech R P, Stein M 1986 Methylxanthines. Clin Chest Med 7: 331–340

Molfino N A, Nannini L J, Martelli A N et al 1991 Respiratory arrest in near-fatal asthma. N Engl J Med 324: 285–288

Morgan M D L, Singh B V, Frame M H et al 1982 Terbutaline aerosol given through pear spacer in acute severe asthma. Br Med J 285: 849–850

Morrison P J, Bradbrook I D, Rogers H J 1977 Plasma prednisolone levels from enteric and non-enteric coated tablets estimated by an original technique. Br J Clin Pharmacol 4: 597–603

National Asthma Education Panel 1991 Guidelines for the diagnosis and management of asthma. J Allergy Clin Immunol 88 (suppl): 425–534

Nowak R M, Tomlanovich M C, Sarkar D D et al 1983 Arterial blood gas and pulmonary function testing in acute bronchial asthma. JAMA 249: 2043–2046

O'Driscoll B R, Taylor R J, Horsley M G et al 1989 Nebulized salbutamol with and without ipratropium bromide in acute airflow obstruction. Lancet 1: 1418–1420

O'Rourke P P, Crone R K 1982 Halothane in status asthmaticus. Crit Care Med 10: 341–343

Ormerod L P, Stableforth D E 1980 Asthma mortality in Birmingham 1975–1977: 53 deaths. Br Med J 1: 687–690

Palmer K N V, Diament M L 1969 Effects of salbutamol on spirometry and blood gas tensions in bronchial asthma. Br Med J 1: 31–32

Popa V 1986 Beta-adrenergic drugs. Clin Chest Med 7: 313–329

Ramirez-R J, Obenour W H Jr 1971 Bronchopulmonary lavage in asthma and chronic bronchitis: Clinical and physiologic observations. Chest 59: 146–152

Ratto D, Alfaro C, Sipsey J et al 1988 Are intravenous corticosteroids required in status asthmaticus? JAMA 260: 527–529

Rebuck A S, Braude A C, Chapman K R 1982 Evaluation of the severity of the acute asthmatic attack. Chest 82 (Suppl): 28S–29S

Rebuck A S, Chapman K R, Abboud R et al 1987 Nebulized anticholinergic and sympathomimetic treatment of asthma and chronic airways disease in the emergency room. Am J Med 82: 59–64

Rebuck A S, Read J 1971 Assessment and management of severe asthma. Am J Med 51: 788–798

Rees H A, Millar J S, Donald K W 1968 A study of the clinical course and blood gas tensions in patients with status asthmaticus. Q J Med 37: 541–561

Robertson C E, Steedman D, Sinclair C J et al 1985 Use of ether for life-threatening acute severe asthma. Lancet 1: 187–188

Rosseel P, Lauwers L F, Baule L 1985 Halothane treatment in life-threatening asthma. Intensive Care Med 11: 241–246

Rossing T H, Fanta C H, Goldstein D H et al 1980 Emergency therapy of asthma: Comparison of the acute effects of parenteral and inhaled sympathomimetics and infused aminophylline. Am Rev Respir Dis 122: 365–371

Rossing T H, Fanta C H, McFadden E R 1981 A controlled trial of the use of single versus combined drug therapy in the treatment of acute episodes of asthma. Am Rev Respir Dis 123: 190–194

Rossing T H, Fanta C H, McFadden E R 1983 Effect of outpatient treatment of asthma with beta agonists on the response to sympathomimetics in the emergency room. Am J Med 75: 781–784

Roussos C 1982 The failing ventilatory pump. Lung 160: 159–184

Rubinfield A R, Pain M C F 1976 Perception of asthma. Lancet 1: 882–888

Rudnitsky G S, Eberlein R S, Schoffstall J M et al 1993 Comparison of intermittent and continuously nebulized salbutamol for treatment of asthma in an urban emergency department. Ann Emerg Med 22: 1842–1846

Salmeron S, Brochard L, Mal H et al 1994 Nebulized versus intravenous salbutamol in hypercapnic acute asthma. Am J Respir Crit Care Med 149: 1466–1470

Schuh S, Reider M J, Canny G 1990 Nebulized salbutamol in acute childhood asthma: comparison of two doses. Pediatrics 86: 509–513

Schwartz S H 1984 Treatment of status asthmaticus with halothane. JAMA 251: 2688–2689

Sears M R, Rea H H, Rothwell R P G 1986 Asthma mortality: comparison between New Zealand and England. Br Med J 293: 1342–1345

Shim C S, Williams M H 1980 Evaluation of the severity of asthma: patients versus physicians. Am J Med 68: 11–13

Shiue S-T, Gluck E H 1989 The use of helium-oxygen mixtures in support of patients with status asthmaticus and respiratory acidosis. J Asthma 26: 177–180

Shivaram U, Donath J, Khan F A et al 1987 Effects of continuous positive airway pressure in acute asthma. Respiration 52: 157–162

Siegel D, Sheppard D, Gelb A et al 1985 Aminophylline increases the toxicity but not the efficacy of an inhaled beta-adrenergic agonist in the treatment of acute exacerbations of asthma. Am Rev Respir Dis 132: 283–286

Skobeloff E M, Spivey W H, McNamara R M et al 1989 Intravenous magnesium sulfate for the treatment of acute asthma in the emergency department. JAMA 262: 1210–1213

Sly R M 1988 Mortality from asthma, 1979–1984. J Allergy Clin Immunol 82: 705–717

Spector S L 1985 The use of corticosteroids in the treatment of asthma. Chest 87 (suppl): 73S–79S

Speizer F E, Doll R, Heaf P et al 1968 Investigation into use of drugs preceding death from asthma. Br Med J 1: 339–343

Stalcup S A, Mellins R B 1977 Mechanical forces producing pulmonary edema in acute asthma. N Engl J Med 297: 592–596

Stein L M, Cole R P 1990 Early administration of corticosteroids in acute asthma in the emergency department. Ann Intern Med 112: 822–627

Summer W R 1985 Status asthmaticus. Chest 87 (suppl): 87S–94S

Uden D L, Goetz D R, Kohen D P et al 1985 Comparison of nebulized terbutaline and subcutaneous epinephrine in the treatment of acute asthma. Ann Emerg Med 14: 229–232

Ward M J, Macfarlane J T, Davies D 1985 A place for ipratropium bromide in the treatment of severe acute asthma. Br J Dis Chest 79: 374–378

Westerman D E, Benatar S R, Potgieter P D 1979 Identification of the high risk asthmatic patient. Am J Med 66: 565–572

Ziment I 1986 Steroids. Clin Chest Med 7: 341–354

Ziment I, Au J P 1986 Anticholinergic agents. Clin Chest Med 7: 355–366

Zimmerman J L, Dellinger R P, Shah A N et al 1993 Endotracheal intubation and mechanical ventilation in severe asthma. Crit Care Med 21: 1727–1730

Ventilated asthan : mortality > 10%   — cardiography out
                                              prior to intubation

                                        → hyperam (dynamic
High Paw peak   hyperinflation)

Dynamic hyperinflation — iatrogenic morbidity + mortality in ventilated asthmatics?

Prefukls —   70%   Acute severe asthma — ass. c̄ Hx of poor control
                      — patent airway oedema
                      — slow response to Rx
                      — Q

          30%   Hyperacute fulminant asthma
                 — rapid deterioration — rapid response to Rx
                 — paucity well-controlled
                 — highly reactive airways (allergen exposure,
                                                  stress)
                 — Q

8. Mechanical ventilation in asthma

David V. Tuxen

Mechanical ventilation for life-threatening asthma was first described by Leonhardt (1961) in five patients, all of whom survived without reported complications. Leonhardt noted that high inspiratory pressures were not only tolerated but also required for good results. Since that time, mortality has not always been as low and numerous strategies and controversies relating to mechanical ventilation have arisen. There are currently over 35 reported series of patients requiring mechanical ventilation for asthma, from which the overall mortality is 12.4% (Table 8.1). Modest reductions in mortality have been achieved over the last three decades (Table 8.1), but rates exceeding 25% have continued to be reported in every decade.

Table 8.1 Summary of mortality from reported series of patients mechanically ventilated for asthma. Mortality shown per episode of mechanical ventilation

Decade	No. papers	No. episodes	No. dead	Mortality		
				Mean	Minimum	Maximum
1960s	8	125	18	14.4%	0%	27%
1970s	7	183	31	16.9%	6%	38%
1980s	10	382	46	12.0%	0%	36%
1990s	12	571	61	10.7%	0%	26%
TOTAL	37	1261	156	12.4%	0%	38%

References
1960s: (Leonhardt 1961, Bates et al 1965, Ambiavagar & Riding 1966, Marchand & Van Hesselt 1966, Misuraca 1966, Riding & Ambiavagar 1967, Williams & Crook 1968, Iisalo et al 1969)
1970s: (Sheehy et al 1972, Karetzky 1975, Cornil et al 1977, Scoggin et al 1977, Crompton et al 1979, Webb et al 1979, Westerman et al 1979)
1980s: (Halttunen et al 1980, Petheram & Branthwaite 1980, Santiago & Klaustermeyer 1980, Chopin et al 1982, De Coster et al 1983, Picado et al 1983, Darioli & Perret 1984, Higgins et al 1986, Lissac et al 1986, Lukska et al 1986)
1990s: (Braman & Kaemmerlen 1990, Ferrer et al 1990, Limthongkul et al 1990, Mansel et al 1990, Moss et al 1990, Pouw et al 1990, Grunberg et al 1991, Lam et al 1992, Marquette et al 1992, Tokioka et al 1992, Kallenbach et al 1993, Tuxen et al 1993)

The most common cause of death (Table 8.2) was hypoxic cerebral injury, usually sustained as a result of cardio-respiratory arrest prior to mechanical ventilation; followed by hypotension or circulatory failure, pneumonia and/or septicaemia (Table 8.2). Approximately one-third of deaths were associated with hypotension. Morbidity was reported less commonly, especially the presence or absence of hypotension, but when reported it occurred in 23% of patients. Pulmonary barotrauma of any type was reported in 12% of episodes of mechanical ventilation and pneumothorax in 10% of episodes where it was responsible for 6% of deaths. Gas trapping or dynamic hyperinflation is now recognized as a significant cause of hypotension and pulmonary barotrauma in mechanically ventilated asthmatics (Darioli & Perret 1984, Tuxen & Lane 1987, Bone & Burch 1991, Williams et al 1992) and is a risk factor for mortality (Rosengarten et al 1990, Kollef 1992). In this context, it is interesting that almost none of the reported morbidity and mortality (Table 8.2) was attributed to dynamic hyperinflation. However, papers using ventilatory strategies to reduce dynamic hyperinflation had a lower mortality and rarely reported complications that caused hypotension. It appears likely that mechanical ventilation itself contributes to the morbidity and mortality of ventilated asthmatics.

Table 8.2 Reported cause of death and morbidity in patients undergoing mechanical ventilation for asthma

MORTALITY	Papers (No.)	Patients (Total No.)	Admissions (Total No.)	Mortality (No. % of Admiss.)
Papers reporting cause	22	672	755	93 (12.3%)
Cerebral hypoxic injury or vascular accident				36 (39%)
Hypotension/circulatory failure				15 (16%)
Pneumonia and/or septicaemia				10 (11%)
Ventilator malfunction or technical complications				6 (6%)
Pneumothorax				6 (6%)
Cardiac arrhythmia				4 (4%)
Premature extubation				3 (3%)
Suspected pulmonary embolus				3 (3%)
Gastrointestinal complication (perforated DU, peritonitis, haemorrhage)				3 (3%)
Miscellaneous (aspiration, tracheostomy insertion, sputum plug, unspecified)				4 (4%)
All illness potentially associated with hypotension				26 (28%)

MORBIDITY
Hypotension and barotrauma reported in all mechanically ventilated patients

	Admissions (Total No.)	Complication (No. % of Admiss.)
Papers reporting morbidity		
Hypotension	404	94 (23%)
Pneumothorax	508	51 (10%)
Pulmonary barotrauma	508	63 (12%)
Cardiac arrhythmia	220	21 (9.6%)

ASTHMA PRODROMES TO MECHANICAL VENTILATION

The apparent severity of the asthma attack and the duration of deterioration prior to the instigation of mechanical ventilation varies considerably between patients. Two patterns have emerged.

1. Acute severe asthma

This group is the most common (70% of patients) (Tuxen & Oh 1990, Wasserfallen et al 1990), is predominantly female (Wasserfallen et al 1990) and usually has a history of poorly controlled asthma — either prolonged and refractory to standard therapy or with recurrent episodes of poor control (Wasserfallen et al 1990). Such patients commonly have a background of persisting moderate to severe airflow obstruction but may have minimal symptoms because of underperception, denial and behaviour modification. This can lead to an underestimation of severity by both patient and doctor and, as a result, undertreatment. The airflow obstruction has a large chronic component including airway wall oedema, hypertrophy and inspissated mucus. The component of bronchospasm may not be large because of the generous use of inhaled beta-agonist prior to presentation.

Such patients usually have a limited response to beta-agonists on presentation, and require high-dose intravenous steroid therapy. The response to treatment is usually slow and several days or more of mechanical ventilation may be required (Wasserfallen et al 1990, Tuxen et al 1992, Kallenbach et al 1993). Improvement in asthma may be heralded by increased production of secretions (Tuxen et al 1992).

This group of patients may have normal, low or only modestly elevated arterial CO_2 tensions ($PaCO_2$) at presentation (Rees et al 1968). Their requirement for mechanical ventilation may arise after presentation as a result of deterioration due to fatigue and failure to respond to treatment (Wasserfallen et al 1990), which may be accompanied by an increasing $PaCO_2$. Although the resultant level may not be excessive ($PaCO_2$ 50–60 mmHg), the trend is an important warning of the need for ventilatory assistance.

Severity ass. c↑ing $PaCO_2$

2. Hyperacute fulminating asthma

This less common group of patients is younger, predominantly male and progresses rapidly to respiratory arrest or near arrest within 3 hours of symptom onset and occasionally within minutes (McDonald et al 1976, Johnson et al 1984, Ferrer et al 1990, Wasserfallen et al 1990, Kallenbach et al 1993). This entity has also been called acute asphyxic asthma (Wasserfallen et al 1990).

Symptoms may appear mild and asthma control can be relatively good prior to the attack but bronchial reactivity is usually heightened (Pouw et al 1990). The stimulus for the attack may appear innocuous or not be identified, although major antigen exposure (Ferrer et al 1990, Wasserfallen et al 1990) and stress (Wasserfallen et al 1990) have also been identified as precipitants.

Because of the rapid onset of the attack, these patients commonly have mechanical ventilation initiated urgently following a respiratory arrest or rapid deterioration. This may occur in the community, in transit to or shortly after arrival at hospital (Rosengarten et al 1990, Wasserfallen et al 1990, Kollef 1992, Williams et al 1992, Kallenbach et al 1993). Respiratory arrest prior to intubation and complications of artificial ventilation place this group at risk of ischaemic and/or hypoxic cerebral injury (Rosengarten et al 1990, Kollef 1992) with its associated morbidity and mortality (Table 8.2).

These attacks are believed to be dominated by acute bronchospasm, with little chronic inflammatory change present in the airways (Wasserfallen et al 1990, Kallenbach et al 1993) and patients may have had little or inadequate beta-agonist therapy prior to presentation. Mechanical ventilation may be averted in quite severe attacks by rapid, aggressive treatment with bronchodilators. Because the response to such therapy is usually prompt, when mechanical ventilation is required, its duration is significantly shorter than that of the severe asthma group and prompt resolution with little sputum production is common (Ferrer et al 1990, Wasserfallen et al 1990, Kallenbach et al 1993). Patients in this group with asthma that requires mechanical ventilation, may be moribund at presentation, yet be extubated and appear normal within 12 hours.

During severe attacks, the minute ventilation (V_E) required to maintain normocapnia is usually high (16 ± 2 l/min) (Tuxen & Lane 1987) and may be very high (up to 22 l/min) because of high CO_2 production and ventilation-perfusion mismatching. However, the dynamic hyperinflation that results from quite a modest V_E (e.g. 10–12 l/min) can result in an end-inspiratory total lung volume (TLV_{EI}) at or slightly above total lung capacity (TLC) (Tuxen & Lane 1987, Tuxen et al 1992). Higher levels of V_E dictate a higher lung volume, which the patient is incapable of achieving. Thus, dynamic hyperinflation from severe airflow obstruction places a physical limitation on the maximum V_E a patient can achieve (e.g. 12 l/min) irrespective of respiratory muscle strength and if the V_E required for normocapnia is higher (e.g. 20 l/min) then hypercapnia must ensue, even if muscle fatigue is not present.

Thus, the decision to intubate cannot be made on $PaCO_2$ alone, because such patients with asthma may be capable of sustaining a low level of V_E (at least for a short time) despite quite high levels of $PaCO_2$ (e.g. >80 mmHg) without immediate risk of respiratory arrest, provided hypoxaemia is not present and airflow obstruction does not increase further. As this patient group may respond rapidly to aggressive bronchodilator therapy, preparation for intubation should be made, but not necessarily undertaken immediately.

Severity n not correlate c̄ $PaCO_2$

Table 8.3 List of respiratory abbreviations

Abbreviation	Scientific Term
$PaCO_2$	arterial CO_2 tension
SaO_2	arterial O_2 saturation
FRC	functional residual capacity
TLC	total lung capacity
V_T	tidal volume (inspired)
V_{EI}	volume of the lung at the end of inspiration (above FRC) = V_T + trapped gas
TLV_{EI}	total lung volume at the end of inspiration = V_{EI} + FRC
V_E	minute ventilation
V_I	inspiratory flow during mechanical ventilation
R	respiratory rate
F_IO_2	fractional inspired O_2 concentration
PIP	peak inspiratory pressure
P_{plat}	plateau airway pressure - measured during transient end-inspiratory airway occlusion
PEEP	positive end-expiratory pressure during mechanical ventilation
PEEPi	intrinsic or auto-PEEP – the end-expiratory alveolar pressure due to gas trapping
CPAP	continuous positive airway pressure
BiPAP	biphasic positive airway pressure
"apnoea test"	a period of apnoea (usually 30–60 sec) during assisted ventilation in which the blood pressure response is assessed
FEV_1	volume expired in 1 second during voluntary forced expiration
PEF	peak expiratory flow — maximum flow during voluntary forced expiration

THE DECISION TO INTUBATE — resp/arrest. GCS ↓

Patients who have suffered a respiratory arrest, who are comatose or drowsy (not due to sedation) or who are undergoing rapid respiratory deterioration require urgent intubation. The decision to perform less urgent intubation must be undertaken carefully. The desire to avoid mechanical ventilation with its difficulties and dangers (Rosengarten et al 1990, Kollef 1992) should be balanced against the need to avoid further deterioration requiring emergency intubation.

Decisions to intubate based on threshold criteria for measurements such as FEV_1, peak expiratory flow (PEF), $PaCO_2$ or respiratory rate are not useful in isolation and have never gained credibility in clinical practice because of individual variability and the different asthma prodromes. The decision to undertake non-urgent intubation is based largely on two criteria.

1. Assessment of the degree of respiratory distress by an experienced clinician. This is an 'end of the bed' assessment, requires no quantitative measurement and is the single most important factor in the decision to intubate. With a little experience, patients can be graded into severity categories such as 'increased respiratory effort without distress' (requiring close observation), 'respiratory distress

but patient coping' (not requiring immediate intubation), 'severe distress and fatigue' (requiring prompt but elective intubation) and finally 'severe respiratory decompensation with slowed gasping respiration' (requiring urgent intubation). Asking the patient whether their breathing feels adequate or whether they feel they need help with their breathing may form a useful part of this assessment.

2. Deteriorating status despite adequate treatment. This includes decreasing PEF, rising $PaCO_2$ or increasing respiratory rate. Deterioration is more important than the absolute values of these variables and can be an important adjunct to clinical assessment. Because of the different mechanisms of hypercapnia, one patient with fatigue and $PaCO_2$ rising from 40 to 50 mmHg despite aggressive treatment may need intubation, whereas another patient presenting with hyperacute asthma and a $PaCO_2 > 80$ mmHg may be coping despite respiratory distress and may avoid intubation with aggressive treatment.

PRINCIPLES OF MECHANICAL VENTILATION

All patients with significant airflow obstruction undergo some degree of dynamic hyperinflation during mechanical ventilation. This is a result of the airflow obstruction which slows expiratory gas flow and causes expiration of the inspired tidal volume ($\dot{V}_T$) to be interrupted by the onset of the next tidal breath (Fig. 8.1) A proportion of each successive $\dot{V}_T$ is trapped in this manner causing the lungs to progressively hyperinflate until an equilibrium point is reached where all the inspired $\dot{V}_T$ can be expired in the time available. This equilibrium point occurs because the increase in lung volume increases the elastic recoil pressure of the lungs and small airway calibre, both of which improve expiratory airflow.

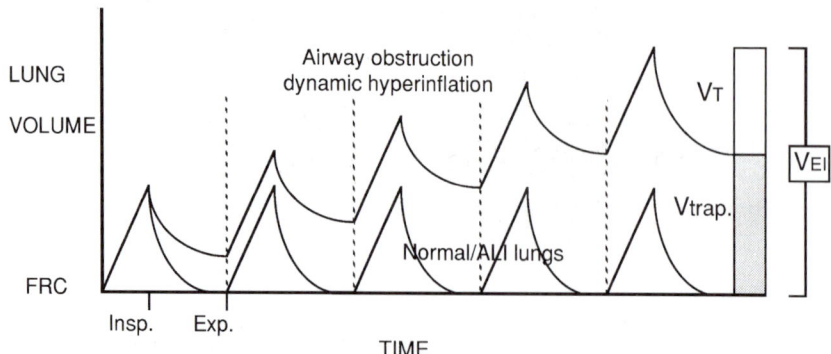

Fig. 8.1 Mechanism of dynamic hyperinflation during mechanical ventilation. Airway obstruction compared with normal lungs or lung with acute lung injury (ALI). Trapped gas volume ($\dot{V}_{trap}$) and $\dot{V}_T$ add to form the end-inspiratory lung volume ($\dot{V}_{EI}$) above functional residual capacity (FRC). Modified from Tuxen & Oh (1990).

$\dot{V}_{EI} > 20 ml/kg$ ann. $=$ dangerous dynamic hyperinflation ($\equiv TL\dot{V}_{EI} > TLC$!!)

In mild airflow obstruction, this process is adaptive as it allows the required $\dot{V}_E$, which could not be achieved at functional residual capacity (FRC), to be achieved at a higher lung volume despite some reduction in inspiratory muscle efficiency due to muscle shortening. However, when airflow obstruction is severe, the lung volume required to achieve normocapnia may be well in excess of TLC (Tuxen et al 1992). A spontaneously breathing patient will be incapable of achieving this, but injudicious mechanical ventilation can readily result in lung volume 2–3 times greater than TLC with a significant risk of inducing hypotension and pneumothorax (Tuxen & Lane 1987, Tuxen et al 1992, Williams et al 1992). During mechanical ventilation for severe asthma, Williams et al (1992) have shown that an end-inspiratory lung volume ($\dot{V}_{EI}$) exceeding 20 ml/kg (1.4 l) above FRC was associated with an increased risk of hypotension and barotrauma. In a subsequent study where FRC was measured (Tuxen et al 1992), the sum of $\dot{V}_{EI}$ and FRC (i.e. TL$\dot{V}_{EI}$), was shown to correlate closely with predicted TLC (Fig. 8.2). This suggested that ventilatory patterns causing TL$\dot{V}_{EI}$ to exceed TLC resulted in a risk of hypertension and barotrauma. Ventilatory patterns that maintained $\dot{V}_{EI} < 20$ ml/kg have been shown to significantly reduce the risk of these two complications (Tuxen et al 1993b).

There are three prime determinants of the level of dynamic hyperinflation: the volume inspired ($\dot{V}_T$), the time available for expiration (t_e) and the

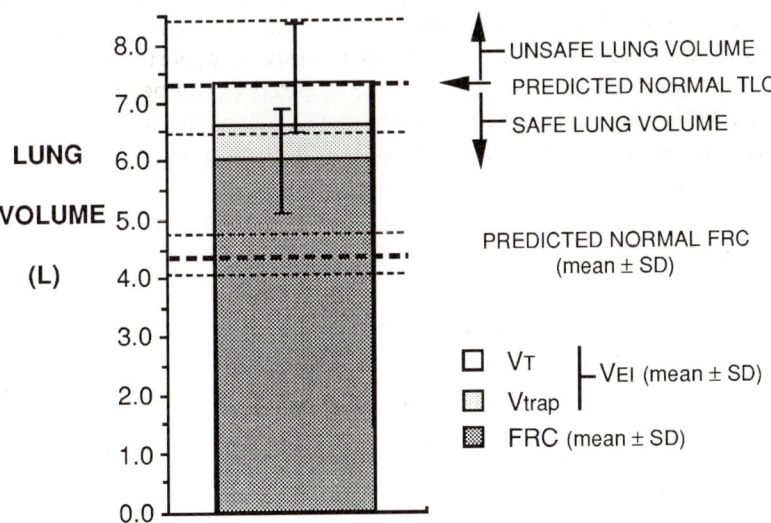

Fig. 8.2 Radiologically measured functional residual capacity (FRC) and the total end-inspiratory lung volumes (TL$\dot{V}_{EI}$) in mechanically ventilated patients with severe asthma whose initial ventilation was regulated to a previously established safe level of dynamic hyperinflation ($\dot{V}_{EI}$ 20 ml/kg). Measured FRC was well above predicted normal FRC and the safe TL$\dot{V}_{EI}$ corresponded almost exactly with predicted normal total lung capacity (TLC) for the same patients. Modified from Tuxen et al (1992).

Handwritten top margin: DYNAMIC HYPERINFLATION = $f(V_T \cdot t_e \cdot capliane')$

Handwritten: capliae = $f(obstruction)$

severity of airflow obstruction. Thus, V_{EI} is minimized by low V_T, high inspiratory flow (V_I) and a low respiratory rate (R), resulting in a low V_E (Tuxen & Lane 1987). These ventilatory patterns result in hypercapnia in the majority of acute asthmatics and form the basis for the controlled hypoventilation for asthma patients proposed by Darioli and Perret (1984).

For the majority of patients with severe asthma, airflow obstruction is worst at the commencement of mechanical ventilation and some patients develop complications immediately (Rosengarten et al 1990, Kollef 1992). Approximately one-third of patients may continue to deteriorate after intubation for up to 6–12 hours (Williams et al 1992). The mean time to detection of hypotension or pneumothorax in one study (Williams et al 1992) was 10 ± 15 hours after mechanical ventilation commenced, with all complications (except one) occurring within the first 24 hours.

Handwritten: ∴ best ventilation strategy = $V_T \downarrow$; $V_{insp} \uparrow$; RR $\downarrow$ → low V_E

VENTILATION MANAGEMENT

Handwritten: ↳ permissive hypercapnia

Mechanical ventilation should be managed in the following manner:

A Initial mechanical ventilation

1. Sedation and paralysis

May not be required in a minority of patients with rapidly resolving asthma but the majority benefit from continuous intravenous infusion of sedatives and muscle relaxants in order to ensure immediate tolerance of controlled hypoventilation during the critical early phase; CO_2 production is reduced thereby limiting the degree of hypercapnic acidosis that results from any given ventilator setting, and it can aid in the quantification of dynamic hyperinflation. Non-depolarizing paralysing agents (especially vecuronium and pancuronium) are currently believed to be significant contributing factors toward acute steroid myopathy (Douglass et al 1992, Hansen-Flaschen et al 1993) and the dose and duration should be minimized for this reason. Muscle relaxants should be withdrawn within 24 hours and recommenced only if there are problems that cannot be controlled with sedation alone.

Handwritten: Sedation
Paralysis — acute steroid myopathy related to non-depolarizing relaxants?

2. V_T

Although some early papers recommended or used a high V_T (Misuraca 1966, Scoggin et al 1977), a low V_T (8–10 ml/kg) is now considered appropriate (Petty 1978, Darioli & Perret 1984, Lukska et al 1986, Tuxen 1989, Bone & Burch 1991, Tuxen et al 1992).

Handwritten: low V_T — 8-10 ml/kg

low $\dot{V}_E$ ≤ 115 ml/kg/min — hypercapnia ok.^rate 10-12/min [handwritten annotation]

3. Respiratory rate (R)

This must be set to achieve a low V_E. Although some have recommended the early normalization of $PaCO_2$ (Scoggin et al 1977, Higgins et al 1986), the vast majority (Williams & Crook 1968, Darioli & Perret 1984, Lissac et al 1986, Tuxen & Lane 1987, Branthwaite 1990, Hall & Wood 1990, Limthongkul et al 1990, Bone & Burch 1991, Tuxen et al 1992) of authorities recommend low V_E. This is the basis of controlled hypocapnia, a technique initially recommended by Darioli and Perrett (1984) and now widely accepted. Williams and Tuxen (Tuxen et al 1992, Williams et al 1992) have recommended an initial $V_E \leq 115$ ml/kg/min (8 l/min). In 22 ventilated asthmatics, they calculated that this would result in an initial $PaCO_2$ of 77 ± 23 mmHg (range 40–134 mmHg) and that 18% of patients would have dynamic hyperinflation that exceeded a limit of $V_{EI} > 20$ ml/kg, but not to a dangerous degree. An initial respiratory rate of 10–12 breaths/min is recommended.

4. Inspiratory flow rate (V_I)

The choice of inspiratory flow rate is controversial. A number of authors (Misuraca 1966, Webb et al 1979, Darioli & Perret 1984, Lukska et al 1986, Branthwaite 1990) recommend a low V_I, mainly to support the goal of low peak inspiratory pressure (PIP). This contention has been seriously questioned by Tuxen & Lane (Tuxen & Lane 1987) who demonstrated that although decreasing V_I reduced PIP, expiratory time was reduced, leading to an increase in alveolar pressures and volumes (V_{EI}). As V_{EI} was subsequently shown to be a better discriminator than PIP for risk of hypotension and pneumothorax (Williams et al 1992), reducing V_I potentially increased the risk of complications.

Connors et al (1981) have shown that increasing V_I improves gas exchange, shunt and dead space in patients with chronic airflow obstruction. High V_I is now recommended by an increasing number of authors (Petty 1978, Connors et al 1981, Tuxen & Lane 1987, Hall & Wood 1990, Bone & Burch 1991). The effect of V_I on the distribution of ventilation between high and low resistance lung units is controversial. Opponents of high V_I argue that it redistributes more ventilation to low resistance lung units thereby increasing their inflation pressures and the risk of barotrauma. Proponents of high V_I argue that the risk of barotrauma is highest in the high resistance lung units which have the most dynamic hyperinflation and that increasing t_e (by increasing V_I) will reduce this risk. While opinion is divided, the weight of evidence favours the use of high V_I to shorten inspiratory time and thereby prolong t_e. V_I 80–100 l/min is recommended (Petty 1978, Connors et al 1981, Tuxen & Lane 1987, Hall & Wood 1990, Bone & Burch 1991, Tuxen et al 1992).

$\dot{V}_I$ — rel. high, to minimi I/E ratio — prolongation of exp'y time — improve ventilation of low-resistance lung units [handwritten annotation]

5. Oxygenation support ↑FiO₂ . ? PEEP ? hyperinflation v. recruitment of both-resistive u

Increasing FiO_2 without the application of PEEP is sufficient to achieve $SaO_2 \geq 95\%$ in nearly all patients. Although continuous positive airway pressure (CPAP) may reduce the work of breathing during spontaneous ventilation, PEEP is potentially harmful during controlled mechanical ventilation as it increases lung hyperinflation (Tuxen 1989). If asthma is complicated by pneumonia or other acute lung injury which results in severe hypoxaemia despite FiO_2 of 1.0, and PEEP must be used, then its effect on lung inflation should be assessed and compensated for by reductions in V_T or R or both.

B Subsequent regulation of mechanical ventilation

Approximately 80% of patients have some degree of hypercapnic acidosis using the above initial ventilatory settings, but this is well-tolerated with few adverse effects. By contrast, there is now considerable evidence that dynamic hyperinflation is a major cause of immediate morbidity. Thus, the level of dynamic hyperinflation should be assessed and ventilation should be regulated accordingly. There are several methods of achieving this:

Permissive hypercapnia ✓   Dynamic hyperinflation ✗

1. Empirical hypoventilation

Empirical hypoventilation can be used, using the initial ventilatory settings with weaning on clinical recovery of asthma. Although safe for the majority of asthmatics, this does not allow for the large variations that occur in the severity and duration of asthma. Patients with less severe or rapidly resolving asthma may have unnecessary hypoventilation, whereas patients with more severe disease may have inadequate hypoventilation (Rosengarten et al 1990).

? hypoventilation — difficult to match degree of hyperinflation to lung capacitance

2. PIP limit

Some authors have recommended either keeping PIP low or maintaining it below an arbitrary limit — commonly 50 cmH_2O (Chopin et al 1982, Darioli & Perret 1984, Lissac et al 1986, Lukska et al 1986, Limthongkul et al 1990). This approach has limited merit because of the tenuous relationship between PIP and dynamic hyperinflation when V_I is not constant. PIP has two components — the pressure required for alveolar inflation (estimated from the plateau airway pressure, P_{plat}), and the pressure expended in the airways to maintain gas flow. The latter may be large when airflow obstruction is present, but there is no evidence that the pressure expended in the airways has any relationship to barotrauma. As previously discussed, PIP does not provide a reliable guide to dynamic hyperinflation (Tuxen & Lane 1987), nor to the risk of complications (Williams et al 1992) in asthma.

Airring PIP? Variable relationship to dynamic hyperinflation .
a) Alveolar inflation press ≈ Pplat
b) Flow-generation — variable, c degree of airway destruction

Thus, PIP cannot be recommended as a guide for adjusting mechanical ventilation, unless V_I rate and waveform is specified and the relationship with P_{plat} and lung volume is measured. Thus, the 'safe limit' of PIP depends on the V_I being used.

'safe' PIP depd a $\dot{V}_I$, waveform, compliance ....

3. P_{plat} and intrinsic PEEP (PEEPi)

These airway pressures relate directly to the level of dynamic hyperinflation in individual patients and are better indicators of risk than PIP. However, respiratory compliance varies between patients and barotrauma has been shown to correlate with lung volume (V_{EI}) and not with these pressures (Williams et al 1992). These findings limit the use of absolute values of P_{plat} and PEEPi, although P_{plat} may be of some value once the relationship between V_{EI} and P_{plat} has been established. (Williams et al 1992) found that the P_{plat} that corresponded with a safe level of dynamic hyperinflation was 22 ± 7 cmH$_2$O), but there have been no studies using or recommending either of these variables to regulate mechanical ventilation.

Volutrauma . Pplat d V_{EI} .   Pplat 15 - 30 cmH$_2$O ?

4. Circulatory responses

An unsafe level of dynamic hyperinflation, where TLV$_{EI}$ exceeds TLC, is associated more commonly with high central venous pressures and hypotension than barotrauma (Tuxen & Lane 1987, Williams et al 1992, Tuxen 1993). Increased blood pressure and reduced central venous pressure during a period of cessation of mechanical ventilation (e.g. for one minute) is strongly suggestive of excessive dynamic hyperinflation and the need to reduce V_E. Because such hypotension can also be overcome with fluid loading, the latter may mask excessive dynamic hyperinflation and risk of barotrauma.

— dynamic hyperinflation — CVP↑ SBP↓

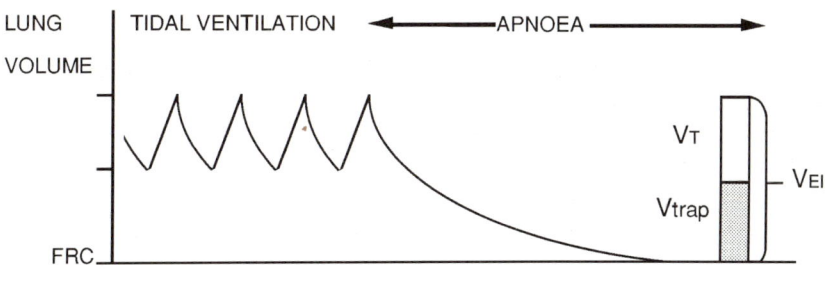

LUNG VOLUME | TIDAL VENTILATION ←——————APNOEA——————→

VT
VEI
Vtrap
FRC

TIME

Fig. 8.3 Measurement of end-inspiratory lung volume (V_{EI}) above FRC in a paralysed patient during controlled mechanical ventilation measured as the total exhaled gas volume during a period of apnoea long enough for all visible expiratory gas flow to cease (usually 40–60 sec). Modified from Tuxen & Oh (1990).

(cf. Used periodic apnea to release Vtrap and produce movement along the phly P-V curve)

5. V_{EI}

V_{EI} is the most direct measurement of dynamic hyperinflation, has been used to quantify the effect of different ventilatory patterns (Tuxen & Lane 1987), has been shown to correlate well with TLV_{EI} (Tuxen et al 1992) and with the risk of hypotension and barotrauma (Williams et al 1992) and has been used to regulate the level and duration of mechanical ventilation (Tuxen et al 1992). Ventilation regulated in this manner has been shown to have a reduced incidence of hypotension and barotrauma (Tuxen 1993b). The measurement of V_{EI} requires pharmacological paralysis, a volumetric spirometer on the expiratory line and a period of apnoea long enough (usually 40–60 sec) for all visible expiratory gas flow to cease (Fig. 8.3). This allows deflation of the lung to FRC, is a highly reproducible measurement, causes no significant hypoxia or hypercapnia and allows the concurrent observation of circulatory response.

Although advantageous, the technique is complex and labour-intensive and for these reasons has not been widely used. If linear compliance is assumed V_{EI} can also be calculated, without paralysis, apnoea or a volumetric spirometer, from measurements of P_{plat} and PEEPi using the formula: compliance $= V_T/(P_{plat} - PEEPi) = V_{EI}/P_{plat}$. However, V_{EI} calculated in this manner has not been validated. Inductance plethysmography has also been used to monitor lung volume but this also is complex and labour-intensive.

Tuxen et al (1992) proposed that mechanical ventilation could be regulated by regular measurements of V_{EI} and adjusting R to maintain V_{EI} near a safe limit of 20 ml/kg (1.4 l, Fig. 8.4). Once normocapnia was achieved with $V_{EI} < 20$ ml/kg, then sedation and paralysis were withdrawn and the patient weaned. Using this method, 20% of patients with rapidly resolving asthma were normocapnic on initial ventilation and could be weaned immediately. The remaining 80% required more prolonged ventilation with levels of support remaining well below the ventilatory requirement for normocapnia (Fig. 8.4). The weaning point was reached by both improved airflow obstruction and decreased ventilatory requirement for normocapnia. Asthma recovery was associated with a period of accelerated improvement (Fig. 8.4), often with increased sputum production (Tuxen et al 1992, Kallenbach et al, 1993). Ventilation regulated in this manner was slightly longer than that of a control group, but the incidence of hypotension and barotrauma was reduced (Tuxen 1993b).

MANAGEMENT OF HYPOTENSION

Hypotension developing during mechanical ventilation is most commonly due to dynamic hyperinflation, sedation or pneumothorax and occasionally due to arrhythmia or other causes (Tuxen & Lane 1987, Tuxen et al 1992, Williams et al 1992). Hypovolaemia may aggravate hypotension attributable to other factors, but is rarely a primary cause. The mechanism

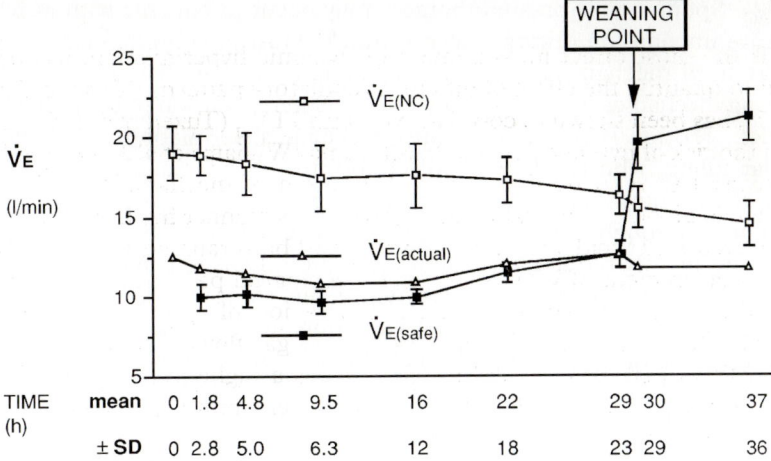

Fig. 8.4   Time course of 8 patients who required mechanical ventilation for severe asthma. The $\dot{V}_E$ actually given ($\dot{V}_{E(actual)}$) is shown compared with the calculated levels of $\dot{V}_E$ required to achieve a $\dot{V}_{EI}$ of 20 ml/kg ($\dot{V}_{E(safe)}$) and to achieve normocapnia ($\dot{V}_{E(NC)}$). The time axis has been standardized to coincide with the commencement of mechanical ventilation and the weaning point (when $\dot{V}_{E(safe)}$ exceeded $\dot{V}_{E(NC)}$). Modified from Tuxen et al (1992).

of hypotension is probably a combination of impaired venous return from high intrathoracic pressures and increased pulmonary vascular resistance from alveolar overdistension. Hypotension may range from mild to life-threatening (Rosengarten et al 1990, Kollef 1992) but should always be avoided as up to one-third of intubations follow respiratory and/or cardiac arrest with a concomitant risk of cerebral injury which could be worsened by subsequent hypotension. Mild hypotension may respond to fluid load-ing, but a favourable response does not exclude dynamic hyperinflation. Occasionally, with very severe airflow obstruction, profound hypotension, apparent electromechanical dissociation and cardiac arrest may occur from excessive dynamic hyperinflation despite conservative mechanical ventila-tion (Rosengarten et al 1990, Kollef 1992). Failure of early identification of dynamic hyperinflation as the cause can lead to inappropriate and inef-fective management with serious consequences. Initial management should exclude dynamic hyperinflation by an 'apnoea test'. If blood pressure im-proves and central venous pressure falls during apnoea this strongly sug-gests dynamic hyperinflation as the cause and ventilation should be resumed at a lower rate. Fluid loading may also be required. *APNOEA TEST*

MANAGEMENT OF PNEUMOTHORACES

The most common causes of pneumothorax in acute severe asthma are excessive dynamic hyperinflation from mechanical ventilation and accidental lung laceration during central venous catheter insertion (Williams et al

1992). Spontaneous pneumothoraces may occur in patients with asthma, but are uncommon during a severe attack. Most pneumothoraces do not occur until mechanical ventilation is commenced (Williams et al 1992). During mechanical ventilation, the risk of bilateral, tension pneumothoraces is high. Tension is common because mechanical ventilation continues alveolar filling, whilst airflow obstruction impedes normal alveolar emptying, encouraging gas to escape through a lower resistance (abnormal) channel. Although lung collapse may not be great, tension may be significant and greatly reduces ipsilateral ventilation. During constant mechanical ventilation, this must increase V_E to the contralateral lung, thereby increasing its level of dynamic hyperinflation and the risk of a second tension pneumothorax. Pneumothoraces have caused 6% of reported deaths (Table 8.2) (Karetzky 1975, Scoggin et al 1977, Webb et al 1979, Westerman et al 1979, Limthongkul et al 1990).

Signs:

HYPOTENSION

Pneumothoraces during mechanical ventilation are most commonly detected following hypotension, but clinical signs can be hard to distinguish from the underlying asthma as hyperinflation, hyperresonance and reduced breath sounds are present in both conditions. Asymmetry of breath sounds can be hard to distinguish during mechanical ventilation, tracheal shift can be difficult to interpret with confidence and subcutaneous emphysema can occur without pneumothorax. Blind intercostal catheter insertion in the absence of a pneumothorax carries a significant risk of lung injury with potentially serious consequences.

(CxR unless severe symptoms)

If mild hypotension is present, respiratory rate should be reduced and an urgent chest X-ray obtained prior to the insertion of an intercostal drain. Serious hypotension dictates a reduction in respiratory rate and urgent intercostal catheter insertion on the suspected side. Under either circumstance, blunt dissection should precede the insertion of the drain which should be inserted either without the stilette or with the stilette withdrawn from the tip and not entering the thoracic cavity, to minimize risk of lung injury.

CPAP, BIPAP AND EXTERNAL CHEST COMPRESSION

CPAP has been reported to decrease dyspnoea and reduce work of breathing in chronic airflow obstruction (Petrof et al 1990) and asthma (Tenaillon et al 1983, Weng et al 1984, Mathieu et al 1987), both in non-intubated patients and in those breathing spontaneously during mechanical ventilation. This is believed to occur as a result of CPAP overcoming intrinsic or auto-PEEP (PEEPi, the end-expiratory alveolar pressure resulting from gas trapping) which would otherwise have to be overcome by the patient's inspiratory effort before inspiration could commence (Martin et al 1982, Rossi et al 1985, Gottfried et al 1986).

CPAP may be used in patients with marginal ventilatory status to reduce the necessity for intubation or in patients experiencing difficulty weaning.

CPAP equal to the level of PEEPi has been recommended. Under either circumstance, the effect of CPAP on dyspnoea, respiratory rate, blood gas tensions and circulation should be carefully assessed and CPAP withdrawn if no benefit is detected.

Biphasic positive airway pressure (BiPAP) can provide ventilatory assistance in non-intubated patients by delivering a higher pressure during inspiration than expiration (i.e. CPAP with pressure support). It may provide helpful ventilatory assistance or may be detrimental by increasing hyperinflation. It requires further evaluation in severe asthma before it can be recommended.

External chest compression has been proposed to assist spontaneous ventilation in non-intubated patients with severe asthma and marginal respiratory status (Fisher et al 1989). External chest compression in dogs with dynamic hyperinflation induced by an added expiratory airflow resistor reduced hyperinflation but caused a deterioration in circulatory status (Van der Touw et al 1993). With fixed expiratory resistance, a reduction in hyperinflation would be expected with chest compression. However, a similar effect could not be expected in patients with small airway obstruction where chest compression may cause dynamic airway compression and no improvement in expiratory flow. In our unit, external chest compression applied to four patients with severe asthma during controlled mechanical ventilation caused an elevation in central venous pressure but no changes in blood pressure, dynamic hyperinflation or gas exchange. The value of this technique is uncertain and further studies are required.

DRUG THERAPY

1. Nebulized beta$_2$-agonists

These should be given 2-hourly, whether mechanical ventilation is being used or not. On initial presentation this may be increased in frequency to 1-hourly or continuously. The agent most commonly used is salbutamol 5–10 mg per dose.

2. Ipratropium bromide

Although a weak bronchodilator in its own right, there is now sufficient evidence of small but significant additional benefit when combined with salbutamol to warrant routine administration of ipratropium bromide 0.5–1.0 mg 4-hourly in severe asthma (Bryant 1985, Editorial 1986).

3. Steroids

Parenteral steroids are central to the treatment of severe asthma and several new insights into this administration have occurred. Previously, parenteral steroids were only given when prolonged bronchodilator therapy had failed and admission to hospital was indicated. One or two early intravenous doses of hydrocortisone have been shown to avert a hospital admission and are now recommended if there has been an inadequate response to initial bronchodilator therapy (Kelly & Murphy 1991, McFadden 1993). There has also been increasing recognition of acute steroid myopathy following high dose intravenous steroids, particularly when combined with non-depolarizing paralysing agents (Douglass et al 1992, Hansen-Flaschen et al 1993). This has stimulated a search for the lowest dose and duration of parenteral steroids that are adequate for the treatment of asthma. Hydrocortisone 250 mg intravenously 6-hourly for 24 h, with dosage reductions each 24 h thereafter is recommended. Occasional patients with refractory asthma may require high, more prolonged doses. Nebulized budesonide 1 mg 12-hourly should also be given to assist parenteral steroid dose minimization. Serum creatine kinase (CK) levels should be measured daily to monitor for steroid myopathy.

4. Aminophylline

The role of aminophylline in the management of acute asthma has been controversial (Fanta 1982, Woodcock et al 1983) because of scarce evidence of benefit once full-dose beta-agonists and steroids have been given and the risk of toxicity (Josephson et al 1979, Fanta et al 1986, Coleridge et al 1993). However, a recent randomized study (Huang et al 1993) has found a significant benefit from aminophylline when added to full-dose beta-agonists and steroids with no difference in adverse effects. We believe that use of aminophylline is justified provided it is administered in a manner that minimizes the risk of toxicity. Toxicity most commonly occurs from the administration of a loading dose to a patient who already has significant aminophylline levels or from an intravenous infusion with inadequate monitoring of serum levels in patients with impaired drug clearance. Loading doses should be low (≤ 3 mg/kg) and should be avoided in patients who have received any theophylline therapy in the preceding 48 h. Infusions should be commenced at conservative levels (≤ 0.5 mg/kg/hr) with the objective of increasing to a therapeutic level over 24 h. Lower infusion rates should be used in congestive cardiac failure, hepatic or renal impairment, chronic airways disease, high fever or with concurrent cimetidine or erythromycin therapy. If there is uncertainty about previous theophylline therapy, a serum level should be taken prior to any drug administration. Serum levels should be taken after the loading dose and 18–24 h after initiating a constant infusion.

5. Parenteral salbutamol

Parenteral salbutamol may be given as an intravenous bolus of 100–300 μg and, during respiratory arrest without intravenous access, the same dose may be given via the endotracheal tube. Salbutamol may be given by infusion, at a rate of 2–10 μg/min. It is our practice to give a salbutamol infusion to all patients who require intensive care. Side-effects include tremor, tachycardia, arrhythmias, hyperglycaemia, hypokalaemia and lactic acidosis (Braden et al 1985, Douglass et al 1992). Serum bicarbonate levels need to be observed closely during salbutamol infusions and serum lactate should be measured if serum bicarbonate levels are low or falling. If lactic acidosis occurs, the salbutamol infusion should be reduced or stopped.

6. Adrenaline

Adrenaline has the theoretical advantage over pure beta-agonists of combining a bronchodilator effect with alpha-mediated vasoconstriction, with the potential for a reduction in mucosal oedema. There have been anecdotal reports of impressive improvement in patients refractory to beta-agonists (Appel et al 1989) but controlled studies have shown adrenaline to be as good as, not superior to, beta-agonists (Baughman et al 1984, Tinkelman et al 1986, Spiteri et al 1988). Adrenaline is not recommended for routine use in asthma, but may benefit patients who are refractory to standard therapy. Adrenaline may be nebulized 0.5–1 mg every 30 min, given subcutaneously 0.1–0.5 mg every 30 min to a maximum of three doses, or may be given intravenously as a dose of 10 μg followed by an infusion of 1–10 μg/min.

7. Other agents

Numerous other therapies have had reported success in acute severe asthma. These include magnesium, ketamine (Betts & Parkin 1971, Fisher 1977), barbiturates (Grunberg et al 1991), droperidol (Prezant & Aldrich 1988) and inhalational anaesthetic agents with bronchodilator properties such as halothane, insofluorane and enfluorane (O'Rourke & Crone 1982, Schwartz 1984, Echeverria et al 1986, Parnass et al 1987). All these agents, with the exception of magnesium, can only be given safely during mechanical ventilation. All have some evidence of benefit, but none have an established place in standard therapy.

8. Helium

Helium is not a bronchodilator but its low density and viscosity improve airflow. It has been shown to reduce the work of breathing and improve dyspnoea during spontaneous respiration in asthma (Gluck et al 1990) and would, no doubt, reduce dynamic hyperinflation during mechanical ventilation.

He – reduction in dynamic hyperinflation...

LACTIC ACIDOSIS

Lactic acidosis has been reported a number of times in association with severe asthma (Roncoroni et al 1976, Shires et al 1979, Appel et al 1983, Braden et al 1985, Douglass et al 1992). We found lactic acidosis in 34/47 (72%) of patients who required mechanical ventilation for asthma with maximum levels of 5.5 ± 2.3 mmol/l (range $2-12$ mmol/l). It has been variously ascribed to asthma, hypoxia and anaerobic muscle activity and beta-agonists. In our experience, it only occurred following high-dose intravenous beta-agonists and was not associated with hypotension or hypoxia. We observed 2 patterns. Some patients developed lactic acidosis during emergency ambulance transport in which they received $500-750$ µg of intravenous salbutamol in divided doses over $15-30$ min. Some of these patients had clinical resolution of severe asthma, but marked dyspnoea due to metabolic acidosis. A second group arrived with a normal serum bicarbonate level and developed lactic acidosis within $4-6$ h of commencing intravenous salbutamol $5-20$ µg/min. In both groups, lactate and bicarbonate levels returned to normal within $4-8$ h provided intravenous salbutamol was reduced or stopped. In a small number of patients, a mild lactic acidosis resolved despite continuation of the salbutamol infusion. Lactate production is believed to result from direct beta-adrenergic stimulation of glycolytic pathways, without anaerobic metabolism, mainly in muscle. Salbutamol infusions should be limited to 10 µg/min and serum bicarbonate levels should be closely monitored in severe asthma, especially following any parenteral agents with beta-adrenergic activity. Serum lactate levels should be measured if serum bicarbonate levels are ≤ 22 mmol/l or fall by ≥ 2 mmol/l. Lactate production has also been reported following intravenous adrenaline, but not noradrenaline, after cardiac surgery (Totaro & Raper 1994), and hence could also occur following adrenaline administration in asthma.

lactate ↑

high dose β-agonists

(stimⁿ of glycolysis in muscle)

ACUTE STEROID MYOPATHY

Acute necrotizing myopathy is now recognized with increasing frequency following mechanical ventilation in asthma (Macfarlane & Rosenthal 1977, Williams et al 1988, Danon & Carpenter 1991, Margolis et al 1991, Douglass et al 1992, Griffin et al 1992, Hirano et al 1992, Barrett et al

[Handwritten annotations at top of page: "Rix: CK — acute necrotizing myopathy — global weakness — ask. c hijdne puretard steroids, + ? ventilate + ? paralysis + ? lactic. acidosis"]

1993, Lacomis et al 1993). In one study of 25 patients ventilated for asthma, a rise in CK was detected in 76% and clinical myopathy in 36% (Douglass et al 1992).

It may range in severity from an asymptomatic rise in CK, through clinically detectable limb weakness without serious functional deficit, to marked muscle weakness producing mild prolongation of hospital stay, to profound global weakness delaying weaning from mechanical ventilation and requiring a prolonged hospital stay and active rehabilitation. Functional quadraparesis with incomplete recovery after 12 months has been observed in a small number of patients (Williams et al 1988, Hirano et al 1992). The onset is usually within 5 days of presentation. The weakness is global and includes limb and facial muscles but difficulty in weaning from mechanical ventilation is usually only encountered in the more severe forms. Reflexes are reduced or absent depending on severity and sensation is intact.

Serum CK levels are invariably elevated, the peaks ranging from as low as $300-400$ IU/l to $> 10\ 000$ IU/l occurring 3.6 ± 1.5 days from onset of treatment (Douglass et al 1992). A second CK peak has been observed in a small percentage of patients undergoing prolonged steroid therapy and was associated with the most profound weakness (Douglass et al 1992). The electromyogram (EMG) is usually markedly abnormal with myopathic changes. In some patients, the EMG may also show neuropathic changes (Margolis et al 1991, Hirano et al 1992, Lacomis et al 1993), but whether or not this is artifactual is uncertain. Muscle biopsy usually shows extensive non-inflammatory muscle necrosis (Douglass et al 1992).

The aetiology has not been fully clarified and a number of factors may contribute. However, myopathy is rarely (if ever) seen in the absence of high-dose parenteral steroids. The most severe forms occur in mechanically-ventilated patients where paralysing agents and acidosis may have contributed, but we have observed CK rises and mild myopathy in non-ventilated patients with severe asthma, in 2 patients who were re-challenged with steroids following recovery from myopathy, and in patients with subarachnoid haemorrhage receiving high-dose steroids.

Paralysing agents (especially pancuronium and vecuronium) have also been implicated as an aggravating factor (Douglass et al 1992, Hansen-Flaschen et al 1993), but it is uncommon for myopathy to occur in the absence of concomitant steroid therapy. Paralysis may increase the number of steroid receptors on muscle cells, possibly increasing their sensitivity to steroids (DuBois & Almon 1980, 1981).

Lactic acidosis may also be a contributory, but not essential, factor. Rapid lactate production in muscle profoundly lowers its intracellular pH and this may, in its own right, initiate muscle injury. If this is a factor, then hypercapnic acidosis may also contribute to intracellular acidosis and aggravate injury.

The role of motor neuropathy, if any, in association with myopathy is unclear. Neuropathic features on EMG have been reported in association with steroid myopathy (Margolis et al 1991, Hirano et al 1992, Lacomis et al 1993) and motor neuropathy has been described, based on EMG findings, in similar patients who have had steroids and paralysing agents (Gorson & Ropper 1993). In our experience of this condition (Williams et al 1988, Douglass et al 1992), features of acute denervation are common on needle EMG examination but much of this, if not all, can be attributed to extensive muscle membrane injury due to the presence of severe myopathy. The presence of myopathy has been established by muscle biopsy, but there has been no histological evidence for neuropathy. Whether motor neuropathy does coexist in some patients and compounds myopathy by denervation (DuBois & Almon 1980, 1981) remains to be established. Because EMG can be misleading, motor neuropathy should not be diagnosed by EMG alone without performing serial CK levels and a muscle biopsy (Tuxen 1993a).

CK levels should be measured daily in all patients with severe asthma receiving parenteral steroids. Although myopathy can occur with CK levels <1000 IU/l, the highest risk occurs with levels >1000 IU/l and this necessitates cessation of paralysis, if not already done, and a reduction in parenteral steroid dosage provided asthma control is reasonable. Careful neurological assessment should be undertaken after sedation and paralysis (if used) have ceased and EMG should be performed if weakness is detected.

LONG-TERM OUTCOME AND FOLLOW-UP

In 37 papers reporting mechanical ventilation for asthma (Table 8.1), repeated mechanical ventilation was required in approximately 9% of cases, despite the serious nature of asthma presumably having been appreciated following the first episode.

Long-term follow-up of patients who required mechanical ventilation for severe asthma reveals a high mortality. Following 147 episodes of mechanical ventilation, Marquette et al (1992) reported a 10% mortality at 1 year, 14% at 3 years, and 22% after 6 years. Maynard & Hillman (1993) followed 96 patients aged between 10 and 50 years who had been admitted to intensive care for asthma and found an 8% mortality after 1–7 years. Richards et al (1993) reported a 7.5% 2-year mortality in 413 patients following admission to intensive care with asthma. Seddon & Heaf (1990) followed 17 children who survived mechanical ventilation and found a 24% mortality after 12 months. These observations highlight the need for careful follow-up.

Special services to identify and treat high-risk asthma patients, especially those who have required mechanical ventilation, are to be recommended and their management should include:

1. More aggressive treatment.
2. Regular medical follow-up.
3. Regular monitoring of lung function by both doctor (spirometry) and patient (PEF).
4. Management plans for deteriorating status including additional medications kept and understood by the patient and early medical attendance.
5. Emergency action plans including ambulance priority, as well as rapid emergency department attendance and response.

KEY POINTS FOR CLINICAL PRACTICE

- Mechanical ventilation of patients with severe asthma has a significant associated risk of morbidity and mortality from dynamic hyperinflation.
- The decision to intubate should be based on clinical assessment of respiratory distress and deteriorating status, rather than arbitrary values of $PaCO_2$ or PEF.
- Mechanical ventilation should commence with sedation, paralysis, V_T 6–8 ml/kg, V_I 80–100 l/min and rate 10–14 breaths/min to maintain V_E < 115 ml/kg/min
- Mechanical ventilation should be regulated by adjusting the rate to maintain dynamic hyperinflation at or below a safe level and not according to $PaCO_2$ or pH.
- Myopathy should be minimized by monitoring CK levels daily, as well as minimizing the dose and duration of both paralysing agents and parenteral steroids, with early introduction of nebulized steroids.
- Serum lactate levels should be monitored if serum bicarbonate levels are low (<22 mmol/l) or falling and if lactate is elevated, salbutamol infusions should be reduced or ceased.
- Any hypotension, circulatory failure or apparent electromechanical dissociation occurring in a mechanically-ventilated patient with airflow obstruction should first have dynamic hyperinflation excluded as the cause by an apnoea test.
- Following mechanical ventilation for asthma, patients should have careful management including aggressive therapy, deterioration or crisis management plans and priority access to emergency services.

REFERENCES

Ambiavagar M, Riding W D 1966 Treatment of status asthmaticus. Lancet 1: 363
Appel D, Karpel J P, Sherman M 1989 Epinephrine improves expiratory flow rates in patients with asthma who do not respond to inhaled metaproterenol sulfate. J Allergy Clin Immunol 84: 90–98
Appel D, Rubernstein R, Schrager K et al 1983 Lactic acidosis in severe asthma. Am J Med 75: 580–584

Barrett S A, Mourani S, Villareal C et al 1993 Rhabdomyolysis associated with status asthmaticus. Crit Care Med 21: 151–153

Bates D V, Klassen G A, Broadhurst C A et al 1965 Management of respiratory failure. Ann N Y Acad Sci 121: 781–787

Baughman R P, Ploysongsang Y, James W 1984 A comparative study of aerosolized terbutaline and subcutaneously administered epinephrine in the treatment of acute bronchial asthma. Ann Allergy 53: 131–134

Betts E K, Parkin C E 1971 Use of Ketamine in an asthmatic child. Anesth Analg 50: 420–421

Bone R C, Burch S G 1991 Management of status asthmaticus. Annals of Allergy 67: 461–469

Braden G L, Johnston S S, Germain M J et al 1985 Lactic acidosis associated with the therapy of acute bronchospasm. N Engl J Med 313: 890

Braman S S, Kaemmerlen J T 1990 Intensive of status asthmaticus a 10-year experience. JAMA 264(3): 366–368

Branthwaite M A 1990 An update on mechanical ventilation for severe acute asthma. Clin Int Care 1: 4–6

Bryant D H 1985 Nebulised ipratropium bromide in the treatment of acute asthma. Chest 88: 24–29

Chopin C, Mangalaboyi J, Dubois D et al 1982 L'etat de mal asthmatique. Rev Prat 32: 681–691

Coleridge J, Epstein J, Cameron P et al 1993 Intravenous aminophylline confers no benefit in acute asthma treated with intravenous steroids and inhaled bronchodilators. Aust NZ J Med 23: 348–354

Connors A F, McCaffree D R, Gray B A 1981 Effect of inspiratory flow rate on gas exchange during mechanical ventilation. Am Rev Respir Dis 124: 537–543

Cornil A, De Troyer A, Thys J P et al 1977 Asthme grave et reanimation a propos de 120 observations. Intensive Care Med 3: 114(Abs)

Crompton G K, Grant I W B, Bloomfield P 1979 Edinburgh emergency asthma admission service: report on 10 years' experience. Br Med J ii: 1199–1201

Danon M J, Carpenter S 1991 Myopathy with thick filament (Myosin) loss following prolonged paralysis with vecuronium during steroid treatment. Muscle & Nerve 14: 1131–1139

Darioli R, Perret C 1984 Mechanical controlled hypoventilation in status asthmaticus. Am Rev Respir Dis 129: 385–387

De Coster A, Naeije R, Cornil A 1983. Asthme grave et reanimation a propos de 120 observations. Care of the critically ill patient, Springer-Verlag, Berlin, pp 359–369

Douglass J A, Tuxen D V, Horne M et al 1992 Myopathy in severe asthma. Am Rev Respir Dis 146(2): 517–519

DuBois D C, Almon R R 1980 Disuse atrophy of skeletal muscle is associated with an increase in number of glucocorticoid receptors. Endocrinology 107: 1649–1651

DuBois D C, Almon R R 1981 A possible role for glucocorticoids in denervation atrophy. Muscle & Nerve 4: 370–373

Echeverria M, Gelb A W, Wexler H R et al 1986 Enflurane and halothane in status asthmaticus. Chest 89: 152–154

Editorial 1986 Acute asthma. Lancet 1: 131–133

Fanta C H, Rossing T H, McFadden E R 1986 Treatment of acute asthma. Is combination therapy with sympathomimetics and methylxanthines indicated? Am J Med 80: 5–10

Fanta C H, Venugopalan C S, Lacouture P G et al 1982 Inhibition of bronchoconstriction in the guinea pig by a calcium channel blocker, nifedipine. Am Rev Respir Dis 125: 61

Ferrer A, Torres A, Roca J et al 1990 Characteristics of patients with soybean dust-induced acute severe asthma requiring mechanical ventilation. Eur Respir J 3: 429–433

Fisher M M, Bowe J, Ladd-Hudson K 1989 External chest compression in acute asthma: A preliminary study. Crit Care Med 17: 686–687

Fisher M McD 1977 Ketamine hydrochloride in severe bronchospasm. Anaesthesia 32: 771–772

Gluck E H, Onorato D J, Castriotta R 1990 Helium-oxygen mixtures in intubated patients with status asthmaticus and respiratory acidosis. Chest 98: 693–698

Gorson K C, Ropper A H 1993 Acute respiratory failure in neuropathy: A variant of critical illness polyneuropathy. Crit Care Med 21: 267–271

Gottfried S B, Rossi A, Milic-Emili J 1986 Dynamic hyperinflation, intrinsic PEEP and the mechanically ventilated patient. Intens Crit Care Digest 5: 30–33

Griffin D, Fairman N, Coursin D et al 1992 Acute myopathy during treatment of status asthmaticus with corticosteroids and steroidal muscle relaxants. Chest 102: 510–514

Grunberg G, Cohen J D, Keslin J et al 1991 Facilitation of mechanical ventilation in status asthmaticu with continuous intravenous Thiopental. Chest 99: 1216–1129

Hall J B, Wood L D H 1990 Management of the critically ill asthmatic patient. Med Clin North Am 74(3): 779–796

Halttunen P K, Luomanmaki K, Takkunen O et al 1980 Management of severe asthma in an intensive care unit. Ann Clin Res 12: 109–111

Hansen-Flaschen J, Cowen J, Raps E C 1993 Neuromuscular blockade in the Intensive Care Unit. More than we bargained for. Am Rev Respir Dis 147: 234–236

Higgins B, Greening A P, Crompton G K 1986 Assisted ventilation in severe acute asthma. Thorax 41: 464–467

Hirano M, Ott B R, Raps E C et al 1992 Acute quadriplegic myopathy: A complication of treatment with steroids, nondepolarizing blocking agents, or both. Neurology 42: 2082–2087

Huang D, O'Brien R G, Harmen E et al 1993 Does aminophylline benefit adults admitted to the hospital for an acute exacerbation of asthma? Ann Intern Med 119: 1155–1160

Iisalo E U, Iisalo E I, Vapaavuori M J 1969 Prolonged artificial ventilation in severe status asthmaticus. Acta Med Scand 185: 51–55

Johnson A J, Nunn A J, Somner A R et al 1984 Circumstances of death from asthma. Br Med J 288: 1870–1872

Josephson G W, MacKenzie E J, Lietman P S et al 1979 Emergency treatment of asthma: a comparison of two treatment regimens. JAMA 242: 639–643

Kallenbach J M, Frankel A H, Lapinski S E et al 1993 Determinants of near fatality in acute severe asthma. Am J Med 95: 265–272

Karetzky M S 1975 Asthma mortality associated with pneumothorax and intermittent positive pressure breathing. Lancet 1: 828–829

Kelly H W, Murphy S 1991 Corticosteroids for acute, severe asthma. DICP 25: 72–79

Kollef M H 1992 Lung hyperinflation caused by inappropriate ventilation resulting in electromechanical dissociation: a case report. Heart Lung 21: 74–77

Lacomis D, Smith T W, Chad D A 1993 Acute myopathy and neuropathy in status asthmaticus: case report and literature review. Muscle & Nerve 16: 84–90

Lam K N, Mow B M, Chew L S 1992 The profile of ICU admissions for acute severe asthma in a general hospital. Singapore Med J 33(5): 460–462

Leonhardt K O 1961 Resuscitation of the moribund asthmatic and emphysematous patient. N Engl J Med 264: 785–790

Limthongkul S, Udompanich V, Wongthim S et al 1990 Status asthmaticus: an analysis of 560 episodes and comparison between mechanical and non-mechanical ventilation groups. J Med Assoc Thai 73: 321–327

Lissac J, Labrousse J, Tenaillon A et al 1986 Traitment des asthmes aigus graves de l'adulte. Ann Med Interne 137(1): 34–37

Lukska A R, Smith P, Coakley J et al 1986 Acute severe asthma treated by mechanical ventilation: 10 years experience from a district general hospital. Thorax 41: 459–463

Macfarlane I A, Rosenthal F D 1977 Severe myopathy after status asthmaticus. Lancet ii: 615

McDonald J B, Seaton A, Williams D A 1976 Asthma deaths in Cardiff 1963–1974: 90 deaths outside hospital. Br Med J 1: 1493–1495

McFadden E R 1993 Dosages of corticosteroids in asthma. Am Rev Respir Dis 147: 1306–1310

Mansel J K, Stogner S W, Petrini M F et al 1990 Mechanical ventilation in patients with acute severe asthma. Am J Med 89: 42–48

Marchand P, Van Hesselt H 1966 Last-resort treatment of status asthmaticus. Lancet 1: 227–230

Margolis B D, Khachikian D, Friedman Y et al 1991 Prolonged reversible quadriparesis in mechanically ventilated patients who received long-term infusions of Vecuronium. Chest 100: 877–878

Marquette C H, Saulnier F, Leroy O et al 1992 Long-term prognosis of near-fatal asthma. Am Rev Respir Dis 146: 76–81

Martin J G, Shore S, Engel L A 1982 Effect of continuous positive airway pressure on respiratory mechanics and pattern of breathing in induced asthma. Am Rev Respir Dis 126: 812–817

Mathieu M, Tonneau M C, Zarka D et al 1987 Effects of positive end-expiratory pressure in severe acute asthma. Crit Care Med 15: 1164

Maynard R, Hillman K 1993 Intensive care asmission as a predictor of asthma mortality. Anaes Int Care 21: 712

Misuraca L 1966 Mechanical ventilation in status asthmaticus. N Engl J Med 257: 318–320

Moss S F, Rudolf M, Owen R et al 1990 Mechanical ventilation for acute severe asthma in a district general hospital (DGH) in the United Kingdom in the 1980s. Am Rev Respir Dis 141: A398

O'Rourke P P, Crone R K 1982 Halothane in status asthmaticus. Crit Care Med 10: 341

Parnass S M, Feld J M, Chamberlin W H et al 1987 Status asthmaticus treated with isoflurane and enflurane. Anesth Analg 66: 193–195

Petheram I S, Branthwaite M A 1980 Mechanical ventilation for pulmonary disease. Anaesthesia 35: 467–473

Petrof B J, Legare M, Goldberg P et al 1990 Continuous positive airway pressure reduces work of breathing and dyspnoea during weaning from ventilation in severe chronic obstructive pulmonary disease. Am Rev Respir Dis 141: 281–289

Petty T L 1978 Oxygen and mechanical ventilation in status asthmaticus. In: Weiss E B (ed) Status asthmaticus. Univ Park Press, Baltimore, MD, pp 285–292

Picado C, Montserrat J M, Roca J et al 1983 Mechanical ventilation in severe exacerbation of asthma. Eur J Respir Dis 84: 102–107

Pouw E M, Koeter G H, deMonchy J G R et al 1990 Clinical assessment after a life-threatening attack of asthma; the role of bronchial reactivity. Eur Respir J 3: 861–866

Prezant D J, Aldrich T K 1988 Intravenous droperidol for the treatment of status asthmaticus. Crit Care Med 16: 96–97

Rees H A, Millar J S, Donald J W 1968 A study of the clinical course and arterial blood gas tensions of patients in status asthmaticus. Q J Med 37: 234–243

Richards G N, Kolbe J, Fenwick J et al 1993 Demographic characteristics of patients with severe life threatening asthma: comparison with asthma deaths. Thorax 48: 1105–1109

Riding W D, Ambiavagar M 1967 Resuscitation of the moribund asthmatic. Postgrad Med J 43: 234–243

Roncoroni A J, Adrogue H J A, DeObrutsky C W et al 1976 Metabolic acidosis in status asthmaticus. Respiration 33: 85–94

Rosengarten P, Tuxen D V, Dziukas L et al 1990 Circulatory arrest induced by intermittent positive pressure ventilation in a patient with severe asthma. Anaes Int Care 19: 118–121

Rossi A, Gottfried S B, Zocchi L et al 1985 Measurement of static compliance of the total respiratory system in patients acute respiratory failure during mechanical ventilation: the effect of intrinsic positive end-expiratory pressure. Am Rev Respir Dis 131: 672–677

Santiago S M, Klaustermeyer W 1980 Mortality in status asthmaticus: 9 year experience in a respiratory intensive care. J Asthma Res 17: 75–79

Schwartz S 1984 Treatment of status asthmaticus with halothane. JAMA 251: 2688–2689

Scoggin C H, Sahn S A, Petty T L 1977 Status asthmaticus. A nine year experience. JAMA 238: 1158–1162

Seddon P C, Heaf D P 1990 Long term outcome of ventilation asthmatics. Arch Dis Child 65: 1324–1328

Sheehy A F, Dibenedeto R, Lefrak S et al 1972 Treatment of status asthmaticus. Arch Intern Med 130: 37–42

Shires R, Joffe B I, Heding L G et al 1979 Metabolic studies in acute asthma before and after treatment. Br J Dis Chest 73: 66–70

Spiteri M A, Millar A B, Pavia D et al 1988 Subcutaneous adrenaline vs terbutaline in the treatment of acute severe asthma. Thorax 43: 19–23

Tenaillon A, Salmona J P, Burdin M 1983 Continuous positive airway pressure in asthma. Am Rev Respir Dis 127: 658

Tinkelman D G, Webb C S, Vanderpool G E et al 1986 The use of ketotifen in the prophylaxis seasonal allergic asthma. Ann Allerg 56: 213–217

Tokioka S, Saito S, Takahashi T et al 1992 Effectiveness of pressure support ventilation for mechanical ventilatory support in patients with status asthmaticus. Acta Anaesthesiol Scand 36: 5–9

Totaro R J, Raper R 1994 Lactic acidosis post cardiopulmonary bypass. Randomised prospective study of adrenaline and noradrenaline as causative factors. Anaes Int Care 11: 220

Tuxen D V 1989 Detrimental effects of positive end-expiratory pressure during controlled mechanical ventilation of patients with severe airflow obstruction. Am Rev Respir Dis 140: 5–9

Tuxen D V, Lane S 1987 The effects of ventilatory pattern on hyperinflation, airway pressures and circulation in mechanical ventilation of patients with severe airflow obstruction. Am Rev Respir Dis 136: 872–879

Tuxen D V, Oh T E 1990 Acute severe asthma. In: Oh T E (ed) Intensive Care Manual. 3rd edn. Butterworths, Sydney, pp 192–199

Tuxen D V, Williams T J, Scheinkestel C D et al 1992 Use of a measurement of pulmonary hyperinflation to control the level of mechanical ventilation in patients with severe asthma. Am Rev Respir Dis 146(5): 1136–1142

Tuxen D V, Day B, Scheinkestel C D 1993a Letter to the Editor regarding Acute respiratory failure neuropathy: a variant of critical illness polyneuropathy. Crit Care Med 21: 1986

Tuxen D V, Williams T J, Scheinkestel C D et al 1993b Limiting dynamic hyperinflation in mechanically ventilated patients with severe asthma reduces complications. Anaes Int Care 21 (5): 718

Van der Touw T, Tully A, Amis T C et al 1993 Cardiorespiratory consequences of expiratory chest wall compression during mechanical ventilation and severe hyperinflation. Crit Care Med 21: 1908–1914

Wasserfallen J B, Schaller M D, Feihl F et al 1990 Sudden asphyxic asthma: A distinct entity? Am Rev Respir Dis 142: 108–111

Webb A K, Bilton A H, Hanson G C 1979 Severe bronchial asthma requiring ventilation. A review of 20 cases and advice on management. Postgrad Med J 55: 161–170

Weng J T, Smith D E, Graybar G B et al 1984 Hypotension secondary to air trapping treated with expiratory flow retard. Anesthesiology 60: 350–353

Westerman D E, Benatar S R, Potgieter P D et al 1979 Identification of the high-risk asthmatic patient. Experience with 39 patients undergoing ventilation for status asthmaticus. Am J Med 66: 565–572

Williams N E, Crook J W 1968 The practical management of severe status asthmaticus. Lancet i: 1081–1083

Williams T J, O'Hehir R E, Czarny D et al 1988 Acute myopathy in severe asthma treated with intravenously administered corticosteroids. Am Rev Respir Dis 137: 460–463

Williams T J, Tuxen D V, Scheinkestel C D et al 1992 Risk factors for morbidity in mechanically ventilated patients with acute severe asthma. Am Rev Respir Dis 146(3): 607–615

Woodcock A A, Johnson M A, Geddes D M 1983 Theophylline prescribing, serum concentrations, and toxicity. Lancet 2: 610–612

Outcome : short-term (28/7) mortality

- multiple risk-factors for 28/7 - mortality.

Interventions : marginal benefits only in certain patient groups →

- difficult to study if these groups are either small, or difficult to define.

Selection of patient groups -

1) LARGE database
2) SEVERITY SCORING
3) RISK ASSESSMENT

Knaus - overall assessment of patient risk

- model casting (physiological) severity scores can account for much of the variation in mortality between different ICU's. Increasingly possible to estimate prognosis of particular disease entities

- categorical definitions (e.g. "sepsis syndrome") - too broad, contain a range of severities

- study is more likely to show a benefit if the risk of death is high: an impact is more difficult to detect if there are a large no. of subjects with low risk (low "signal to noise ratio")

- potential for harm of a treatment is more important if the severity of the condition, the risk of death, is low

9. The use of severity scoring in clinical investigations of seriously ill patients

W. A. Knaus

INTRODUCTION

The repeated failure of recent clinical trials of immunotherapy to demonstrate reductions in mortality dramatically illustrates the complex new challenges associated with the design and completion of clinical trials in seriously ill patients. One of the most important challenges is that seriously ill patients have multiple risk factors for short-term (e.g. 28-day) mortality, the most frequently used endpoint in current investigations. These many risk factors must be taken into consideration in order to correctly interpret the results of clinical trials and to measure benefit with assurance. Another challenge relates to the nature and potential impact of the new therapies being tested. Many new compounds, especially those directed at sepsis and inflammation, aim to modify intrinsic biological host responses (Bone 1991). This implies that the best indicators of drug efficacy may be patient characteristics rather than the primary disease process or, in the case of sepsis, the infecting organism. New pharmacological and biological approaches to treatment, such as immunotherapy, as well as others such as novel modes of mechanical ventilation or patient monitoring, may bring important, but marginal benefits only to certain subsets of seriously ill patients. These benefits can be difficult to detect using current methods of patient description. Finally, once a new therapy is available, deciding on the most efficient and appropriate use for an individual patient is an increasingly important, but difficult clinical judgement.

We believe these challenges require a new approach to the methods used to select patients for clinical trials and the appropriate methods for analysis. This chapter will describe how the use of large databases, severity scoring and risk assessment can address these challenges by improving patient identification, study entry criteria, trial design, data interpretation, and eventually, development of indications for the use of these new therapies.

BACKGROUND ON RISK FACTORS AND PREDICTIVE MODELS

The current challenges for new clinical evaluations are related to large changes in the type and severity of illness of hospitalized patients. We are treating more severely ill patients, at later stages of diseases, and the majority have complex illnesses, usually with both acute and chronic components. In response, the speciality of critical care medicine has pioneered the development of new methods of patient description, including measurement of severity of illness and incorporation of this, together with other patient characteristics into an overall assessment of patient risk (Knaus et al 1981, 1985, 1991a, 1991b). This capability has been made possible by the availability of large, contemporary, clinically-accurate databases along with more biologically appropriate statistical models (Knaus et al 1991a). These databases, combined with research over the past decade, have demonstrated that patient severity is best determined by measuring acute physiological abnormalities. Severity data, combined with a knowledge of patient age, chronic health status, primary disease, and length of time the patient was ill prior to treatment can be used to estimate mortality risk (Knaus et al 1991b).

Severity scoring or risk prediction (the terms will be used interchangeably in this chapter) has proved very useful for evaluating the utilization of intensive care units (ICUs) (Knaus et al 1993a). Current risk prediction models that incorporate severity measurement based on physiological derangement can account for the majority of variations found in outcome across different intensive care units (ICUs) (Knaus et al 1993a, Zimmerman at al 1993) and as a result it is now possible to monitor risk-adjusted outcomes among ICUs with a variety of different patient populations. Such risk assessments have been very useful in the evaluation of ICUs, as well as to refine intensive care utilization and are increasingly being recommended for use as adjuncts to clinical decision-making (Knaus et al 1991a). As a result of these efforts, the clinical databases are growing in size and it is now possible to collect data and outcomes from a large number of patients within specific diagnostic groups. These disease-specific predictions are becoming increasingly more accurate and are able to identify patients' acute risk for mortality throughout the entire range of severity of illness (Knaus et al 1993b). This capability, in turn, has implications for the design and evaluation of clinical trials.

CURRENT CHALLENGES IN CLINICAL TRIALS

Reliance on categorical definitions for patient identification

Clinical trials have necessarily relied on categorical, or textual descriptions for primary patient identification and eligibility, i.e. the inclusion and exclusion criteria. It is in the best interests of trial sponsors to try to make these definitions for eligibility clinically meaningful, inclusive and capable of capturing a significant proportion of the more severely ill patient population, i.e. those most at risk for the endpoint under study. In this way, it is hoped that patients will be reliably identified and that the power of the trial will be increased. For example, for a trial whose endpoint is mortality, the greater the proportion of patients enrolled in the study who are at risk of death, the greater the statistical power to detect a benefit of the experimental treatment. This also means that fewer patients will need to be enrolled, thereby saving costs. An additional advantage is that fewer patients who are at low risk for mortality will be exposed to any potential risk of the new treatment.

For example, recent trials of immunotherapy have used the categorical definition of sepsis syndrome as an entry criteria. This definition uses a combination of clinical signs and symptoms to identify candidates prospectively for clinical trials (Bone et al 1989, Ziegler at al 1991, Greenman et al 1991, Fisher et al 1994a,b). The categorical definition — sepsis syndrome — identifies patients with a mean mortality risk that is generally higher than that found among all patients hospitalized with sepsis, but there is a substantial variation in the placebo mortality rate between studies. Moreover, it has been demonstrated recently that the definition of sepsis syndrome is neither very sensitive nor specific (Bone et al 1992, Knaus et al 1992) in regard to the level of risk of the patient. There are also many patients with a clinical diagnosis of sepsis who fail to meet the precise physiological criteria and are excluded from trials (Knaus et al 1992).

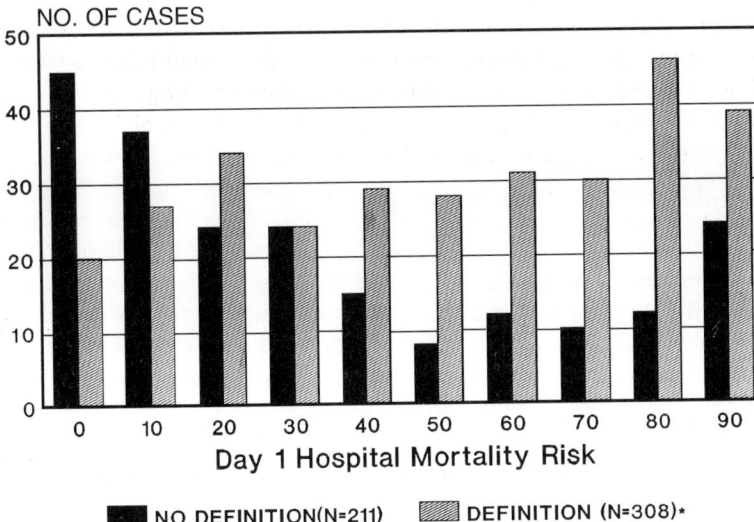

Fig. 9.1 Distribution of predicted risk of hospital mortality for patients with a definition of sepsis syndrome or with no definition of sepsis syndrome for 519 ICU admissions with a clinical diagnosis of sepsis. Note the wide distribution of mortality risk. See Knaus et al 1992 for additional explanation. Reproduced with permission from Knaus et al 1992.

This raises two significant difficulties with regard to clinical studies. First, categorical definitions capture only a portion of patients with clinical or physiological characteristics consistent with a particular diagnosis such as sepsis and who may benefit from a new treatment. Second, there is a wide risk distribution of patients enrolled. This is illustrated in Figures 9.1 and 9.2. Figure 9.1 examines the risk distribution of 519 patients admitted to ICUs with a clinical diagnosis of sepsis according to whether or not they met the categorical criteria for sepsis syndrome. The figure illustrates that this categorical definition frequently excludes clinically septic patients from treatment who, in terms of risk for hospital mortality and other important characteristics, may be identical to those patients accepted. This figure also illustrates that patients with a wide distribution of severity and risks, ranging from 0 to 99%, meet the entry criteria and qualify for trials using sepsis syndrome criteria. Figure 9.2 shows the distribution according to risk of mortality for patients with sepsis syndrome who also meet criteria for septic shock. While the addition of a criteria for shock shifts the distribution of patients to the more severely ill, there is still a wide distribution of individual risks (Fig. 9.2). These findings are true regardless of the categorical definition chosen — sepsis syndrome, sepsis syndrome with shock, or adult respiratory distress syndrome with severe hypoxemia (Knaus et al 1994). Each of these categories will contain patients with a wide range of severity and predicted risk of death. For example, Figure 9.3 shows the wide risk distribution for patients meeting two different physiological (PaO_2/FiO_2) categorical cut-offs for acute lung injury (Knaus et al 1994). Similar figures have been produced for other categorical definitions.

Variations in baseline mortality risk

This variation in the distribution of baseline mortality risk explains the now widely recognized observation that the same categorical definitions can result in large differences in the placebo death rates in different trials. Since many trials involving seriously ill patients are designed and sized to detect a reduction in mortality based on the anticipated death rate in the placebo group, the admission of many patients at low risk of death can reduce this rate. This may make it impossible to detect a significant improvement in mortality from a beneficial treatment, despite having enrolled the expected number of patients. For example, the ability of recent clinical trials of immunotherapy to detect efficacy may have been reduced, since reliance on the sepsis syndrome definition permitted the admission of a substantial numbers of patients at low risk of death.

Another reason variations in severity of illness are important is that the relative benefit of many new therapies may be related directly to the underlying risk of the patient. In general, the more sick the patient, the more likely they will be to benefit from the therapy. If the patient is at low risk

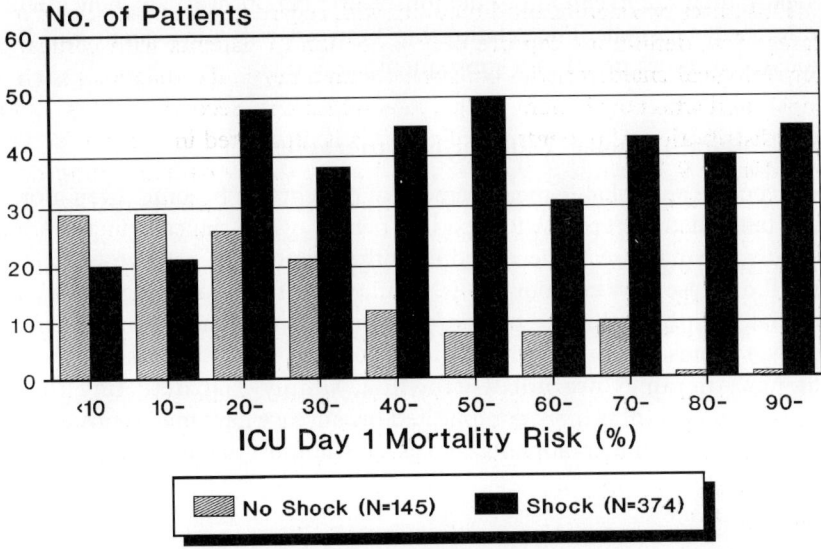

Fig. 9.2 Distribution of predicted risk of hospital mortality for 519 ICU admissions with a clinical diagnosis of sepsis according to whether they met a categorical definition for shock, defined as a systolic blood pressure ≤90 mmHg or a mean blood pressure ≤60 mmHg. Note the wide distribution of mortality risk.

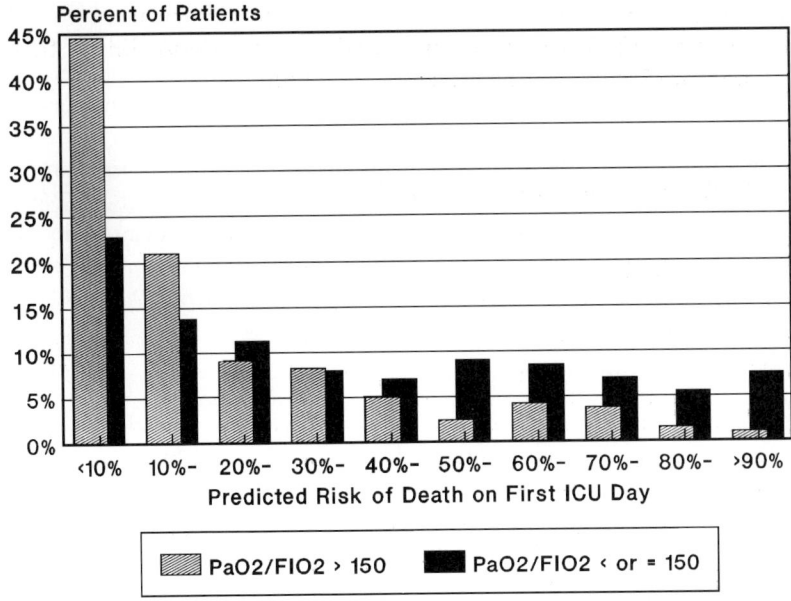

Fig. 9.3 Distribution of predicted risk of hospital mortality for 423 ICU admissions with acute lung injury and a hospital discharge diagnosis of adult respiratory distress syndrome according to whether they meet criteria for moderate (PaO_2/FiO_2 ratio >150) or severe (PaO_2/FiO_2 ratio <150) hypoxaemia. See Knaus et al 1994a for additional explanation. Reproduced with permission from Knaus et al 1994a.

of death, then the likelihood of demonstrating benefit with any new inter-vention will be small. The relationship between risk and benefit will be discussed in more detail in a subsequent section.

Small 'signal-to-noise' ratio for new therapies

The accurate and reliable measurement of patient risk becomes even more important when therapies whose patient benefit, while clinically important, is relatively small are to be tested. In other words, the relative effect or 'signal' of these new compounds is small, while the underlying 'noise' in the trial, i.e. the influence of confounding but unalterable patient risk factors, such as severity, co-morbidities, etc. is large. This does not mean that new therapies are not worthwhile, simply that detecting their incremental bene-fit is more complicated because we have made substantial progress with existing treatments, and as a result most therapies are working at 'the margin'.

Risk, randomization balance, and power to detect drug effects

If a trial's entry criteria permit selection of patients at widely varying levels of risk, randomization can fail to distribute the many risk factors equally among the treatment groups; this may reduce or eliminate the ability of the study to detect the impact of new therapy. This problem is substantial in Phase II clinical trials where sample sizes may be small and multiple treatment arms are needed for dose range determination. Phase II trials with limited numbers of patients frequently have imbalances in important patient risk factors between arms of the trial that can confound any con-clusions about the effects of the drug. This can lead to interpretation er-rors with under- or overestimation of potential benefit (Fisher et al 1994b) and/or harmful effects. Mis-estimation of treatment effects can seriously skew the hypothesis generated from the initial clinical trials for validation in subsequent larger (and costlier) Phase III studies (Fisher et al 1994a).

Assessing the potential for harm

Another major concern with evaluations of some new therapies is their potential for harm. A recent meta-analysis of cholesterol-lowering drugs, for example, suggested that when low-risk patients are treated, they have an increased death rate (Davey Smith et al 1993). With regard to the evalu-ation of immunotherapy, experimental animal data suggests that the de-gree of the biological or inflammatory response to disease may be appropriate and beneficial at certain levels, but inadequate or too high at others (Dinarello et al 1993). In sepsis, for example, an appropriate level of interleukin-1, tumour necrosis factor, and other pro-inflammatory cytokines is essential for an adequate inflammatory response to combat infection and for tissue healing (Cross et al 1989, Schwab et al 1991, Fisher et al 1992, Airua et al 1993, Mancilla et al 1993). On the other hand, it also has been demonstrated that these mediators can cause tissue damage and multiple organ failure. The administration of new immunotherapy or biological response modifiers ideally should therefore take into account the magnitude and appropriateness of the immunological response, although currently we do not have readily available, accurate and reliable markers of the magnitude and appropriateness of this host response. Measuring the level of the mediators would be a good starting point, but this is limited by a short half-life, intermittent appearance in the blood and extensive tissue compartmentalization (Hack et al 1989, Waage et al 1989, Calandra et al 1990, Hamilton et al 1992, Casey et al 1993, Dinarello et al 1993, Dinarello & Cannon 1993). Concurrently, concerns have been expressed regarding the optimal timing and duration of some forms of anticytokine therapy, as well as the appropriate selection of patients (Warren et al 1992, Wenzel 1992).

ROLE FOR DATABASES AND RISK MODELS

Identification of patients - database (ICNARC?)

Patient identification and trial design

Recent advances in the storage and retrieval of clinically-accurate data have resulted in the development of large contemporary databases. From these objective information is now available regarding various patient groups which might be considered for investigation. The utility of this prior knowledge for clinical researchers is substantial and broad (see Knaus et al 1994b). The major applications of clinical databases in clinical trial planning and design are listed below:

- Study population profile
- Estimate recruitment rates
- Pre-specify subgroup identification
- Select endpoints (mortality, morbidity, resources)
- Refine inclusion/exclusion criteria; optimize event frequency
- Estimate sample size; power calculations
- Select time points
- Choose most appropriate statistical models
- Identify rates of adverse events

Using the steps outlined below, these databases can be used as large contemporary control groups which can be used to investigate, confirm and compile risk factors for outcome. As the size and representativeness of these databases expand, efforts at risk prediction can be revisited and improved. If similar data collection procedures are followed consistently, then as indicated below the risk prediction may also enable comparison of the efficacy of combinations of new therapeutic approaches.

Step 1   Apply exact study selection criteria, e.g. sepsis syndrome, severe sepsis, SIRS to large clinically-accurate database of severely ill hospitalized patients to select cohort of patients for risk assessment.

Step 2   Analyse cohort of patients meeting exact study entry criteria to create comprehensive risk assessment model. Investigate various approaches to modeling and risk assessment.

Step 3   Develop and validate risk model prior to analysis of clinical trial data.

Step 4   Apply independent risk prediction on patients at time of study qualification. Use risk assessment to check for imbalances in risk between treatment and control groups, and to investigate relationship between risk and drug efficacy.

Step 5   Use results from clinical trial to refine entry criteria for next trial, or to develop indications for use.

Note   As clinical trials are performed and the clinical databases described in Step 1 expand, Steps 2–4 can be repeated to improve risk prediction, and to investigate indications for specific compounds or combinations of compounds.

Risk factors and risk models

[handwritten annotation: BASELINE risk in prospective studies 'Qualitative risk prediction' → (accurate) prospective models]

Simultaneous advances in the ability to analyse and model risk factors for outcome from an acute illness, like sepsis, have created a new technical and intellectual basis for risk adjustment in clinical evaluations of new therapeutic compounds. Databases can also be used to develop predictive models or equations that are extremely accurate for predicting baseline risk of patients currently being enrolled into clinical trials (Knaus et al 1993b). Quantitative risk predictions are more accurate for selecting a group of patients with a predictable death rate when compared to categorical definitions, such as sepsis syndrome or the degree of organ system dysfunction (Goris et al 1985, Bone et al 1992).

Risk predictions also describe all patients on a continuum of severity from very low through intermediate to high (Figs 9.1, 9.2, 9.3). Compared to subgroup analyses using organ system dysfunction definitions, which apply to approximately two-thirds of most patients entered into clinical trials (Greenman et al 1991, Ziegler et al 1991, Fisher et al 1994a), an analytic approach based on risk assessment analyses all patients randomized.

In the future, risk prediction may also be useful for providing some insight regarding the degree of the inflammatory response. There is some initial evidence that severity scoring, as determined by the patient's acute physiological status at the time of the patient's entry to the trial, correlates with cytokine activity, as measured by IL-6 levels or soluble TNF receptors (Damas et al 1992, Werden, personal communication). As such, risk scoring may represent a useful adjunct to the determination of mediator levels or other measures of the host response. One could imagine, for example, that patients at low risk of death could have comparatively low (and appropriate) levels of mediators. Knowing this, the clinician would leave well alone. In another scenario, a patient may have an exaggerated immune response and might, therefore, benefit from mediator blockade. Some patients at high risk of death may have an inadequate inflammatory response and might benefit from augmentation of their immune system. The simultaneous measurement of mediator levels (or other measures of inflammatory activity), in conjunction with risk assessment may help to describe these relationships. Such initial efforts are now underway (Knaus et al 1995) and we hope others will soon follow.

APPLICATION OF RISK SCORING AS ENTRY CRITERIA FOR CLINICAL TRIALS

A good way to illustrate this concept might be to follow an example of how such an approach might be used to design and complete an analysis of a new compound for patients with sepsis. As previously discussed, sepsis is an excellent example of a disease that contains patients at various levels of risk as a result of a wide variety of risk factors, i.e. the severity of the acute physiological response, the origin of the infection, the length of time prior to treatment, and the presence or absence of co-morbidities (Knaus et al 1992, 1994b). This multiplicity of risk factors means that there really is no typical patient with sepsis entering a clinical trial. Candidates can vary from a young patient with a relatively uncomplicated urinary tract infection to an elderly patient recovering from an abdominal aortic aneurysm repair who develops an intra-abdominal abscess. Such patients have very different risk profiles and may respond very differently to new adjunctive therapies. The interaction of these many different risk factors for an individual patient results in the wide variation in risk distribution previously discussed (Figs 9.1, 9.2 and 9.3).

Risk thresholds as entry criteria (patient identification)

The calculation of a risk prediction at the time of recruitment would increase the power of a trial to detect a significant clinical benefit by quantitatively selecting those patients most likely to respond favourably as illustrated in Figure 9.4. This approach also enables the investigator to analyse all patients randomized, thereby reducing or eliminating the need for subgroup analysis and multiple testing.

To address this problem of patient diversity, we recently developed a mortality risk model for patients with sepsis syndrome who are currently entered into clinical trials for immunotherapy (Knaus et al 1993b). This independent risk model was created by assembling, from a large dataset, a cohort of 1195 patients who met criteria for sepsis syndrome. These

[handwritten annotation: Increased relative benefit — high-risk patients ?]

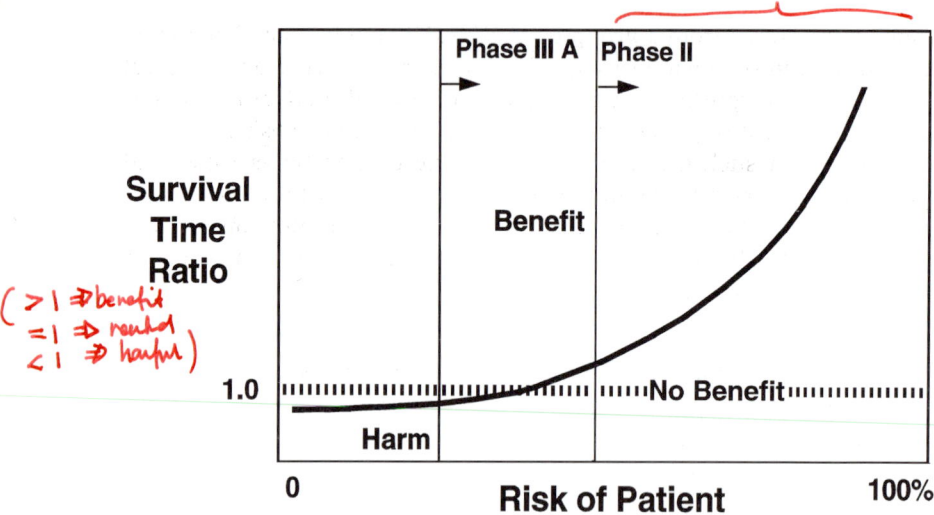

[handwritten annotation: (>1 ⇒ benefit / =1 ⇒ neutral / <1 ⇒ harmful)]

Fig. 9.4 Relationship between baseline risk of death of patient on admission to a clinical trial and relative benefit as measured by increases in the survival time ratio of patients who receive placebo versus treatment. Patients with low baseline risks receive little benefit and could theoretically be harmed by new therapy. Relative benefit of treatment increases directly with risk. Phase II trials that wish to maximize power to detect efficacy of new compound could screen and admit patients that meet risk criteria. Once a Phase II trial had demonstrated efficacy, a subsequent Phase III trial could use a lower risk threshold (Phase IIIA), if there were safety concerns at low risk. If there were no safety concerns, the trial could enrol patients independent of risk. See text for further explanation.

[handwritten annotation: (What is the evidence that the curve has this shape? None?) (Relative power (to reduce mortality) related to risk (% mortality).)]

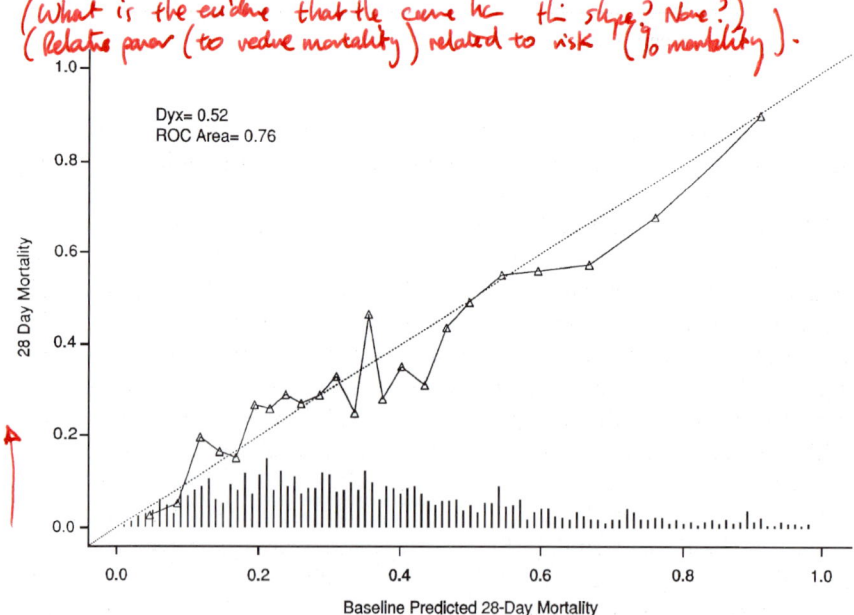

[handwritten annotation: Risk frequency]

Fig. 9.5 Relationship between predicted baseline risk of 28-day mortality with sepsis-specific risk model and actual 28-day mortality for 1195 patients who met criteria for sepsis syndrome. Each represents 50 patients. The diagonal line is the line of identity which would represent perfect agreement between predicted and observed 28-day mortality. The histogtram provides the risk of distribution of patients. See Knaus et al 1993 for additional explanation. (Reproduced with permission from Knaus et al 1993.

patients were drawn from a group of 65 000 ICU admissions. The model uses information on a wide variety of risk factors, i.e. acute physiological abnormalities, diagnosis, length of time in hospital, and other patient factors to risk stratify patients who meet the traditional sepsis syndrome entry criteria for such trials. Table 9.1 lists the prognostic variables and their relative importance within the prognostic model. Each of these prognostic factors has been identified as being influential in previous studies (Knaus et al 1993b). What our model did was to assemble them into a summary index of prognosis.

Table 9.1 Listing of prognostic factors in sepsis. All prognostic factors were obtained from examining 1195 patients meeting clinical criteria for sepsis syndrome. Relative importance of each variable is expressed as its contribution to the overall predictive model. See Knaus et al 1993b for additional explanation.

General APACHE III factors	Relative importance*
Acute physiology score	71.5%
Age	5.7%
Chronic health (cirrhosis)	0.4%
Disease	6.3%
Lead time (no. days in hosp/ICU)	5.2%
Sepsis-specific physiology	
Serum pH	6.3%
White blood cell count	4.6%

* As percentage of total chi-square

The predictive accuracy of this sepsis-specific risk model is tailored specifically for patients meeting certain entry criteria for clinical trials and, used for this purpose, is substantially more accurate than the general APACHE III and APACHE II equations, which are for all patients with sepsis admitted to an ICU. In Figure 9.5, the ability of this model to place patients accurately at varying levels of risk is illustrated on the observational database of 1195 patients used to create the predictive model. This figure also provides the risk distribution of the patients. Note that once again patients meeting categorical criteria for sepsis syndrome have varying levels of risks, with many patients being at low risk of 28-day mortality. This predictive model enables the investigator to design a more targeted approach that would reduce or eliminate low risk patients from trials. Specifically, after initial Phase I testing, a targeted Phase II trial could use a risk threshold for mortality that would include patients at highest risk for mortality. This approach would increase the ability to detect efficacy of the drug by increasing the statistical power of the trial. As illustrated in Figure 9.4, the relative power to detect efficacy is directly related to risk in the control group and eliminating patients at low risk using the sepsis-specific risk model would ensure a sufficient baseline mortality rate for efficacy testing.

The other benefit of this approach would be that patients at low risk would not need to be exposed to the new drug until there was some evidence of efficacy. It appears that in testing new compounds there is the possibility that we have increased death rates in some subgroups (Fisher et al 1993). Such results may be inevitable given our limited knowledge of these compounds, but the approach illustrated in Figure 9.4 deserves consideration for its potential to both increase power for detecting efficacy and to reduce the risks for patients who enter early clinical evaluations of new therapies.

Withhold new Rx from low-risk patients - phase II trials.

Safety assessment and monitoring

One important goal of initial Phase II evaluations is to evaluate safety. How would a risk assessment approach affect our ability to test safety? First, it is important to appreciate that most Phase II evaluations enrol relatively small numbers of patients (Fisher et al 1993, 1994b) and that, therefore, only serious safety problems, especially in regard to mortality, will be detected. Most Phase II studies are also designed to achieve a high placebo death rate, but categorical entry criteria permit the enrolment of substantial numbers of patients at low baseline risk of death. This can decrease the power of the study to detect adverse effects, since the frequency of the outcome is low.

An approach to Phase II as suggested in Figure 9.4 would result in a trial design with more power to detect a reduction in mortality. This approach would therefore permit clinical evaluations to be halted at a relatively early stage in a drug's development with greater confidence that efficacy was not present. Obviously, if the initial Phase II trial was equivocal, a repeat trial targeted on the risk spectrum most likely to be of benefit could follow. Large scale clinical testing, however, would require more definitive evidence of efficacy before exposing large numbers of low-risk patients to the new compound. On the other hand, if the evidence from an initial trial was positive, then the initial Phase III evaluation could expand the risk profile for admission. If there were no safety concerns then the next evaluation could adopt an unrestricted entry criteria to fully evaluate the compound using all potential candidates for the drug. Alternatively, a restriction on risk could still remain part of the trial's entry criteria (Phase IIIA on Figure 9.4) and might, eventually, become part of labelling for indications for use.

Choice of appropriate analytic model

Another major advantage that risk prediction drawn from large clinically-accurate databases provides is an enhanced ability to choose the most appropriate statistical model and analytic plan. Because so little is known about the exact mechanism and duration of action of many of the new

Modely – Cox proportional hazard model – equal efficacy on safe period
– accelerated failure time models – efficacy greater initially

SEVERITY SCORING IN THE SERIOUSLY ILL   203

compounds now undergoing human testing, traditional statistical models, such as the Cox proportional hazard or the accelerated failure time generalized Wilcoxin models, have been the primary analytic models used in initial trials (Gore et al 1984, Greenman et al 1991, Ziegler et al 1991). While the choice of an analytic model may be of only passing interest to a clinical investigator, all these mathematical models contain assumptions regarding how the patient will respond to the new therapy. The Cox proportional hazards model, for example, makes the assumption that the new therapy will be just as successful in reducing mortality the 27th day following drug administration as it was on the first or second. This is why it is used frequently in clinical trials of cancer chemotherapy where the beneficial effect of treatment on survival is prolonged over months or years.

In contrast, the Wilcoxin and other models are collectively termed *accelerated failure time* models. They assume that the impact of the therapy will be greater immediately following its administration, and then will fade quickly over time (Lawless 1982). Data from a number of clinical trials of immunotherapy in sepsis and shock suggests that this may indeed be the case (Greenman et al 1991, Ziegler et al 1991, Fisher et al 1993, 1994a). Some of the compounds tested appear to lower mortality immediately following infusion and then maintain an increased survival rate over time. There are a number of such accelerated failure time models from which to choose. Choosing the statistical model that most closely replicates the mechanism of action of a new compound is essential. A model whose assumptions do not match the data may underestimate the value of a new compound. Fortunately, with large contemporary clinical databases, the appropriateness of different statistical models can be more carefully evaluated before actual trial data are collected (Knaus et al 1993b).

For example, most trials within a specific disease area, such as sepsis or ARDS, use very similar entry criteria. These criteria can be applied to a contemporary database of seriously ill patients and a cohort of patients isolated that will be very similar to those that will be enrolled in the trial. The timing or pattern of mortality in this population can then be studied. If, as in sepsis, most deaths occur relatively soon following study entry, then a statistical model can be pre-specified for the study's analytic plan. There are a number of ways the fit or appropriateness of a model can be tested but description of these techniques is beyond the scope of this chapter. The important concept, however, is that the analytic approach can be tailored to the type of patients being studied.

Detecting drug efficacy — risk relationships

The use of risk assessment also provides the opportunity to test for drug efficacy-risk interactions. If, as previously illustrated, there is a direct relationship between patient risk and drug efficacy (Fig. 9.4), then specification of this relationship as part of the primary analytic plan, will increase statistical power to detect drug efficacy. The pre-specification on the analytic model, the risk-adjustment technique and model, along with an interaction between new therapy and baseline risk is a very different approach than that currently followed by most trials of new compounds (Greenman et al 1991, Ziegler et al 1991, Fisher et al 1993, 1994b).

Most of these trials have been designed from scratch, assuming little prior knowledge of patient risk factors or appropriate statistical models. This has frequently resulted in a failure to demonstrate a benefit for all patients treated, the intent-to-treat principle, with benefit limited to a retrospectively defined subgroup (Greenman et al 1991). This subgroup then becomes the focus of a new confirmatory trial which frequently fails to confirm efficacy. These failures could have been due to either actual failure of the compound to reduce mortality or the inability to detect efficacy, because multiple testing of the original trial dataset resulted in identification of an inconsistent group of patients (Warren et al 1992, Wenzel 1992). Prior risk assessment can help standardize patient identification and avoid this problem (Mills 1993).

Retrospectively defined benefit to subgroups often illusory. Minimize with false +ve's. Prior risk assessment?

Point mortality versus survival time as end-points

Twenty-eight day mortality traditionally has been used as the end-point of most trials in the critically ill. Mortality end-points are problematic because the exact time period chosen, i.e. 14, 28, 30, 45, 60 days is a relatively arbitrary choice. A death on day 27 is a failure, but a death on day 29 is a success. The exact day chosen can influence the statistical significance of the result because the P value varies according to the exact distribution of the deaths. The exact day of death can be influenced by the exact timing of DNR orders. In response, some trials are using survival time — a continuous measure — as the primary end-point. Survival time uses the entire length of time the patients in the control group survive compared to placebo. Survival time has the advantage that it mirrors the likely mechanism of action of many new compounds under testing, i.e. improvements in outcome as the result of prolongation of survival through the initial inflammatory cascade. Survival time also requires fewer patients to demonstrate statistical evidence of efficacy and it correlates with mortality. Survival time can also be influenced by decisions to limit or reduce therapy, but not as severely as point mortality. The disadvantage of survival time is that it can achieve statistical significance by prolonging survival for a few days without substantially improving the patient's final outcome. This is why we recommend that if a statistically significant increase in survival time is used as the major end-point of clinical evaluations, there should also be an associated clinically important improvement in short-term, i.e. 28-day mortality. There is also a discussion regarding changes in the exact timing of any proposed mortality end-point. While, as mentioned, 28-day mortality is an historical rather than scientific choice, its use in virtually all pre-

Survival time — statistically can be sh important, but may be unrelated to final outcome.

vious clinical trials in sepsis will give it a continued presence. This will make future trials challenging, but mortality at any given time point, i.e. 7, 14, 28 or 60-day is preferable to mortality at ICU or hospital discharge. Both of these end-points are arbitrary and vary greatly among individual hospitals and across different countries. Because of these variations, the use of either ICU or hospital discharge is not recommended.

Changes in risk scores as end-points

As the number of new compounds increases, and especially after one or more new drugs are approved for use, design of clinical trials will become even more complex. If a new product is determined to be broadly, albeit marginally, efficacious, it may be adopted as the standard of care and placebo patients will become very scarce. As a result, it will be increasingly difficult to rely on short-term mortality or even survival time as the primary end-point, since very large sample sizes will be required to demonstrate an impact on these end-points. In these situations, looking at improvements in health status or changes in risk scores, i.e. physiological responses over time, may be essential as sensitive initial guides to the efficacy of new compounds. Improvements in daily risk scores would be a very sensitive way of detecting drug activity, and certainly more sensitive than counting the number of organ system failures. The acute improvement of risk scores over time between the placebo and treatment arms of a clinical trial may also be an early indication of a new compound's efficacy. Acute physiological changes have been closely correlated to ultimate short-term outcome (Wagner et al 1994). As is the case with survival time, short-term mortality rates can be simultaneously examined for trends toward improvement in the treatment versus placebo group but evidence of biological activity can reside with daily risk reduction as a clinically meaningful end-point.

Application of severity scoring to a recent anticytokine clinical trial — a case example

A risk assessment approach was recently prospectively applied to a randomized clinical trial of an anticytokine interleukin-1 receptor antagonist (rhIL-1ra) (Fisher et al 1994a). This was a trial of 893 patients randomized to placebo (N = 302), low dose 1 mg/kg/h (N = 298), or high dose 2 mg/kg/h rhIL-1ra (N = 293). The trial used traditional sepsis syndrome entry criteria. The prespecified sepsis-specific risk prediction previously described was applied to the trial data and was able to accurately risk stratify and predict outcome for patients receiving placebo with a predicted 28-day mortality rate of 35%, compared to 34% observed. The discriminatory power of this model was identical in the data from this independent trial to its performance in the original database (ROC = 0.76 in both)

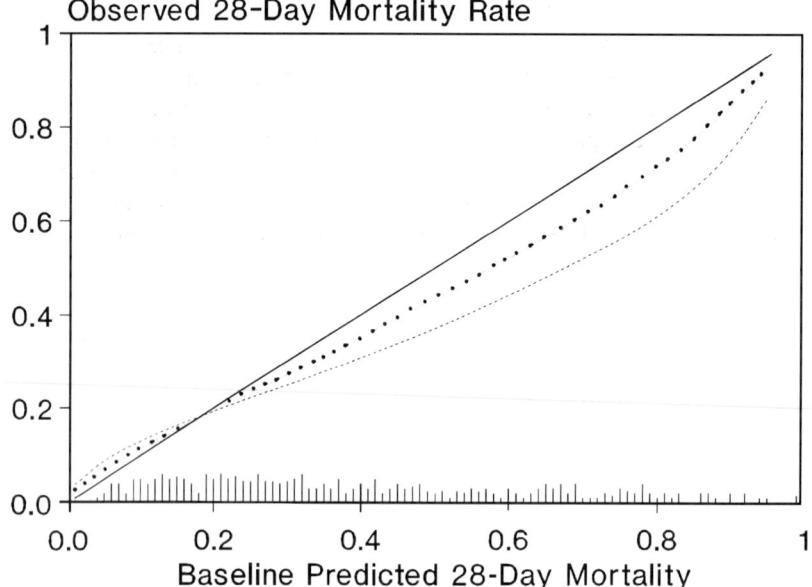

Fig. 9.6   Observed versus predicted risk of 28-day mortality outcomes of three treatment groups in the Phase III evaluation of rhIL-1ra using log-normal regression analysis. This analysis assumes linearity for dose and baseline patient risk. Placebo [——] is contrasted with low [...] and high [----] dose treatment arms. The histogram demonstrates the distribution of patients. See Fisher et al 1994a for additional explanation.

(Fig. 9.6). The distribution of individual patient risks was also similar in the trial to that observed in the independent database used to create the predictive model. Risk distribution was also equivalent across the three treatment groups (Fisher et al 1994a).

When the risk distribution was applied to the trial data using a log-normal analytic model and specifying an interaction between the patient's baseline risk estimate and the efficacy of rhIL-1ra, a significant increase in survival time was demonstrated for all patients randomized (N = 893, log-normal $P < 0.02$). As anticipated from the relationship illustrated in Figure 9.4, however, benefit was not uniform for all patients. Patients at low baseline risk of death did not receive benefit from rhIL-1ra (Fig. 9.6). A retrospective analysis limited to those patients at or above a 24% predicted risk of mortality at study entry demonstrated a very significant benefit from rhIL-1ra (N=580, log-normal $P=0.005$). For patients at or above a 40% predicted risk of 28-day mortality, there was 95% confidence that the patient would have an increase in survival time. Such patients would make good candidates for a Phase II trial that would focus on high risk patients (Fig. 9.4).

The results from this trial further demonstrated that while traditional categorical descriptors, such as having one or more organ system failures, also identified groups of patients with significant increases in survival time

(N=563, log-normal P=0.009) individual risk assessment was more specific. Patients with three of four predefined organ system failures — adult respiratory distress syndrome, disseminated intravascular coagulation, or renal dysfunction — had significant increases in survival time using rhIL-1ra. For all of these patients as well as for all patients with one or more organ systems in failure, significant increases in survival time were limited to patients at or above a 24% predicted risk of 28-day mortality as described in Table 9.2. These results are also summarized for patients meeting criteria for the adult respiratory distress syndrome in Table 9.3. In each case, patients defined as being at less than 24% risk of mortality either have no reduction in 28-day mortality or an increase in placebo death rate compared to high dose rhIL-1ra (Fisher et al 1994a). In other words, all of the benefit observed in these subgroups appeared to be limited to patients at 24% predicted risk or above. These results demonstrate the potential value of an individual predicted risk of mortality, as compared to categorical definitions in defining patients most likely to benefit from new therapies.

Table 9.2 Relationship between predicted risk of 28-day mortality on admission to randomized clinical trial of recombinant human interleukin-1 receptor antagonist (rhIL-1ra) and presence of one of four predefined organ system failures. Clinical benefit, as determined by increases in survival time, were limited to patients at or above a 24% predicted risk. See Fisher et al 1994a for additional explanation.

Risk	Placebo	IL-1ra 2.0 mg/kg/h	P-value
All (563)	43%	33%	0.009
≥0.24 (411)	52%	36%	0.002
<0.24 (152)	18%	24%	0.67

Table 9.3 Relationship between predicted risk of 28-day mortality and benefit for patients randomized to clinical trial of recombinant human interleukin-1 receptor antagonist (rhIL-1ra) with adult respiratory distress syndrome. Clinical benefit, as determined by increases in survival time, were limited to patients at or above a 24% predicted risk. See Fisher et al 1994a for additional explanation

Risk	Placebo	IL-1ra 2.0 mg/kg/h	P-value
All (223)	49%	34%	0.04
≥0.24 (150)	60%	35%	0.01
<0.24 (73)	21%	32%	0.54

Practical implications of calculating risk scores

When a risk assessment approach to the design and analysis of clinical trials is presented, a frequent question concerns complexity of risk evaluation (Knaus et al 1993b). Is there not a simpler way of identifying patients for entry to trials? First, it is important to emphasize that all of the information necessary for the calculation of the risk estimates described here are already being collected routinely for all patients in most critical care units (see Table 9.1). In the time that it takes a research associate to determine whether a patient meets entry criteria for a clinical trial, a risk estimate can be obtained either through direct calculation of a score or with a hand-held calculator or lap-top personal computer. The calculation is straight forward and uncomplicated. In the near future, the ease and availability of risk calculation will further improve as computerized clinical information systems and electronic interfaces make virtually all data collection and risk calculation electronic. The reluctance to calculate such estimates is also difficult to understand considering that conditions like sepsis involve multiple risk factors that confound subjective interpretations of patient prognosis (Knaus et al 1993b). Reducing patient description in these trials to simple definitions, such as shock or other organ system dysfunction is imprecise and may be misleading. As illustrated in Table 9.2, this has been the experience in most of the clinical trials completed to date, that have relied on simple descriptors of organ system failure (Greenman et al 1991, Ziegler et al 1991, Fisher et al 1993, 1994a).

Developing indications for use

A final argument for the value of risk calculations is their ability to develop precise and useful clinical indications for a particular therapeutic intervention. Earlier in this chapter, we illustrated how the relative benefit of a new compound varies according to the baseline risk of the patient (Fig. 9.4). The absolute mortality benefit for a particular patient is also dependent on risk. In every clinical trial there are patients who are not ill enough to benefit from therapy, there are those in the middle with a moderate degree of illness who can benefit to varying degrees, and there are those who are so ill that the likelihood of benefit diminishes. As illustrated in Figure 9.7, this relationship can be used to directly estimate the degree of benefit a patient is likely to receive from a new drug and the number of patients that would have to be treated to save one life (an estimate based on the patients' condition at the time the drug is being considered for administration). The results can be summarized on one graph, which can easily be referred to prior to a decision to use a new compound. For example, in Figure 9.7, one can estimate potential benefit for future patients who might be considered candidates for this therapy. For a patient with a 50% predicted baseline risk of 28-day mortality, an estimated 10% reduction in 28-day mortality was observed in the clinical trial. This implies that one life would be saved for every 10 such patients treated.

Such a presentation provides information to the prescribing clinician, but not in rigid and inflexible indications for drug utilization. Although the risk model accurately summarizes risk there are other clinical factors not in the model which may influence a particular patients' ability to benefit from a drug. This implies that the physician should combine the estimate, illustrated in Figure 9.7, with their own clinical judgement and personal observations prior to making a final decision to administer the drug. Institutions and groups interested in documenting the pattern of utilization would, however, be able to use the pre-treatment risk as an accurate descriptor of drug use and as a tool to enhance understanding of the drugs' incremental contribution. A 'number needed to treat estimate' also provides a common measurement method to compare the efficacy of new, existing, and competing approaches to care.

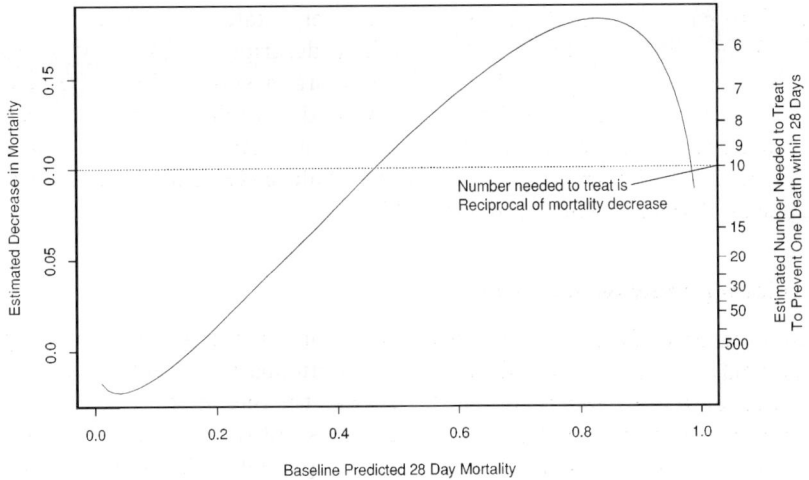

Fig. 9.7   Relationship between baseline risk of 28-day mortality for patients enrolled in a clinical trial and the estimated decrease in 28-day mortality. As patients' baseline predicted risk of 28-day mortality increases, the estimated decrease in mortality increases until the patient risk reaches approximately 90% when it begins to decrease. The estimated decrease in 28-day mortality rate can also be expressed as the number of patients needed to be treated in order to prevent one death. Such comparisons should be useful to compare relative efficacy of various new compounds. See text for further explanation.

FUTURE CONSIDERATIONS FOR CLINICAL TRIALS IN CRITICALLY ILL PATIENTS

With the recent failure of multiple attempts to reduce 28-day mortality with new immunotherapy agents it is appropriate to re-evaluate the basis of conducting these trials, along with their primary design and end-points.

First, it is clear that sepsis is a complex and challenging syndrome to study. It occurs in a wide variety of patients with a broad spectrum of severity ranging from a mild febrile illness to severe shock. Traditional entry criteria for these clinical trials include patients with all levels of disease severity. As previously emphasized, this variation in risk complicates the use of mortality as a primary end-point, since many patients do not have substantial risks of death.

From the results of recent trials, it is also becoming clear that single drug therapy may not be very powerful given the complex interplay of biological and host responses in sepsis. The clinical impact of each of these new compounds appears quite limited. This also makes use of mortality as a primary clinical end-point difficult.

An alternative approach could be for subsequent trials to use more sensitive measures of initial patient response as primary end-points. For example, use of the rapidity of recovery of physiological imbalance as measured by either change in acute physiology score or other severity index or acute risk of death would be good candidates for these primary end-points. Changes in longer term patient outcome could serve as secondary confirmatory indicators of therapeutic efficacy. Adoption of such an approach might permit the incremental introduction of biologically and clinically useful therapies. The use of the large contemporary clinical databases described in this chapter could increase the precision of such analytic efforts. These databases could also serve as a common language across trials and as contemporary controls that could be used to evaluate the value of combinations of model therapies. Perhaps in this way, the complex and deadly syndrome of sepsis may begin to be better understood and more effectively treated.

KEY POINTS FOR CLINICAL PRACTICE

- Categorical definitions, such as sepsis syndrome, sepsis with shock, specific organ system failure or dysfunction, ARDS, etc. include patients with a wide variety of baseline risk. They cannot be used to reliably estimate prognosis for either patient groups or individual patients.
- Critically ill patients enrolled in clinical trials have multiple risk factors for mortality and other outcomes. These risk factors can now be combined in predictive models that provide accurate baseline risk assessment for patients entered into clinical trials.
- There is a direct relationship between a patient's baseline risk and the efficacy of new and existing therapies. Knowledge of this relationship in the design, conduct, and analysis of clinical trials can improve the power of the trial to detect efficacy.

- Clinical trials using risk assessment as part of their analytic design can use the relationship between risk and efficacy to calculate an estimate of the clinical benefit anticipated from the new therapy. This can be used to compare the efficacy of new and existing therapies.
- Clinicians can use the estimated efficacy derived from risk assessment, in combination with their clinical judgement, to determine the appropriateness of new therapy for an individual patient.

REFERENCES

Aiura K, Gelfand J A, Barke J F et al 1993 Interleukin-1 (IL-1) receptor antagonist prevents staphylococcus epidermis-induced hypotension and reduces circulating levels of tumor necrosis factor and IL-1β in rabbits. Infect Immun 61: 3342–3350

Bone R C et al 1989 Sepsis syndrome: a valid clinical entity. Crit Care Med 17: 389–394

Bone R C 1991 The pathogenesis of sepsis. Ann Intern Med 115: 457–469

Bone R C, Balk R A, Cerra F B et al 1992 Definitions of sepsis and organ failure and guidelines for the use of innovative therapies in sepsis. Chest 101: 1644–1655

Calandra T, Baumgartner J D, Grau G E et al 1990 Prognostic values of tumor necrosis factor, interleukin–1, interferon-a, and interferon-y in the serum of patients with septic shock. J Infect Dis 161: 982–987

Casey L C, Balk R A, Bone R C 1993 Plasma cytokines and endotoxin levels correlate with survival in patients with sepsis syndrome. Ann Intern Med 119: 771–778

Cross A S, Sadoff J C, Kelly N et al 1989 Pretreatment with recombinant murine tumor necrosis factor α/cachectin and murine interleukin 1α protects mice from lethal bacterial infection. J Exp Med 169: 2021–2027

Damas P, Ledoux D, Nys M et al 1992 Cytokine serum level during severe sepsis in human IL-6 as a marker of severity. Ann Surg 213: 356–361

Davey Smith G, Song F, Sheldon T A 1993 Cholesterol lowering and mortality: The importance of considering initial level of risk. Br Med J 306: 1367–1373

Dinarello C A, Gelfand J A, Wolff S M 1993 Anticytokine strategies in the treatment of the systemic inflammatory response syndrome. JAMA 269: 1829–1835

Dinarello C A, Cannon C A 1993 Cytokine measurements in septic shock. Ann Intern Med 119: 853–854

Fischer E, Marano M A, VanZee K J et al 1992 Interleukin-1 receptor blockade improves survival and hemodynamic performance in E. coli septic shock, but fails to alter host responses to sublethal endotoxemia. J Clin Invest 89: 1551–1557

Fisher C J, Opal S M, Dhainaut J F et al 1993 Influence of an anti-tumor necrosis factor monoclonal antibody on cytokine levels in patients with sepsis. Crit Care Med 21: 318–327

Fisher C J, Dhainaut J F, Opal S M et al 1994a Recombinant human interleukin-1 receptor antagonist (rhIL-1ra) reduces the mortality of patients with sepsis syndrome as a function of disease severity: A randomized, double-blind, placebo-controlled trial. JAMA 271: 1836–1843

Fisher C J, Slotman G J, Opal S M et al 1994b Initial evaluation of human recombinant interleukin-1 receptor antagonist in the treatment of sepsis syndrome — randomized open-label, placebo controlled trial. Crit Care Med 22: 12–21

Gore S M, Pocock S J, Kerr G R 1984 Regression models and non-proportional hazards in the analysis of breast cancer survival. Applied Statistics 33: 176–195

Goris R J A, te BoeDherst T P A, Nuytinek J K S et al 1985 Multiple organ failure: generalized autodestructive inflammation. Arch Surg 120: 1109–1115

Greenman R L, Schein R M H, Martin M A et al 1991 A controlled clinical trial of E5 murine monoclonal IgM antibody to endotoxin in the treatment of gram-negative sepsis. JAMA 266: 1097–1102

Hack C E, DeGroot E R, Felt-Bersma R J F et al 1989 Increased plasma levels of interleukin-6 in sepsis. Blood 74: 1704–1710

Hamilton G, Hofbauer S, Hamilton B 1992 Endotoxin, TNF-alpha, interleukin-6 and parameters of the cellular immune system in patients with intra-abdominal sepsis. Scand J Infect Dis 24: 362–368

Knaus W A, Zimmerman J E, Wagner D P 1981 APACHE — acute physiology and chronic health evaluation: a physiologically based classification system. Crit Care Med 9: 591–597

Knaus W A, Draper E A, Wagner D P, Zimmerman J E 1985 APACHE II: a severity of disease classification system. Crit Care Med 13: 818–829

Knaus W A, Wagner D P, Lynn J 1991a Short-term mortality predictions for critically ill hospitalized adults: science and ethics. Science 254: 389–394

Knaus W A, Wagner D P et al 1991b The APACHE III prognostic system: Risk prediction of hospital mortality for critically ill hospitalized adults. Chest 100: 1619–1636

Knaus W A, Sun X, Nystrom P O, Wagner D P 1992 Evaluation of definitions for sepsis. Chest 101: 1656–1662

Knaus W A, Wagner D P, Zimmerman J E, Draper E A 1993a Variations in hospital mortality and length of stay from intensive care. Ann Intern Med 118: 753–761

Knaus W A, Harrell F E, Fisher C J et al 1993b The clinical evaluation of new drugs for sepsis. A prospective study design based on survival analysis. JAMA 270: 1233–1241

Knaus W A, Sun X, Hakim R B, Wagner D P 1994a Evaluation of definitions for adult respiratory distress syndrome. Am J Resp Crit Care Med 150: 311–317

Knaus W A, Wagner D P, Harrell F E, Draper E A 1994b What determines prognosis in sepsis? Evidence for a comprehensive individual patient risk assessment approach to the design and analysis of clinical trials. In: Reinhard K, Eyrich K, Sprung C (eds) Sepsis: current perspectives in pathophysiology and therapy. Springer-Verlag I.(18): 23–27

Knaus W A, Wagner D P, Harrell F E Jr, Hedstrom J S 1995 Risk assessment in recent clinical trials in sepsis/SIRS: lessons learned and future directions. J Endo Res 2: 169–175

Lawless J F 1982 Statistical models and methods for lifetime data. Wiley & Sons, New York

Mancilla J, Garcia P, Dinarello C A 1993 The interluekin-1 receptor antagonist can either reduce or enhance the lethality of Klebsiella pneumonial sepsis in newborn rates. Infect Immun 61: 926–932

Mills J L 1993 Data torturing. N Engl J Med 329: 1196–1199

Schwab J H, Anderle S K, Brown R R et al 1991 Pro- and anti-inflammatory roles of IL-1 in recurrence of bacterial cell wall-induced arthritis in rats. Infect Immun 59: 4436–4442

Waage A, Brandtzaeg P, Halstensen A et al 1989 The complex pattern of cytokines in serum from patients with meningococcal septic shock. J Exp Med 169: 333–338

Wagner D P, Knaus W A, Harrell F E et al 1994 Daily prognostic estimates for critically ill adults in intensive care units. Crit Care Med 22: 1359–1372

Warren H S, Danner R L, Munford R S 1992 Anti–endotoxin monoclonal antibodies. N Engl J Med 326: 1153-1156

Wenzel R P 1992 Anti-endotoxin monoclonal antibodies — a second look. N Engl J Med 326: 1151–1152

Werdan K personal communication

Ziegler E J, Fisher C J, Sprung C L et al 1991 Treatment of gram-negative bacteremia and septic shock with HA-1A human monoclonal antibody against endotoxin. N Engl J Med 324: 429–436

Zimmerman J E, Shortell S M, Knaus W A et al 1993 Value and cost of teaching hospitals: A prospective, multicenter, inception cohort study. Crit Care Med 21: 1432–1442

10. Pathogenesis and diagnosis of acute renal failure in the intensive care unit

D. Taube

INTRODUCTION

This chapter deals with acute renal failure (ARF) in the Intensive Care Unit (ICU) and will therefore focus on patients with renal failure in the setting of multiple organ failure (MOF) rather than single organ renal failure, which is usually managed outside the ICU.

DEFINITION OF ARF

For the purposes of this chapter, ARF is simply defined as acute, usually reversible deterioration of renal function often, but not always, associated with a reduction in urine output.

INCIDENCE OF ARF

In the United Kingdom, the incidence of ARF requiring dialysis is 50 cases per million population per year with at least three times as many patients developing ARF not severe enough to warrant dialysis. Approximately 15% of patients admitted to an ICU will have or will develop ARF (Trann et al 1990). However, the relative incidence of ARF in a large multi-disciplinary ICU subserving complex cardiothoracic, vascular and liver transplant surgery will be much higher.

The pattern of ARF is also constantly changing. Thus, improvements in cardiac surgery and obstetrics have reduced the incidence of ARF in these settings, only for new high-risk procedures such as liver and cardiac transplantation to emerge. Acute renal failure in pregnancy is now rare although still associated with a high mortality (Turney et al 1989).

Table 10.1   Common causes of pre-renal ARF

Ischaemic ATN	Hypovolaemia (haemorrhage, excessive use of diuretics, inadequate fluid replacement, diarrhoea and vomiting)
	Low cardiac output states (post-myocardial infarction and cardiac surgery, cardiomyopathies, tamponade)
	Sepsis
	Drugs
	Hepatic failure
	Pancreatitis
	Renal artery and vein thrombosis, embolization, dissection and distal cholesterol embolization
	Hypercalcaemia
Nephrotoxic ATN	Drugs, poisons and X-Ray contrast media
	Pigments (myoglobin and haemoglobin)
	Myeloma and light chains

CLASSIFICATION OF THE CAUSES OF ARF IN THE ICU

The causes of ARF are summarized in Tables 10.1–10.4. The standard, robust classification of pre-renal, intrinsic renal and ARF due to obstruction is still very useful and clinically effective. Pre-renal ARF includes causes related to reduction in renal blood flow (RBF) and the development of acute tubular necrosis (ATN). Intrinsic renal failure encompasses the various forms of rapidly progressive glomerulonephritis (RPGN) and acute tubulointerstitial nephritis (ATIN), whereas post-renal refers to ARF caused by obstruction of the urinary tract. In a multidisciplinary ICU, particularly in the setting of multiple organ failure, ARF is usually pre-renal.

Not all causes fit comfortably into this classification. Acute renal failure at the bedside is usually multifactorial, often complicated, if not caused by sepsis, hypovolaemia and drugs, and the aetiology of a particular patient's renal failure may therefore change during the course of their ICU stay.

Many patients with ARF in the ICU have pre-existing renal disease, or are old and chronically ill. Although acute renal failure is readily treatable with dialysis and haemofiltration and theoretically reversible, the prognosis of these patients is poor with an overall mortality of approximately 80%.

PATHOGENESIS OF PRE-RENAL ARF

Pre-renal ARF results in ATN which in humans is often multifactorial with a final common pathway of reduced renal blood flow, so called *ischaemic* or *vasomotor* ATN and direct tubular injury referred to as *nephrotoxic* ATN. It is usually impossible at the bedside to dissect out which factor is most clinically relevant. Furthermore, the treatment of the particular cause of the ATN and the development of other associated medical complications may exacerbate matters. For example, patients with low cardiac outputs often receive vasoconstrictors such as noradrenaline, which further reduce renal blood flow, as may sepsis which is a constant hazard and common complication in all ICUs.

PATHOPHYSIOLOGY OF ATN

Although there is a huge volume of literature describing the pathophysiology of ATN, most of this refers to work in experimental animals which is often incorrectly extrapolated to humans and often does not take into account that the initial causes of ATN may be different to those responsible for its persistence. Nevertheless, reduction of renal blood flow and the glomerular capillary ultrafiltration coefficient (K_f), intratubular obstruction and back-leak are experimentally held to be the most important factors responsible for impaired glomerular filtration in ATN (Hostetter & Brenner 1988).

ISCHAEMIC ATN

Experimentally, renal artery occlusion, infusion of vasoconstrictors such as noradrenaline and controlled haemorrhagic shock are used to study this form of ATN. Depending on the experimental method, proximal tubules, particularly the straight segments, are most vulnerable to ischaemia. Tubular cell swelling, bleb formation and vacuolization result in obstruction of tubular lumens with back-leak through the abnormally permeable necrotic tubular cells. Lysis of tubular cells then occurs with granular cast formation and further tubular obstruction (Donohoe et al 1978, Venkatachalan et al 1981). Glomerular epithelial foot process flattening and fusion with a reduction in K_f also occurs in certain animal models (Barnes et al 1981, Williams et al 1981). The intracellular events and processes which take place in these animal models are complex (Weinberg 1991). Intracellular ATP depletion, Ca^{2+} accumulation and phospholipase activation are important interlinked mechanisms of tubular cell injury which may have therapeutic relevance (Bonventre 1993).

NEPHROTOXIC ATN

Mercuric chloride, uranyl nitrate and aminoglycosides are used to induce nephrotoxic ATN in experimental animal models. The patterns of tubular and glomerular epithelial cell injury are similar to those demonstrated in ischaemic ATN (Kreisberg & Venkatachalan 1988).

REPAIR AND RECOVERY IN ATN

One of the hallmarks of ATN in humans is recovery, with renal function normally returning to previous levels. This may take time and can be prolonged by further circulatory or nephrotoxic insults which may be different to the original precipitating cause. Recovery from ATN is not only associated with tubular epithelial cell regeneration but also restitution of nephron continuity (Oliver 1953).

CAUSES OF PRE-RENAL ARF (TABLE 10.1)

Ischaemic ATN — *protective autoregulation in hypovolaemia : PG/NO*

Hypovolaemia and low cardiac output states

The autoregulation of renal blood flow by vasodilatory prostaglandins and nitric oxide protects the kidney during haemorrhage despite systemic vasoconstriction (Vatner 1974) and low blood pressure. Hypovolaemia is now an increasingly rare sole cause of pre-renal ARF, being generally rapidly recognized and treated.

Similarly, established pre-renal ARF due to low cardiac output states associated with myocardial infarction, cardiac surgery, tamponade, valvular dysfunction or cardiomyopathy is relatively rare in clinical practice. This is because the cause of the low cardiac output is either rapidly reversed or the patients die with intractable heart failure before established renal impairment becomes a clinical problem.

Sepsis *local renal hypo-perfusion in sepsis — cortical flow ↓*

Sepsis has been found to precede ARF in up to 50% of patients in the ICU (Trann et al 1990, Groeneveld et al 1991). There are good animal and human data to suggest that despite systemic vasodilatation renal blood flow is reduced during endotoxaemia in animals (Lugon et al 1989, O'Hair et al 1989, Shaer et al 1990) as well as sepsis in humans (Tristani & Cohn 1970, Brenner et al 1990). Intrarenal blood flow is altered, with cortical vasoconstriction and relative preservation of juxtaglomerular and medullary blood flow (Van Lambalgen et al 1991). Cytokines, including tumour necrosis factor, interleukin-1 and platelet activating factor are released in response to endotoxins. They affect renal haemodynamics, activate complement and leucocytes and damage vascular endothelium with intravascular coagulation as well as glomerular and intertubular capillary thrombosis. Endotoxins further reduce renal blood flow by promoting the synthesis and release of the endothelins (Takahashi et al 1990) and thromboxane A_2 (Badr et al 1986). Although the mediators and their interactions in this cascade have yet to be fully identified, this area promises considerable experimental therapeutic potential.

Drugs *Vasoconstriction NAdr/DA ?? rel. balance betw CO/perfusion pressure and RBF/vasodilation*

Noradrenaline and dopamine (at doses greater than 5 µg/kg/min) are renal vasoconstrictors and can cause ischaemic ATN. However, clinically it is often impossible to separate the effects of these agents from the underlying reason (usually sepsis induced hypotension) for which they are being administered.

Non-steroidal anti-inflammatory agents (NSAIDs) and angiotensin-converting enzyme inhibitors (ACEIs) reduce renal blood flow by interfering with autoregulation. NSAIDs inhibit the synthesis of vasodilatory prostanoids and may produce ARF in patients who are already hypovolaemic, septic or have a low cardiac output or pre-existing renal disease (Clive & Stoff 1984). ACEIs, particularly the longer acting variants, characteristically cause ARF in patients with reduced renal blood flow due to renal artery stenosis (Hrickik et al 1983) which may result in irreversible renal failure with renal artery thrombosis. Acute renal failure is not always associated with renal artery disease and may occur in ACEI-treated patients in the presence of hypotension, hypovolaemia and salt restriction (Bridoux et al 1992).

The major side-effect of the two most effective immunosuppressive agents in transplantation, the cyclophilins, cyclosporin A and FK506 is nephrotoxicity. This effect is not necessarily dose or drug level dependent. The cyclophilins reduce renal blood flow by vasoconstriction of the preglomerular afferent arteriole (Bennett et al 1994). In high doses in experimental animals, cyclosporin may be directly tubulotoxic and in humans can cause ARF with a clinical picture resembling that of the haemolytic uraemic syndrome (Bennett et al 1994).

Other nephrotoxic drugs such as amphotericin B may also mediate their effects by renal vasoconstriction (Sawaya et al 1991).

Hepatic failure

ARF in the setting of hepatic failure is often superficially referred to as the hepatorenal syndrome (HRS). Whilst there is no doubt that this entity exists, ARF associated with hepatic failure is often multifactorial and thus reversible without recourse to liver transplantation. Patients with hepatic disease may develop glomerulonephritis, have a higher incidence of sepsis, are often hypovolaemic and receive nephrotoxic drugs. HRS occurs in patients with alcoholic cirrhosis, hepatitis and hepatic malignancy. Patients with HRS behave as if they are hypovolaemic, retain sodium avidly, have evidence of reversible renal vasoconstriction (Epstein et al 1970) and histologically have classical ATN (Solez 1974).

Pancreatitis

Pancreatitis is a frequently missed cause of ARF in the ICU because the diagnosis is overlooked. The ARF is associated with hypotension, sepsis, increased renal vascular resistance and reduced renal blood flow (Werner et al 1974).

Renal artery and vein thrombosis, embolization, dissection and distal cholesterol embolization   [handwritten: Vascular surgery; renal arterial occlusion/stenosis]

Complex vascular surgery and aortic aneurysm repair in frail, elderly patients with pre-existing renal impairment is a common cause of ARF (and multiple organ failure) in the ICU (Svensson et al 1992). Hypotension, sepsis, low cardiac output related to coexistent coronary artery disease, rhabdomyolysis, radiocontrast agents and nephrotoxic drugs complicate the renal impairment caused by dissection and stenosis of the renal arteries, surgical ligation of the renal vein and intrarenal cholesterol embolization. Acute renal failure in this setting can be further exacerbated by the mesenteric ischaemia, bowel infarction and pancreatitis, which are not uncommon complications of major aortic surgery.

Acute renal failure may occur in patients with endocarditis or atrial fibrillation following renal artery embolism. Angiotensin-converting enzyme inhibition (see above) in the presence of renal artery stenosis is now a common cause of renal artery thrombosis and acute renal impairment (Hrikik et al 1983, Kalra et al 1990).

Renal vein thrombosis with other thrombotic complications such as pulmonary embolism may present as acute renal impairment in patients with the nephrotic syndrome (Llach et al 1980)

Cholesterol embolization following aortic or cardiac surgery, coronary, aortic and renal angiography (Lye et al 1993) and streptokinase therapy for myocardial infarction (Schwartz & McDonald 1987) may also present as ARF.

Hypercalcaemia   [handwritten: — tubular + post-renal effects]

Hypercalcaemia secondary to myeloma and other malignant disease, sarcoidosis, hyperparathyroidism and, very rarely, the milk-alkali syndrome can present as ARF. Hypercalcaemia interferes with distal convoluted tubular concentrating ability, resulting in polyuria and hypovolaemia and more chronically, nephrocalcinosis and stone formation (Benabe & Martinez-Maldonado 1978).

Nephrotoxic ATN   [handwritten: aminoglycosides, cephalothin   (paracetamol) chlorthopaste (cisplatin, methotrexate) mitomycin C, high osmolality, ionic contrast media]

For practical purposes, the most important nephrotoxic agents employed in the ICU are antibiotics. Gentamicin and the other aminoglycosides (tobramicin, netilmicin, amikacin) accumulate in high concentrations in proximal convoluted tubular lysosomes and bind to anionic phospholipids causing tubular cell injury and necrosis in 7–36% of patients. Renal impairment is dose and duration of treatment dependent and more common in older patients with pre-existing renal and hepatic disease (Kaloyanides 1994). The early generation of cephalosporins (cephaloridine and to a lesser extent cephalothin and cephalexin) have been reported to be nephrotoxic (Porter & Bennett 1981).

Paracetamol overdose is characteristically associated with liver damage and the ARF that occurs in this setting is part of the multiple organ failure associated with fulminant hepatic failure. However, small numbers of patients recovering from hepatic failure develop ARF as a secondary event. Occasionally patients who have taken heavy metals (mercury, arsenic, lead), organic solvents (carbon tetrachloride, ethylene glycol antifreeze) (Rosa & Brown 1988), paraquat-containing weedkillers or poisonous mushrooms (*Amanita phalloides*) present with acute renal, hepatic and subsequently multiple organ failure in the ICU. Cisplatinum, methotrexate and other chemotherapeutic agents such as mitomycin C also cause acute renal impairment either by direct tubular injury or uric acid deposition; or in the case of mitomycin C, an acute haemolytic uraemic syndrome (Cantrell et al 1985).

Radiocontrast media are long recognized as important causes of ARF (Pendergrass et al 1942), causing initial renal vasodilatation followed by more prolonged constriction (Lund et al 1984) and are directly tubulotoxic (Moreau et al 1975). They can also cause tubular obstruction not only by tubular cell necrosis and sloughing but also by forming insoluble precipitates with urinary proteins such as light chains in myeloma (Cwynarske & Saxton 1969). Patients with pre-existing renal impairment, hypovolaemia, diabetes mellitus and myeloma are more susceptible to contrast-induced renal impairment (Porter 1994). Contrast volume and tonicity are also important determinants of renal failure (Porter 1994). Low osmolality, non-ionic contrast media induce less renal vasoconstriction and are associated with a lower incidence of renal failure (Porter 1994).

Pigment-induced ARF

Myoglobin (from damaged muscle), haemoglobin (haemolysis) and possibly methaemoglobin and bilirubin can cause renal failure in the appropriate circumstances. Myoglobin and haemoglobin are protein bound in the circulation to an $\alpha2$ globulin and haptoglobin respectively, are not directly nephrotoxic and only cause renal failure in the presence of hypovolaemia and acidosis (Dubrow & Flamenbaum 1988). Myoglobin and haemoglobin at a urinary pH of 5.6 or below dissociate into haematin which is nephro- and hepatotoxic (Braun et al 1970). Myoglobin can cause renal vasoconstriction (Ayer et al 1971) and the precipitation of these pigments in renal tubules leading to tubular obstruction may be another important mechanism by which they cause renal failure (Dubrow & Flamenbaum 1988). Clinically, myoglobin-induced ARF or rhabdo-myolysis, is increasingly common whereas haemoglobin-induced ARF following intravascular haemolysis (transfusion reactions, poisons, malaria, prosthetic heart valve dysfunction, paroxysmal nocturnal haemoglobin-uria) is rare.

Table 10.2 Causes of rhabdomyolysis

NB non- traumatic rhabdomyolysis

Traumatic	Non-traumatic
Crush injuries, torture and beatings	Metabolic (hypokalaemia, hypo-
Heavy, unaccustomed exercise	phosphataemia, diabetic ketoacidosis)
Uncontrollable grand mal epilepsy	McArdle's and Tarui's diseases
Ischaemia and vascular surgery	Infections (atypical pneumonias, influenza A,
Snake bite, lightning and electric shock	Legionnaire's disease, tetanus)
Full thickness burns	Recreational drugs: cocaine, heroin,
Dermatomyositis	ecstasy, amphetamines
	Lipid-lowering agents
	Malignant hyperthermia
	Carbon monoxide poisoning

The causes of rhabdomyolysis are diverse and can be divided into traumatic and non-traumatic (summarized in Table 10.2). Traumatic rhabdomyolysis is common in inner city ICUs subserving populations in which drug addition, alcoholism, trauma and torture are frequent (Knottenbelt 1994). Rhabdomyolysis associated with alcohol and recreational drugs may occur in the setting of prolonged coma or immobility and thus widespread tissue or limb ischaemia and necrosis may contribute as well as drug-induced direct muscle injury.

Rhabdomyolysis is often missed as a cause of ARF, particularly in association with the non-traumatic causes listed in Table 10.2, and may be diagnosed only when myoglobin is discovered in renal tubules after renal biopsy.

Myeloma and lights chains

Patients with myeloma and light chain-secreting B-cell lymphomas may present with renal failure which is usually multifactorial in origin. Hypovolaemia, hypercalcaemia, hyperviscosity, sepsis, drug induced hyperuricaemia, NSAID administration for bone pain, chemotherapeutic and radiocontrast agents as well as light chains all contribute towards the renal failure detectable in up to 50% of patients with myeloma (Mallik 1994).

INTRINSIC ACUTE RENAL FAILURE (TABLE 10.3)

Rapidly progressive glomerulonephritis (RPGN) *(inv u. 2° Gr eg. immunoprn*

ARF in the ICU is rarely caused by RPGN, in that such patients generally have single (kidney) organ failure and are not sufficiently ill to be admitted to the ICU as a result of their underlying disease. Their presence on the ICU usually reflects a complication of treatment, often immunosuppression-induced sepsis. Occasionally patients with microscopic polyarteritis,

Wegener's granulomatosis, Goodpasture's syndrome and Henoch–Schönlein purpura develop pulmonary haemorrhage requiring ventilation and therefore ICU admission.

Acute tubulointerstitial nephritis (ATIN)

Similarly, ARF due to ATIN is rare in the ICU. However, antibiotics, NSAIDs and diuretics are frequently prescribed for the critically ill. Patients who develop renal failure whilst receiving these drugs or shortly afterwards should always be suspected of having drug-induced ATIN, particularly in the presence of a rash, fever, arthralgia or lymphadenopathy. Ampicillin, amoxicillin, flucloxacillin, carbenicillin, sulphonamides and rifampicin have all be implicated in ATIN. Considering the frequency with which these agents are prescribed, ATIN is extraordinarily rare and in clinical practice, rifampicin is the commonest cause of this problem. Renal biopsies from patients with rifampicin-induced ARF show interstitial oedema, a tubulointerstitial mononuclear cell infiltrate and tubular epithelial cell necrosis with no significant glomerular changes (Kleinknecht et al 1972).

NSAIDs usually cause renal failure by reducing renal blood flow, but ATIN, occasionally with minimal change nephropathy, has been frequently described (Brezin et al 1980, Curt et al 1980). Diuretic-induced ARF is usually caused by hypovolaemia, but ATIN has been described following the administration of thiazides (Magil et al 1980) and frusemide (Jennings et al 1986).

Although patients with leukaemia and lymphoma rarely present with MOF, the complications of their treatment, particularly sepsis, result in acute renal and multiple organ failure. Leukaemia (Echman & Lynch 1978) and lymphoma (Tsokos et al 1981) may occasionally present with ARF due to ATIN, the kidney being a common extranodal site of involvement in acute lymphoblastic leukaemia and non-Hodgkin's lymphoma.

Table 10.3 Intrinsic causes of ARF

Rapidly progressive glomerulonephritis
Systemic lupus erythematosis, microscopic polyarteritis, Wegener's granulomatosis, Goodpasture's syndrome, Henoch–Schönlein purpura, IgA nephropathy, post-infectious nephritis.

Acute tubulointerstitial nephritis
Drug allergies, infiltrations (leukaemia, lymphoma, sarcoidosis)
Infections (acute pyelonephritis, leptospirosis, candidiasis, Legionnaire's disease)

Acute endothelial cell injury
Haemolytic uraemic syndrome, thrombotic thrombocytopenic purpura, scleroderma, malignant hypertension

Pregnancy

Acute bacterial pyelonephritis in the absence of obstruction and pre-existing renal impairment rarely causes ARF. However, patients with pyelonephritis may become septic and develop acute, multiple organ failure requiring ICU treatment. Other specific infectious causes of ATIN and acute renal and multiple organ failure which present in an ICU setting include leptospirosis, candidiasis and Legionnaire's disease. Acute renal failure occurs in half the cases of leptospirosis and is mainly due to direct invasion of the kidney with consequent ATIN (Sitprija & Evans 1970). Disseminated candidiasis, not an uncommon cause or complication of MOF, affects the kidneys either in the form of a cortical ATIN or proliferation of the organisms with little inflammatory response in the medulla, collecting systems and upper urinary tract (Lehner 1964). Acute renal failure has been described in Legionnaire's disease either as a result of ATIN or rhabdomyolysis.

Acute endothelial cell injury

The haemolytic uraemic syndrome (HUS) and thrombotic thrombo-cytopenic purpura (TTP) occasionally present as acute renal and multiple organ failure with microangiopathic haemolytic anaemia and cerebral involvement. HUS is often associated with infections, particularly verotoxin-producing *E. coli* (Karmali et al 1983), drugs, including high dose cyclosporin A (Bennett et al 1994) and mitomycin C (Cantrell et al 1985). Cerebral involvement and the lack of specific initiating factors distinguish TTP from HUS. Renal biopsy shows widespread small vessel and glomerular intravascular thrombosis, fibrinoid necrosis and fibrin deposition. Scleroderma with widespread visceral involvement and malignant or accelerated hypertension may present as acute renal failure with severe hypertension.

Pregnancy

Fortunately, ARF in pregnancy is now rare (Turney et al 1989). RPGN or ATIN are unusual causes of renal failure during the early or mid stages of pregnancy. In late pregnancy ARF is usually associated with eclampsia, massive post-partum haemorrhage, abruptio placentae, amniotic fluid embolism and acute fatty liver. A proportion of these patients have pre-existing renal disease and hypertension. Patients with eclampsia are hypertensive and have a microangiopathy and renal histopathology similar to patients with HUS and TTP. Occasionally this picture may present in the post-partum period.

Table 10.4   Causes of obstruction leading to ARF

Kidney or upper ureter
Bilateral calculi or calculi in a single kidney
Papillary necrosis (analgesics, diabetes, sickle cell disease)
Blood clot, blocked indwelling stents
Pelviureteric junction stenosis

Ureter
Lymphoma, carcinoma
Idiopathic retroperitoneal fibrosis
Stones, papillae and blood clot
Surgical ligation or trauma

Bladder, bladder neck or urethra
Benign prostatic hypertrophy
Carcinoma of the prostate, bladder, endometrium, cervix or colon
Stones
Urethral stricture, meatal stenosis
Neurogenic bladder

ARF DUE TO OBSTRUCTION

Table 10.4 summarizes the causes of ARF due to obstruction. Obstructive ARF per se is rare in the ICU, although such patients may be admitted following surgery or radiological intervention with sepsis or massive haemorrhage. Occasionally, bilateral papillary necrosis or staghorn calculi with pyelonephrosis and sepsis present as acute renal with multiple organ failure. Obstructive uropathy may occur or complicate ARF on the ICU, particularly if patients do not have indwelling urethral catheters. Relief of urinary obstruction may be followed by a massive diuresis which, if mismanaged, can lead to hypovolaemia and further renal impairment.

DIAGNOSIS AND ASSESSMENT OF PATIENTS WITH ARF ON THE ICU

This is not difficult. Problems usually follow basic errors related to inadequate history taking, scrutiny of the patient's records, simple physical examination and over-emphasis on complex physiological tests which in themselves may be inaccurate. Simple tests such as examination of the urine are often overlooked. Frequent monitoring of renal function and urine output on the ICU usually results in the early recognition of impairment.

Simple tests!   Examination of urine!!

History   NB drugs

Most critically ill patients are ventilated or sufficiently unwell to be unable to give a history. The admitting physician is therefore dependent on the notes, referring doctors or relatives. The former two sources are notoriously unreliable, particularly if a chain of cross-covering medical or surgical teams have been involved in the patient's care prior to the ICU admission. Information from relatives or the nursing notes is often extremely useful. Scrutiny of 'hidden', expired drug or treatment charts may provide the major clue to the cause of the ARF. A history of pre-existing renal impairment, hypertension, abnormal urinary sediment and conditions associated with renal disease such as diabetes mellitus should be sought. If necessary the patient's family doctor should be contacted for vital information relating to past history. The patient's drug history and other treatments should be carefully scrutinized. Factors suggesting multisystem disease should be considered. The circumstances relating to the admission or presentation as well as subsequent course on the ICU, should be carefully thought through. Not all ventilated patients are sufficiently sedated or unwell to be unable to give accurate histories; the process may be time consuming but extremely helpful.

Physical examination — volume status /co — feet + fundi (emboli)

A thorough physical examination should be performed, not only on admission to the ICU but regularly throughout the patient's stay. Careful attention should be paid to clinical signs related to circulating volume and cardiac output (preferred patient posture, peripheral perfusion, skin turgor, pulse, paradox and jugular venous and systemic pressure) and if these signs are at odds with the data from electronic monitoring systems, the accuracy of these, rather than the physical signs, should be questioned. Signs of multisystem disease (cutaneous vasculitis, arthropathy, sclerodactyly, metastatic calcification), poisoning (oropharyngeal desquamation), intravenous drug abuse and ischaemic necrosis of skin and subcutaneous tissues (rhabdomyolysis) should be sought. Examination of the abdomen, peripheral pulses and the feet and fundi for evidence of cholesterol emboli should always be carried out in patients with vascular disease and otherwise unexplained renal failure.

Investigations

1. Tests of renal function and other biochemical tests which may aid diagnosis

The realization that the patient is developing ARF is not usually delayed because urine output, electrolytes and renal function are constantly monitored. However, the severity of the impairment is often underestimated because the relationship between plasma creatinine and GFR is not understood. The plasma creatinine does not rise above the normal range (110–120 μmol/l) until the GFR is approximately 50% of normal. Furthermore, thin patients with little muscle mass who produce relatively less creatine may have plasma levels within the normal range despite severe renal dysfunction. This point is important in ICUs patients, when despite parenteral or enteral feeding, they become increasingly wasted. Notice should therefore be taken of a rising plasma creatinine rather than waiting for it to become abnormally raised.

Despite the above, plasma creatinine is still the most useful, robust and cheapest test of renal function. There are no easily available, rapid tests of GFR although with catheterised patients 24-hour urine collections should be reliable, facilitating creatinine clearances which are a reasonable method.

Measurements of urinary electrolytes and urea, plasma and urinary osmolality are occasionally useful. Patients with the hepatorenal syndrome avidly retain sodium (urinary sodium <10 mmol/l) and this may therefore help diagnostically. Urinary potassium excretion may facilitate the estimation of parenteral replacement in intravenous fluid and feeding regimes, particularly when patients are polyuric. Urinary urea is used to assess nitrogen balance. Plasma and urinary osmolalities are helpful in diagnosing the cause and treatment of hyper- or hyponatraemia.

Measurement of the plasma amylase and creatine phosphokinase (CPK) should always be performed in patients with ARF, especially if the cause is not apparent. Amylase is excreted in the urine and mild hyperamylasaemia is frequently found in ARF. However, a plasma amylase of >1000 μ/l is indicative of either pancreatitis or another intra-abdominal catastrophe such as bowel infarction or upper gastrointestinal perforation. A significantly raised CPK (>10 000 μ/l) is highly suggestive of rhabdomyolysis. A degree of hypocalcaemia (1.8–2.0 mmol/l) is common in ARF but marked hypocalcaemia (<1.5 mmol/l) should prompt a search for either pancreatitis or rhabdomyolysis (damaged muscle is said to take up calcium). Patients with rhabdomyolysis are also frequently very catabolic and persisting hyperkalaemia, hyperphosphataemia and hyperuricaemia in spite of adequate dialysis or filtration should suggest this diagnosis.

Acidosis is a hallmark of renal failure but persistent severe acidosis in ARF (pH <7.0) should alert clinicians to the possibility of lactic acidosis, metformin overdosage or accumulation, bowel infarction, untreated sepsis or ethylene glycol poisoning.

2. Haematological and serological investigations useful in the diagnosis of ARF

Inappropriate anaemia in patients presenting with ARF (Hb <8.0 g/dl) should suggest haemolysis, pulmonary haemorrhage (Goodpasture's syndrome) microscopic polyarteritis, Wegener's granulomatosis or systemic lupus erythematosus (SLE), myeloma or longstanding pre-existing renal impairment.

Patients with SLE may be leucopenic. Although patients with sepsis classically have a leucocytosis, gram-negative sepsis may be associated with leucopenia. Eosinophilia has been described in drug-induced ATIN and cholesterol embolization.

Thrombocytopenia, raised titres of fibrin degradation products and red cell fragmentation on the peripheral film may be found in patients with severe sepsis, HUS, TTP and ARF post partum. Thrombocythaemia is commonly found in patients with active vasculitis.

Complement levels may decrease in patients with RPGN, SLE and cholesterol embolization. Patients with SLE and ARF usually have positive antinuclear factors, DNA binding titres and antibodies to other nuclear antigens. Indirect immunoflourescent tests and solid phase immunoassays for antineutrophil cytoplasmic antibodies are positive in most patients with active MPA, WG and some patients with active Goodpasture's syndrome, SLE, rheumatoid arthritis and subacute bacterial endocarditis. Care must therefore be taken in the interpretation of these tests. Patients with Goodpasture's syndrome have circulating antiglomerular basement membrane antibody. Elevated immunoglobulin levels and light chains in blood and urine are highly suggestive of myeloma, although in ARF light chains may not be excreted in the urine. Serological testing for evidence of recent mycoplasma, Legionella, infleunza and other infections may be helpful in determining the cause of non-traumatic rhabdomyolysis.

3. *Testing the urine*

It is remarkable how often this simple but extremely important procedure is overlooked, despite the increasing reliability and sophistication of urinary testing strips. The presence of large amounts of blood and protein in the urine should alert the clinician to the possibility of glomerulo- or interstitial nephritis as the cause of the patient's renal failure. This simple test may be the only clue to a multisystem disease such as a SLE or MAP. The presence of large amounts of haemoglobin in urine detected by sticks with few red cells on microscopy is highly suggestive of haemolysis or now more commonly, rhabdomyolysis (most sticks are not able to distinguish between myoglobin and haemoglobin) as the cause of the renal impairment. Myoglobinuria resembles black coffee and occurs during the early phase of rhabdomyolysis whilst the patient is still passing urine or during the recovery phase when urine flow is restored. Red or frankly bloody urine may occur after haemolysis or in patients with RPGN or after renal infarction.

4. *Imaging*

There is now no place for intravenous pyelography in ARF. Intravenous contrast, as described above, can be nephrotoxic and if renal function is significantly impaired, the image will be poor. Plain abdominal films may show the renal outline and demonstrate stones.

All patients with ARF should have an abdominal ultrasound examination to establish kidney size, detect stones, tumours and other anatomical abnormalities and to rule out ureteric obstruction. Doppler examination of the renal vasculature will determine whether the kidneys are still perfused. Small shrunken kidneys are suggestive of pre-existing renal impairment. Large kidneys are found in ATN, RPGN, ATIN and the earlier phases of diabetic nephropathy. Asymmetric kidneys should raise the possibility of renal artery stenosis, especially in patients with known vascular disease. Computerizd tomographic (CT) scanning, particularly spiral CT because it is so quick, is often very helpful in the management of patients with acute renal or multiple organ failure. Conventional abdominal ultrasound may be difficult in patients who are fat, have an ileus or extensive retroperitoneal haemorrhage. CT may be the only reliable method of diagnosing pancreatitis, detecting intra-abdominal collections, aortic aneurysms, dissection and elucidating the cause of extrinsic ureteric obstruction. Renal angiography is the best method of diagnosing renal artery stenosis or occlusion.

5. Renal biopsy

Acute tubular necrosis is a histological diagnosis and although the clinical features associated with an episode of ARF may suggest ATN, a renal biopsy should be performed to verify the diagnosis if there is any reasonable doubt in order to exclude other potentially treatable causes. Although patients with renal impairment have prolonged bleeding times and their underlying disease may be associated with a coagulopathy, these difficulties can usually be reversed. With the appropriate help, ventilated patients can also safely undergo percutaneous renal biopsy provided they are haemodynamically stable.

ARF is often multifactorial, the patients are often old and chronically ill with pre-existing renal impairment and the initiating cause may not be the only cause, particularly if patients have a prolonged ICU stay.

KEY POINTS FOR CLINICAL PRACTICE

- Around 15% of patients admitted to a general ICU will develop ARF, although the incidence in certain predisposed groups of critically ill patients (e.g. those with sepsis or liver failure, or with cardiovascular insufficiency) may be much higher.
- The classical classification of prerenal, intrinsic and post renal causes of ARF remains useful in determining aetiology and formulating clinical management.

- Hypovolaemia and nephrotoxicity through inappropriate drug administration are possibly the commonest avoidable causes of ARF in the ICU
  setting. Rhabdomyolysis is often missed as a cause of ARF, particularly
  in cases where trauma is not involved.
- A clinical history should always be obtained from the patient, relatives or
  GP together with careful physical examination repeated at regular inter-
  vals; examination of the urine and simple biochemical tests (serum
  creatinine, creatinine clearance) should be performed. Intravenous
  pyelography should not be performed, but all patients subjected to
  careful ultrasound examination to establish kidney size and detect
  stones, tumors and evidence of ureteric obstruction.
- Acute tubular necrosis (ATN) is a histological diagnosis and although
  the clinical features associated with an episode of ARF may suggest ATN,
  a renal biopsy should be performed to confirm the diagnosis if doubt
  exist.

REFERENCES

Ayer G, Grandchamp A, Wyler T et al 1971 Intrarenal haemodynamics in glycerol-
    induced myoglobinuric acute renal failure in the rat. Circ Res 29: 128
Badr K F, Kelley V E, Rennke H G, Brenner B M 1986. Roles for thromboxane A_2 and
    leukotrienes in endotoxin induced acute renal failure. Kidney Int 30: 474
Barnes J L, Osgood R W, Reineck H J, Stein J H 1981 Glomerular alterations in an
    ischaemic model of acute renal failure. Lab Invest 45: 378
Benabe J E, Martinez-Maldonado M 1978 Hypercalcemic nephropathy. Arch Intern Med
    138: 777
Bennett W M, Burdmann E A, Andoh T F, Houghton D C, Lindsley J, Elzinga L W.
    Nephrotoxicity of immunosuppressive drugs. Nephrol Dial Transplant 9 (suppl 4):
    141
Bonventre J V 1993 Mechanisms of acute renal failure. Kidney Int 43: 1160
Braun S R, Weiss F R, Keller A I et al 1970 Evaluation of the renal toxicity of haem
    proteins and their derivatives. A role in the genesis of acute tubule necrosis. J Exp
    Med 1431: 443
Brenner M, Schaer G L, Mallory D L, Suffredini A F, Parillo J E 1990 Detection of
    renal blood flow abnormalities in septic and critically ill patients using a newly
    designed indwelling renal vein thermodilution catheter. Chest 98: 170
Brezin J H, Katz S M, Schwartz A B, Chinitz J L 1980 Reversible renal failure and
    nephrotic syndrome associated with non-steroidal anti-inflammatory drugs. N Engl J
    Med 301: 1271
Bridoux F, Hazzab N, Pallot J L et al 1992 Acute renal failure after the use of
    angiotensin converting enzyme inhibitors in patients without renal artery stenosis.
    Nephrol Dial Transplant 7: 100
Cantrell J E, Phillips T M, Schein P S 1985 Carcinoma-associated haemolytic uraemic
    syndrome: A complication of mitomycin C chemotherapy. J Clin Oncol 3: 723
Clive D M, Stoff J S 1984 Renal syndromes associated with non-steroidal anti-
    inflammatory drugs. N Engl J Med 310: 563
Cwynarske M T, Saxton H M 1969 Urography in myelomatosis. Br Med J 1: 486
Curt G A, Kaldany A, Whitley L G et al 1980 Reversible rapidly progressive renal failure
    with nephrotic syndrome due to fenoprofen calcium. Ann Intern Med 92: 72
Donohoe J F, Venkatachalan M A, Bernard D B, Levinsky N G 1978 Tubular leakage
    and obstruction in acute ischaemic renal failure. Kidney Int 13: 208
Dubrow A, Flamenbaum W 1988 Acute renal failure associated with myoglobinuria and
    haemoglobinuria. In: Brenner B M, Lazarus J M (eds) Acute renal failure, 2nd edn,
    Churchill Livingstone, p 279

Echman L N, Lynch Ed 1978 Acute renal failure in patients with acute leukaemia. South Med J 71: 382

Epstein M, Berk D P, Hollenberg N K et al 1970 Renal failure in the patient with cirrhosis. The role of active vasoconstriction. Am J Med 49:175

Groeneveld A B J, Tran D D, Van der Meulen J, Nauta J J P, Thijs L G 1991 Acute renal failure in the medical intensive care unit. Predisposing, complicating factors and outcome. Nephron 59: 602

Hostetter T H, Brenner B M 1988 Renal circulatory and nephron function in experimental acute renal failure. In: Brenner B M, Lazarus J M (eds) Acute renal failure, 2nd edn, Churchill Livingstone, p 67

Hrickik D E, Browning P J, Kopelman R et al 1983 Captopril induced functional renal insufficiency in patients with bilateral renal artery stenoses or renal artery stenosis in a solitary kidney. N Engl J Med 308: 373

Jennings M, Shortland J R, Maddocks J L 1986 Interstitial nephritis associated with frusemide. J R Soc Med 79: 239

Kaloyanides G J 1994 Antibiotic related nephrotoxicity. Nephrol Dial Transplant 9 (suppl 4): 130

Kalra P A, Mamtora H, Holmes A M, Waldek S 1990 Renovascular disease and renal complications of angiotensin converting enzyme inhibitor therapy. Q J Med 77: 1013

Karmali M A, Petric M, Steele B T, Lim C 1983 Sporadic cases of haemolytic uraemic syndrome associated with faecal cytotoxin and cytotoxin producing E. coli in stools. Lancet 1: 619

Kleinknecht D, Homberg J C, Decroix G 1972 Acute renal failure after rifampicin. Lancet 1: 1238

Knottenbelt J D 1994 Traumatic rhabdomyolysis from severe beating — experience of volume diuresis in 200 patients. J Trauma 37: 214

Kreisberg J I, Venkatachalan M A 1988 Morphologic factors in acute renal failure. In: Brenner B M, Lazarus J M (eds) Acute renal failure, 2nd edn. Churchill Livingstone, p 45

Lambalgen A A van, Kraats A A van, Bos G C van den et al 1991 Renal function and metabolism during endotoxaemia in rats; role of hypoperfusion. Circ Shock 35: 164

Lehner T 1964 Systemic candidiasis and renal involvement. Lancet 1: 1414

Llach F, Papper S, Massry S G 1980 The clinical spectrum of renal vein thrombosis. Acute and chronic. Am J Med 69: 819

Lugon J R, Boim M A, Ramos O L, Ajzen H, Schor N 1989 Renal function and glomerular haemodynamics in male endotoxaemic rats. Kidney Int 36: 570

Lund G, Einzig S, Rysavy J et al 1984 Role of ischaemia in contrast induced renal damage: an experimental study. Circulation 9: 783

Lye W C, Cheah J S, Sinniah R 1993 Renal cholesterol embolic disease. Case report and review of the literature (review). Am J Nephrol 13: 489

Magil A, Ballon H S, Cameron E C, Rae A 1980 Acute interstitial nephritis associated with thiazide diuretics, Clinical and pathological observations in 3 cases. Am J Med 69: 939

Mallik N P 1994 Acute renal failure and myeloma. Nephrol Dial Transplant 9 (suppl 4): 108

Moreau J F, Droz D, Sabto J et al 1975 Osmotic nephrosis induced by water soluble triiodinated contrast media in man. Radiology 115: 329

O'Hair D P, Adams M B, Tunberg T C, Osborn J L 1989 Relationships among endotoxaemia, arterial pressure and renal function in dogs. Circ Shock 27:199

Oliver J 1953 Correlations of structure and function and mechanisms of recovery in acute tubular necrosis. Am J Med 15: 535

Pendergrass E P, Chamberlin G W, Godfrey E W, Burdick E D 1942 A survey of deaths and unfavorable sequelae following the administration of contrast media. Am J Radiol 48: 741

Porter G A 1994 Radiocontrast-induced nephropathy. Nephrol Dial Transplant 9 (suppl 4): 146

Porter G A, Bennett W M 1981 Nephrotoxic acute renal failure due to common drugs. Am J Physio 241: Fl

Provision of services for adult patients with renal disease in the United Kingdom. November 1991

Rosa R M, Brown R S 1988 Acute renal failure associated with heavy metals and organic solvents. In: Brenner B M, Lazarus J M (eds) Acute renal failure, 2nd edn. Churchill Livingstone, p 353

Sawaya B P, Weiprecht H, Campbell W R et al 1991 Direct vasoconstriction as a possible cause for amphotericin B induced nephrotoxicity in rats. J Clin Invest 87: 209

Schwartz M W, McDonald G B 1987 Cholesterol embolisation syndrome: occurrence after intravenous streptokinase therapy for myocardial function. JAMA 258: 1934

Shaer G L, Fink M P, Chernow B, Ahmed S, Parrillo J E 1990 Renal haemodynamics and prostaglandin E2 excretion in a non human primate model of septic shock. Crit Care Med 18: 52

Sitprija V, Evans H 1970 The kidney in human leptospirosis. Am J Med 49: 780

Solez K 1992 Acute renal failure, hepatorenal syndrome. In: Heptinstall R H (ed) Pathology of the kidney, vol II, 4th edn. Little Brown p 1274

Svensson L G, Crawford S, Hess K R, Coselli J S, Safi H J 1992 Thoracoabdominal aortic aneurysms associated with coeliac, superior mesenteric and renal artery occlusive disease: methods and analysis of results in 271 patients. J Vasc Surg 16: 378

Takahashi K, Silva A, Cohen J, Lam H-C, Ghatei M A, Bloom S R 1990 Endothelin immunoreactivity in mice with gram-negative bacteraemia: relationship to tumour necrosis factor. Clin Sci 79: 619

Trann D D, Groeneveld A B J, Van der Meulen J, Nauta J J P, Strack van Schijndel R J M, Thijs L G 1990 Age, chronic disease, sepsis, organ system failure and mortality in a medical intensive care unit. Crit Care Med 18: 474

Tristani F E, Cohn J N 1970 Studies in clinical shock and hypotension VII; Renal haemodynamics before and during treatment. Circulation 42: 839

Tsokos G C, Balow J E, Seigel R J, Magrath I T 1981 Renal and metabolic complications of undifferentiated and lymphoblastic lymphomas. Medicine 60: 218

Turney J H, Ellis C M, Parsons F M 1989 Obstetric acute renal failure 1956–1987. J Obstet Gynaecol 96: 679–687

Vatner S F 1974 Effects of haemorrhage on regional blood flow distribution in dogs and primates. J Clin Invest 54: 225

Venkatachalan M A, Jones D B, Rennke H G et al 1981 Mechanism of proximal tubule brush border loss and regeneration following mild renal ischaemia. Lab Invest 45: 355

Weinberg J M 1991 The cell biology of ischaemic renal injury. Kidney Int 39: 476

Werner M H, Hays D F, Lucas C E, Rosenberg I K 1974 Renal vasoconstriction in association with acute pancreatitis. Am J Surg 127: 185

Williams R H, Thomas C E, Nava L G, Evan A P 1981 Haemodynamic and single nephron function during the maintenance phase of ischaemic acute renal failure in the dog. Kidney Int 19: 503

1) Renal failure — ITU part of multi-organ failure (i.e. u. a secondary event)
⇒ (a) acute (but ? acute-on-chronic ?) (b) reversible (in principle)

2) At least 15% (potentially more in units with complex admissions) of ITU admissions will develop ARF.

of multifactorial ITU {

Prevent — ischaemic (RBF↓) → ATN
nephrotoxic + rhabdomyolysis
hypercalcaemia (→ tubular / diuretic effects)

Intrinsic — inflammatory, infiltrative d—, endothelial dge, pym—

Obstructive —

3) INV. (creatinine) creatinine clearance, — aufare, CPK (rhabdo.) FBC/film (fns)/
urinalysis; USS ? CT ? Renal angio. if stenosis suspected. Renal Bx — guidance.

4) The initial cause of ATN may be different from the maintaining cause of established ATN.

11. Renal replacement therapy — new developments

P. E. Stevens   S. P. Davies

INTRODUCTION

In 1952, during the Korean war a Renal Insufficiency Centre was established 30 minutes' helicopter flight from the field. Equipped with a laboratory and a Brigham-Kolff rotating drum dialyser this facility reduced the mortality rate in those with traumatic acute renal failure (ARF) from 90% to 60%. ARF was described at that time as a wasting disease, often complicated by infections, poor wound healing, bleeding and anaemia (Smith et al 1955). Dialysis could only be effected by direct cannulation of peripheral vessels, it was performed only intermittently, and starvation during ARF was the rule. The development of the arteriovenous shunt (Quinton et al 1960) subsequently made repeated access to the circulation a practical proposition. More frequent dialysis also allowed the provision of nutrition, but there was still a risk of fluid overload between sessions and cardiovascular instability was inevitable in critically ill patients. Therefore, there was clearly a need to improve on existing techniques of renal replacement therapy.

Interest in ultrafiltration (the convective removal of fluid) dates back to the origins of haemodialysis (Skeggs et al 1952), but it was years later that a technique based solely on the principle of convective solute transport in the treatment of chronic renal failure was first proposed (Henderson et al 1967). In 1976, it was demonstrated that cardiovascular instability could be circumvented by ultrafiltration without dialysis. This rekindled interest in haemofiltration (the convective removal of solute and water) as a technique for treating ARF (Silverstein et al 1974), culminating in the first description of continuous arteriovenous haemofiltration (CAVH) by Kramer in 1977 (Kramer et al 1977).

Spontaneous CAVH is limited by low clearance of small solutes. Since its original description, various methods for enhancing its performance have been described, including suction CAVH (Kaplan et al 1983), predilution CAVH (Kaplan 1985) and pumped CAVH (Lauer et al 1983). The inclusion of a blood pump in the circuit allowed the generation of ultrafiltration rates high enough to control severely catabolic ARF and the use of venovenous access (CVVH). To overcome the potential disadvantages of the need for high ultrafiltration rates, Geronemus & Schneider (1984) described the addition of a slow continuous flow of dialysis fluid through the ultrafiltrate compartment of the haemofilter. This continuous arteriovenous haemodialysis (CAVHD), or its venovenous counterpart (CVVHD), combined diffusive with convective transport and substantially improved the clearance of small solutes.

Since the introduction of CAVH (Dodd et al 1982) and CAVHD (Stevens et al 1988) to the United Kingdom, there has been a proliferation of continuous renal replacement therapy techniques and a reduction in the requirement for conventionally trained haemodialysis staff to be involved in their implementation and management (Stevens & Rainford, 1992). This chapter details the techniques currently available and briefly considers their principles. Advances in membrane technology and their potential advantages are discussed. Strategies for anticoagulation of the extracorporeal circulation and for vascular access are reviewed. Finally, the clinical implications of the use of continuous renal replacement therapy, including the advantages and disadvantages of the available techniques, are discussed.

TECHNIQUES FOR CONTINUOUS RENAL REPLACEMENT THERAPY (TABLE 11.1)

The aim of renal replacement therapy is the removal of uraemic toxins and the correction of fluid, electrolyte and acid–base disturbances. For many years peritoneal dialysis (PD) was the only continuous form of renal replacement therapy available to the intensivist. Although PD still has a place in the management of ARF, its use in critically ill patients is limited by failure to control uraemia, insufficient ultrafiltration, catheter migration, and the potential for respiratory embarrassment. Moreover, the technique is generally contraindicated in those who have undergone abdominal surgery and in patients with peritonitis. The development of CAVH, CVVH, CAVHD, CVVHD, CAVHDF, CVVHDF, and CHFD has considerably widened the choice of techniques for continuous renal replacement therapy. Isovolaemic intermittent conventional haemodialysis for control of uraemia, combined with slow continuous ultrafiltration to maintain isovolaemia between dialysis sessions, is less frequently used.

Table 11.1 Techniques for continuous renal replacement therapy (CRRT)

CAVH	Continuous arteriovenous haemofiltration
CVVH	Continuous venovenous haemofiltration
CAVHD	Continuous arteriovenous haemodialysis (arteriovenous haemodiafiltration)
CVVHD	Continuous venovenous haemodialysis (venovenous haemodiafiltratiion)
CAVHDF	Continuous arteriovenous haemodiafiltration
CVVHDF	Continuous venovenous haemodiafiltration
CHFD	Continuous high flux dialysis
IHD + SCUF	Intermittent haemodialysis + slow continuous ultrafiltration
PD	Peritoneal dialysis

Table 11.2   Typical solute concentrations in blood and filtrate in a patient with ARF undergoing haemofiltration with a polysulfone Amicon Diafilter 20 (Amicon Corporation, Danvers, Massachusetts)

Solute		Blood	Filtrate
Sodium	(mmol/l)	137	143
Potassium	(mmol/l)	5.0	5.0
Urea	(mmol/l)	32.4	35
Creatinine	(mmol/l)	492	500
Calcium	(mmol/l)	2.37	1.5
Phosphate	(mmol/l)	2.16	2.25
Urate	(mmol/l)	0.54	0.55
Protein	(g/l)	68	not detected

Table 11.3   Typical biochemical composition of commercially available haemofiltration replacement solutions

Sodium	140	mmol/l	Potassium	1 mmol/l
Magnesium	0.75	mmol/l	Chloride	101 mmol/l
Lactate	45	mmol/l	Glucose	11 mmol/l
Osmolality	300	mosmol/l		

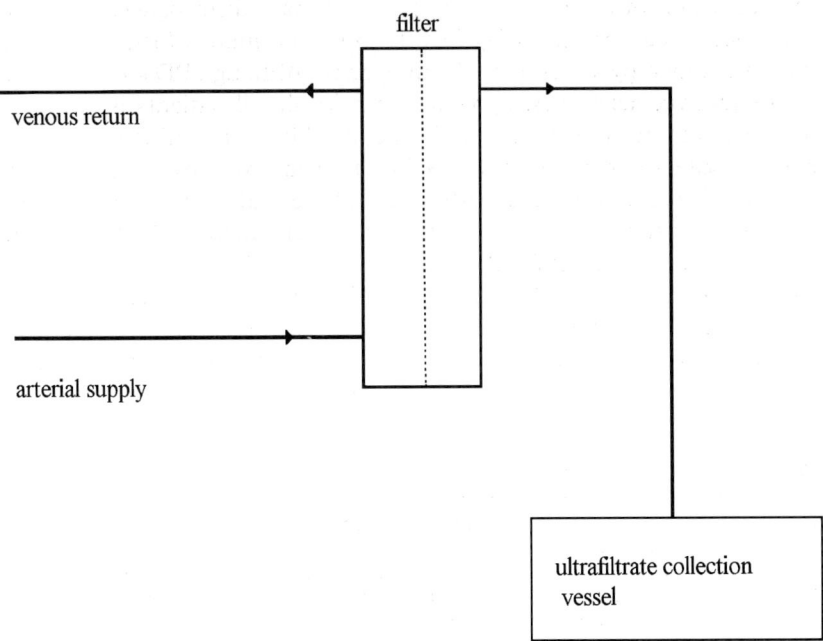

Fig. 11.1   Schematic representation of circuit diagram for CAVH.

PRINCIPLES OF CAVH AND CVVH

The same principles underlie all haemofiltration techniques. Solute and water removal is by convection achieved by filtration of blood (Fig.11.1).

The rate of removal of solute is dependent on the ultrafiltration rate and the concentration of the solute in the ultrafiltrate. This in turn depends on the concentration of the solute in plasma water and its sieving coefficient (i.e. the ratio of the solute concentration in ultrafiltrate to its concentration in plasma water). The sieving coefficient is determined by the relative size of the solute molecule and membrane pores. It follows that the more protein bound a solute, the lower its sieving coefficient. Typical solute concentrations in ultrafiltrate and blood are shown in Table 11.2.

The ultrafiltration rate is determined by the hydraulic conductivity of the membrane, the membrane surface area and the net transmembrane pressure; the latter being determined by the hydrostatic and osmotic pressure gradients across the membrane. For any given filter a linear relationship might be predicted between transmembrane pressure and ultrafiltration rate, but this is not quite the case. Accumulation of proteins and other large molecules occurs at the membrane surface leading to complex interactions which lead to a reduction in ultrafiltration rate (and sieving coefficient) with time (Colton et al 1975). In practice the ultrafiltration rate may be increased by lowering the height of the collection vessel below the ultrafiltrate port, applying a negative pressure to the ultrafiltrate port (Kaplan et al 1983) or by lowering the osmotic pressure opposing ultrafiltration by predilution (Kaplan 1985). Alternatively, the introduction of a pump into the circuit obviates the need for these manoeuvres (Fig. 11.2) and the ultrafiltration rate becomes directly related to blood flow through the filter at flow rates between 90 and 250 ml/min (Lauer et al 1983). With blood flows of 200–300 ml/min, ultrafiltration rates of 35–40 ml/min may be achieved which readily control catabolism, but necessitate considerable care in the replacement of fluid and electrolytes. Commercially-available replacement fluids exist (Table 11.3) and should be employed in a controlled system, such as that described by Mason et al (1985), where the ultrafiltration rate and the rate of replacement of fluid are accurately monitored to achieve the required fluid balance.

PRINCIPLES OF CAVHD AND CVVHD .

The ingenious addition of a slow, continuous flow of dialysate through the filtrate compartment of a haemofilter in a direction countercurrent to blood flow (Geronemus & Schneider, 1984, Fig. 11.3), avoids the requirement for volumes of ultrafiltration greater than those needed to create space for adequate nutrition and drug infusions, or to treat fluid overload. Blood

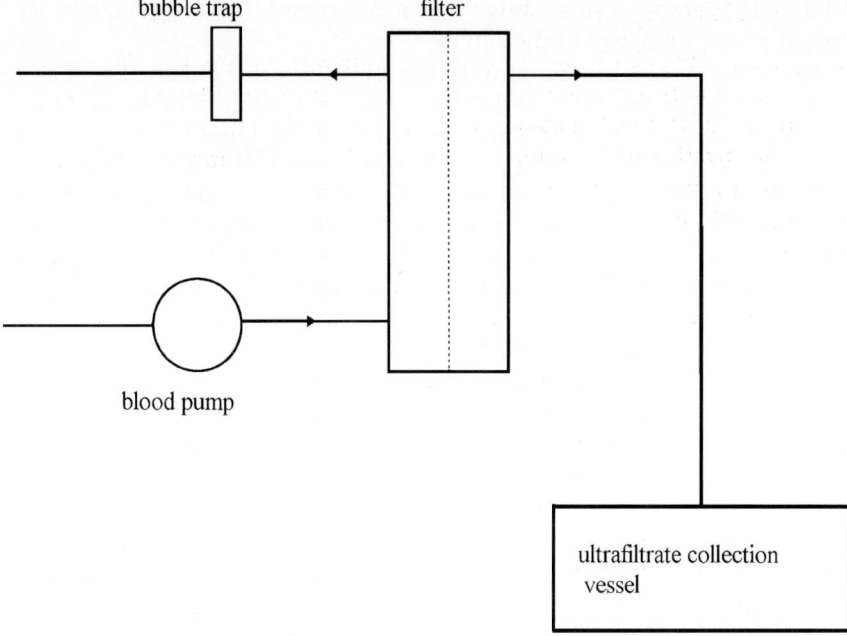

Fig. 11.2   Schematic representation of circuit diagram for CVVH/pumped CAVH.

and dialysate flows are low compared to conventional haemodialysis. Providing blood flow is significantly greater than dialysate flow, almost complete equilibration of small solutes occurs. Over a range of blood flows
between 50 and 190 ml/min using a 0.43 m² flat plate polyacrylonitrile
parallel plate haemodialyser, the clearance of small molecular weight
solutes is roughly equivalent to the sum of the dialysate and ultrafiltrate
flow rates. Thus, with a dialysate flow of 16.6 ml/min (1 l/h) and a mean
ultrafiltration rate of 8 ml/min whole blood clearances of urea, creatinine
and phosphate of 25, 24 and 21 ml/min can be achieved respectively (Sigler
& Teehan 1987). Other investigators have confirmed the higher clearances
of small molecular weight solutes afforded by CAVHD (Raja et al 1986,
Pattison et al 1988, Stevens et al 1988). Increasing dialysate flow to 33.3
ml/min can increase urea clearance from 22 to 33 ml/min, creatine clearance from 20 to 29 ml/min and phosphate clearance from 21 to 29 ml/min
(Stevens & Davies 1990). Clearances also depend on the sieving characteristics and age of the filter employed, increasing age impeding equilibration of solute between dialysate and blood. This can be monitored simply
by comparing blood and spent dialysate/ultrafiltrate urea concentrations.
At dialysate flow rates of 1 l/h there should be no discrepancy, whereas at

2 l/h there is always a small difference of 3–4 mmol/l. Wider discrepancies should prompt renewal of the filter.

The addition of a blood pump to the extracorporeal circuit (Fig. 11.4) ensures adequate blood flow and allows venovenous access if preferred (Tam et al 1988, Bellomo et al 1992a). Small solute clearances are comparable to CAVHD and no complications related to use of the blood pump have been reported (Bellomo et al 1993a).

The dialysate employed may be standard peritoneal dialysis fluid (to which potassium may need to be added) or commercially-available solutions. These may be acetate or lactate buffered, depending on the clinical circumstances (Table 11.4).

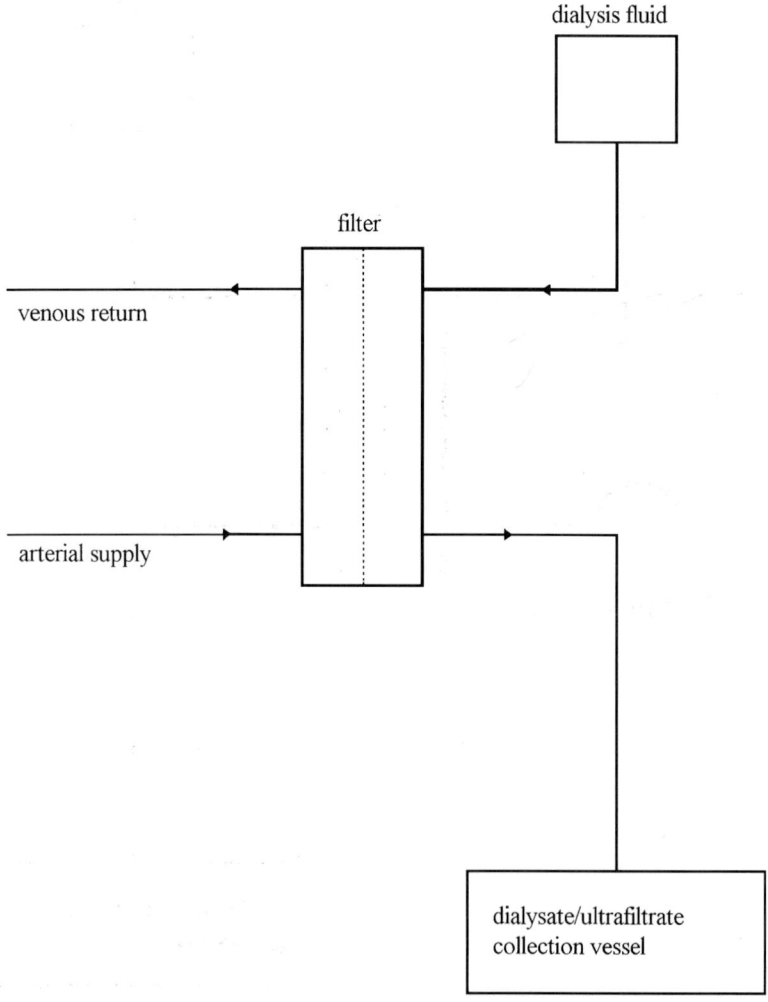

Fig. 11.3   Schematic representation of circuit diagram for CAVHD.

Table 11.4 Biochemical composition of Hemosol (Hospal) sterile dialysates for haemodialysis

LG4			AG4		
Sodium	140	mmol/l	Sodium	140	mmol/l
Potassium	4	mmol/l	Potassium	4	mmol/l
Calcium	4	mmol/l	Calcium	3.5	mmol/l
Magnesium	1.5	mmol/l	Magnesium	1.5	mmol/l
Chloride	109.5	mmol/l	Chloride	119	mmol/l
Lactate	40	mmol/l	Acetate	30	mmol/l
Glucose	6	mmol/l	Glucose	45	mmol/l
Osmolarity	302	mosm/l	Osmolarity	335	mosm/l

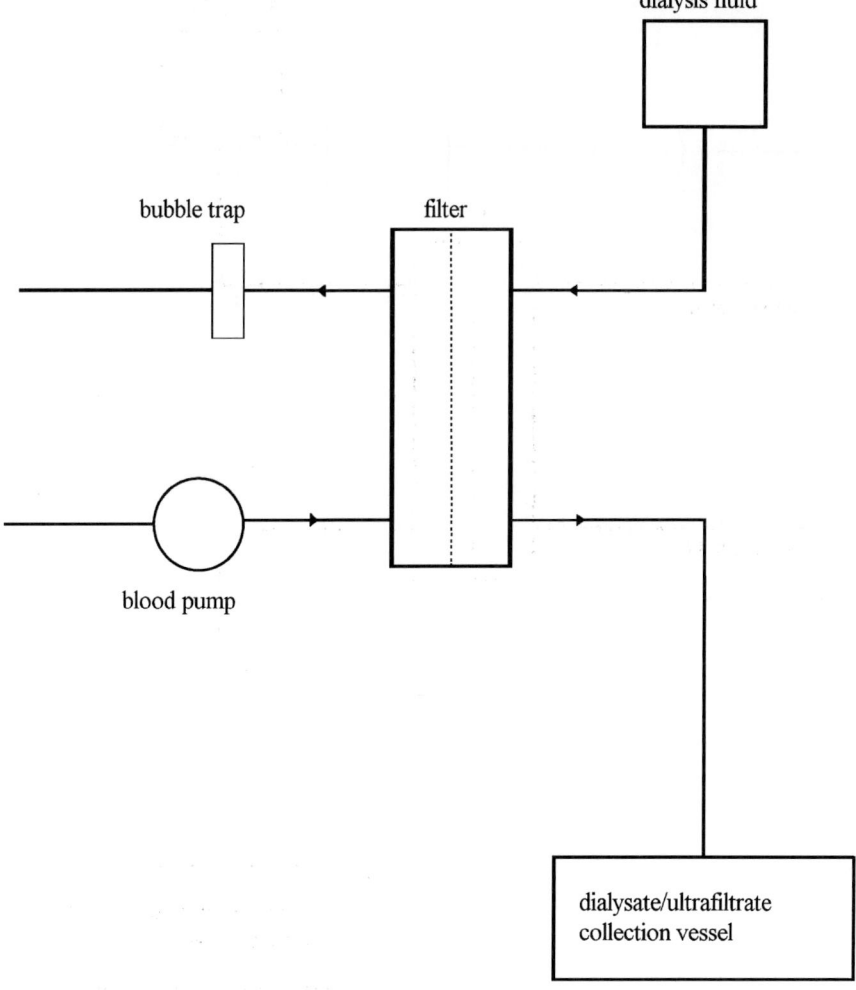

Fig. 11.4 Schematic representation of circuit diagram for CVVHD/pumped CAVHD.

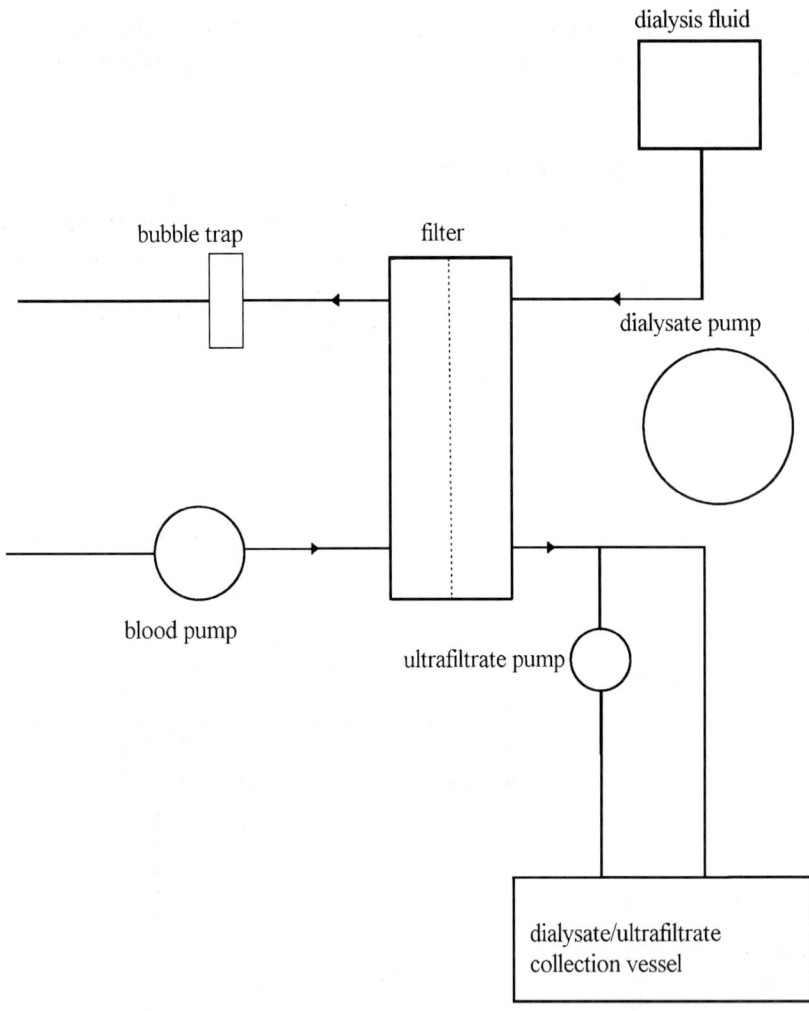

Fig. 11.5 Schematic representation of circuit diagram for CVVHD/pumped CAVHD with the addition of pumps controlling dialysate flow and ultrafiltration rate.

Although ultrafiltration rates with CAVHD and CVVHD are lower than with CAVH and CVVH because of the porosity of the membranes used (see below), they are still generally higher than those required for clinical purposes and fluid replacement is usually necessary. One way of avoiding this is to control the ultrafiltration rate with pumps (Peachey et al 1988, Tam et al 1988). Recently a more sophisticated system has been described incorporating computer monitored and regulated pumps which control the rate of blood and dialysate flow, together with ultrafiltration rates (Fig. 11.5). Using weighing scales for measurement of fluids the overall accuracy of the system is within 3.5 g of fluid (Kitaevich et al 1993). This system therefore has the potential for safe use in children as well as adults. The same equipment may be used for haemofiltration, plasmapheresis and haemoperfusion.

CAVHDF, CVVHDF AND CHFD

Haemodiafiltration, as the name implies, combines the diffusive clearance of CAVHD/CVVHD with convective clearance by deliberately utilising the high ultrafiltration rates which modern highly porous membranes engender. The obvious advantages are enhancement of small solute clearance and much greater middle molecular clearances. The major disadvantage is the requirement for replacement fluid.

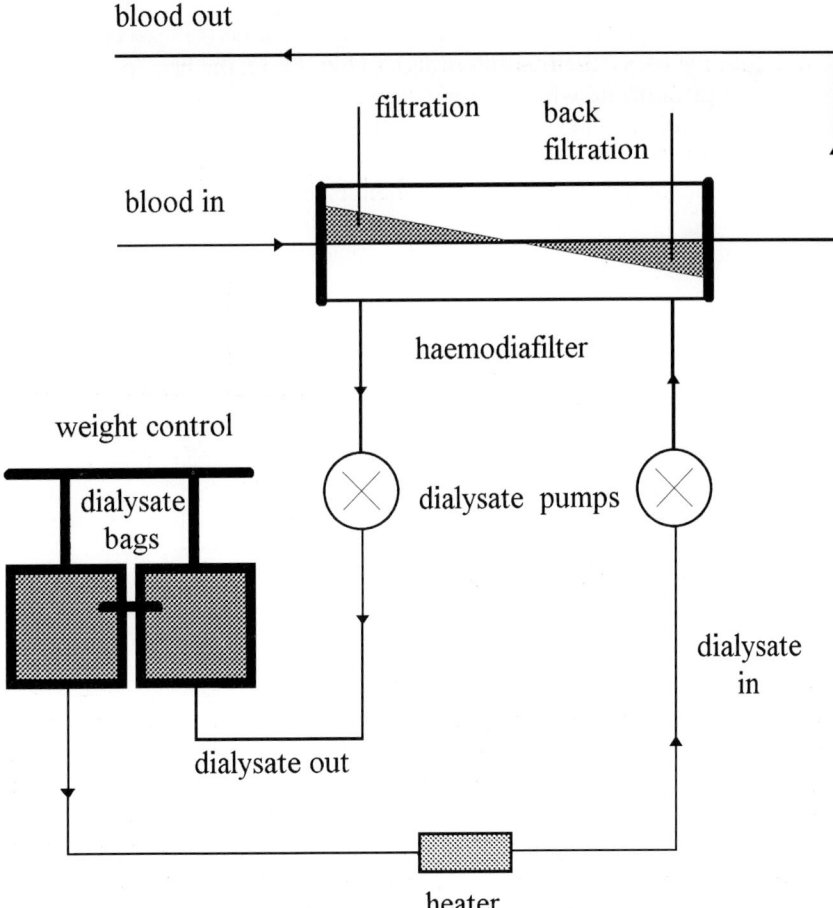

Fig. 11.6 Schematic representation of circuit diagram for continuous high flux dialysis (after Ronco, 1994).

The introduction of continuous high flux dialysis combines the advantages of adequate convection without the disadvantage of the requirement for replacement fluid (Fig. 11.6) The dialysate pumps regulate recirculation of sterile bicarbonate dialysate through the filter at a dialysate flow rate set by the inflow pump. The outflow pump is set at that rate plus the desired ultrafiltration rate. The high permeability of the membrane used (polysulfone) leads to a filtration-backfiltration mechanism. Clearance of higher molecular weight solutes is considerably enhanced by filtration in the proximal part of the filter, whilst the requirement for replacement fluid is avoided by back-filtration of sterile bicarbonate dialysate in the distal part of the filter. Continuous treatment using 10 litres of dialysate recirculating at 100 ml/min, replacing with fresh dialysate every 4 h, will give a daily urea clearance of 60 litres and an inulin clearance of 36 litres.

An alternative approach utilizes a technique described as paired filtration dialysis, in which haemodiafiltration is performed using regenerated ultrafiltrate with added bicarbonate as replacement fluid (Ghezzi et al 1992). The technique uses 2 membranes in series (Fig. 11.7); the first (polysulfone) producing ultrafiltrate which is then regenerated by passing it through an uncoated absorbent charcoal cartridge. This regeneration eliminates both small and medium to large solutes but not the electrolytes, bicarbonate, urea, glucose or phosphates. The regenerated ultrafiltrate is replaced

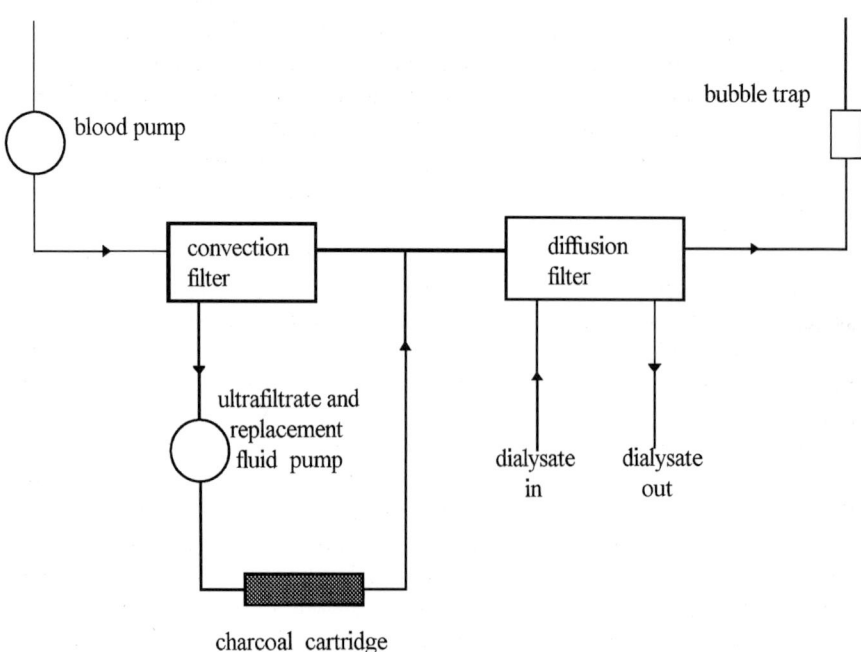

Fig. 11.7   Schematic representation of circuit diagram for paired filtration dialysis.

together with bicarbonate proximal to the second membrane (hemophan) which is used purely as a dialyser. Experimental studies have confirmed that it is possible to perform haemodiafiltration using this approach but clinical trials are awaited.

ISOVOLAEMIC HAEMODIALYSIS AND SLOW CONTINUOUS ULTRAFILTRATION

With the introduction of haemofiltration, several groups have reported the use of intermittent haemodialysis combined with CAVH in the treatment of ARF (Paganini & Nakamoto 1980, Dodd et al 1982, Leung et al 1983). Because the dialysis component of this combination was associated with haemodynamic instability the technique fell out of favour. However, the degree of haemodynamic instability associated with haemodialysis is influenced by a variety of factors. Thus, in 1976 Bergstrom and colleagues demonstrated improved cardiovascular stability, with simultaneous fluid removal, could be achieved by using *recirculating* dialysis. Studies of *isovolaemic*, single pass dialysis have also demonstrated improved cardiovascular stability (Wehle et al 1979, Rouby et al 1980). The choice of *dialysate buffer* may also influence haemodynamic stability, for example ultrafiltration during conventional haemodialysis in ARF appears better tolerated when a bicarbonate rather than an acetate buffer is used (Vincent et al 1982, Hyghebaert et al 1985, Leunissen et al 1986). Early animal experiments suggested that bolus administration of acetate produced peripheral vasodilatation and myocardial depression (Kirkendol et al 1977), although infusion of acetate at a steady rate did not cause myocardial depression (Kirkendol et al 1978, Liang & Lowenstein 1978). Furthermore, in a recent study there were no changes in heart rate, mean arterial pressure, cardiac index, systemic vascular resistance or myocardial oxygen consumption during acetate infusion in 12 patients with chronic renal failure undergoing coronary angiography (Wizemann et al 1993). Finally, in critically ill patients with ARF, acetate-buffered dialysis in a recirculating system *without* ultrafiltration does not compromise cardiovascular stability (Stevens & Rainford 1990). Uraemia is readily controlled with this technique and isovolaemia is maintained by slow continuous ultrafiltration between dialyses.

Another system of recirculating dialysis has been proposed utilizing a closed circuit with a double pump controlling dialysate inflow and outflow through the dialyser, and an additional pump on the dialysate outflow side for control of ultrafiltration (Fig. 11.8) (Kudoh & Iimura 1988). Solute clearance was manipulated by increasing dialysate flow rate, increasing the volume of dialysate in the tank or by more frequent changes of dialysate. This system has been reported to be superior to PD, continuous haemofiltration or conventional haemodialysis in terms of solute removal, volume control and haemodynamic effects.

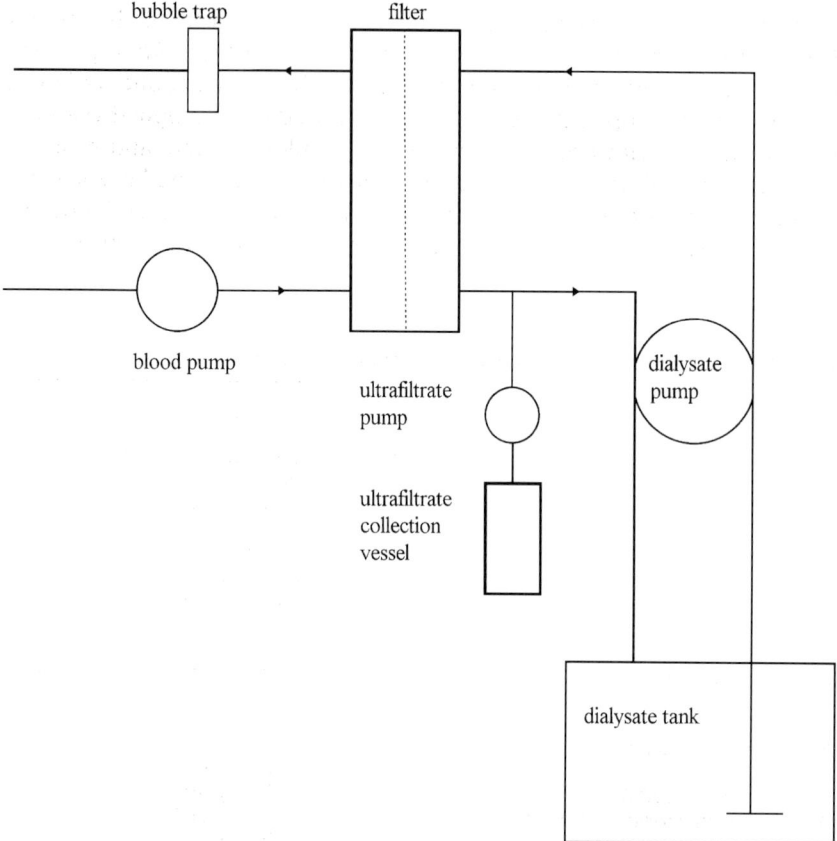

Fig. 11.8   Schematic representation of circuit diagram for continuous recirculating dialysis.

MEMBRANES USED FOR CONTINUOUS RENAL REPLACEMENT THERAPY

For many years the majority of membranes used for dialysis were cellulose-based. These were relatively inexpensive and strong and allowed good clearance of small molecules. The continuing search for increasingly efficient methods of dialysis, the requirements for improved biocompatibility, and the need to remove middle molecules, together with the increased variety of treatment options for ARF, has seen a proliferation in the number and type of membranes, which can have a considerable influence on the physiological consequences of dialysis.

Currently available membranes may be broadly divided into *cellulosic* and *synthetic* (Table 11.5). Traditional cellulose membranes are hydrogels which have high diffusive fluxes for small, but not for larger (500–1000 daltons) solutes and possess low hydraulic permeabilities. They activate complement via the alternative pathway (Chenoweth 1988), probably by binding C3b to free hydroxyl groups on the membrane surface. Attempts have therefore been made to mask the presence, or change the configuration, of these hydroxyl groups either by substitution with diethyl aminoethyl groups (hemophan) or with acetate or triacetate (cellulose acetate and cellulose triacetate). Simultaneous attempts to improve diffusive flux have led to a progressive reduction in membrane wall thickness, higher hydraulic permeabilities and more effective removal of molecules up to 12 000 daltons in size.

Table 11.5   Types of haemodialysis and haemofiltration membranes

A. Cellulosic membranes	Structure
Cellulose	Polysaccharide units with free hydroxyl groups on the membrane surface
Cuprophan	Regenerated cellulose by the cuprammonium process (dissolution of purified cellulose in an ammonia solution of cupric oxide)
Haemophan	Cellulose with substitution of 1% of hydroxyl groups with diethylaminoethyl (DEAE) groups
Cellulose acetate	Cellulose with substitution of 80% of hydroxyl groups with triacetate
Cellulose triacetate	Cellulose with substitution of hydroxyl groups with triacetate

B. Synthetic membranes	Structure
Polyacrylonitrile (PAN)	Hydrophobic
Polymethylmethacrylate (PMMA)	Hydrophobic
Polyamide	Hydrophobic
Polysulfone (PS)	Hydrophobic
Ethylvinylalcohol	Hydrophilic
Polyetherpolycarbonate	Hydrophilic

Synthetic membranes are either hydrophobic or hydrophilic. Hydrophobic membranes are more porous and have higher ultrafiltration coefficients. They also adsorb proteins, a property which may be beneficial in terms of removal of circulating cytokines. Because of their high hydraulic permeabilities, these membranes are ideally suited to techniques such as CAVH and CVVH which rely on ultrafiltration and convective solute transport for their efficacy (Lysaght et al 1986).

BIOCOMPATIBILITY

When blood comes into contact with foreign surfaces, such as the components of an extracorporeal circuit and membranes, several reactions are triggered including activation of the complement and coagulation cascades. Cellular mechanisms may also be activated both by direct contact of cells with the membrane (Betz et al 1988) and by complement. There may be activation of neutrophils, monocytes and platelets with release of a host of enzymes and cytokines including histamine, proteinases, leukotrienes, platelet activating factor, interleukin-1, tumour necrosis factor and thromboxane B2 (Hakim 1993). These mediators may produce smooth muscle contraction and increased vascular permeability and may be partly responsible for the 'first use syndrome' which affects 5–10% of patients dialysed with a new cellulosic membrane.

Biocompatibility may influence the duration of ARF and the incidence of associated infection. These may be interrelated since persistent sepsis is known to perpetuate renal impairment and continued dialysis dependence may prolong the length of stay in the intensive care unit, thereby increasing the risk of further infective episodes (Masterton 1990).

Experimentally-activated neutrophils have been shown to inhibit recovery from ARF (Hakim 1993), particularly in ischaemic kidneys, and recovery of ARF in the rat has been shown to be significantly better in animals exposed to a polyacrylonitrile membrane rather than cuprophan (Schulman et al 1991). A prospective clinical study of 72 patients with ARF revealed earlier recovery and reduced mortality in those treated with polymethylmethacrylate (PMMA) membranes compared to those treated with cuprophan (Hakim et al 1994). 23 of 37 patients treated with PMMA membranes recovered renal function after a median of 5 dialysis treatments; only 13 of 35 patients treated with cuprophane membranes recovered renal function, requiring a median of 17 treatments. Survival in the PMMA group was 57%, compared with a survival of only 37% in the cuprophane group. At the time of initiation of dialysis the 2 groups were comparable in terms of age, APACHE II scores, prevalence of oliguria, and biochemical indices of renal failure.

Repeated exposure of blood to biologically incompatible material causes recurrent complement, neutrophil and monocyte activation. This may compromise the ability of the white cell population to respond to infection. Various studies have demonstrated the deleterious effects of cellulosic compared with more biocompatible membranes on leucocyte chemotaxis, adherence and phagocytosis (Descamps-Latscha et al 1991, Spertini et al 1991, Vanholder et al 1991, Himmelfarb et al 1992, Ilvento et al 1992). These effects, together with depression of cell-mediated immunity, may be clinically relevant in the critically ill patient where host defence is already compromised.

MIDDLE MOLECULES, CYTOKINES AND POROUS MEMBRANES

Currently available membranes have differing properties in terms of hydraulic conductivity, porosity and biocompatibility but, providing the correct type is selected with the right technique, small solute clearances are adequate for clinical needs. The synthetic, highly-porous membranes allow clearance of molecules up to 30 000 daltons, although recently there has been considerable interest in the clearance of middle molecules and cytokines. It has been postulated on the basis of experimental studies of haemofiltration in endotoxic shock that cytokine removal by high flux membranes may be beneficial in sepsis and multiple organ failure (Gomez et al 1990, Stein et al 1990, Grootendorst et al 1992). Although clearance of tumour necrosis factor and interleukin-1 has been demonstrated in septic patients (using polyacrylonitrile filters), clinical benefit has yet to be confirmed (Bellomo et al 1993c). Thus, despite substantial clearance of cytokines no significant changes in serum levels were demonstrated. Strategies aimed at switching off the inflammatory response by eradicating the underlying cause, rather than removing the products of the inflammatory cascade may yield more significant gains.

Increased porosity of membranes may confer some disadvantages. Endotoxin fragments lie well within the middle molecule range (1000 and 10 000 daltons) and their back diffusion into the blood has been demonstrated both in vitro and in vivo (Vanholder et al 1992, Urena et al 1992). Also, a number of drugs not appreciably removed by more conventional membranes may be cleared by those more porous. Protein-layering effects and membrane charge may also influence drug transport (Golper & Ward 1990).

ANTICOAGULATION OF THE EXTRACORPOREAL CIRCUIT

The problem of anticoagulation of the extracorporeal circuit in haemodialysis and haemofiltration therapies represents a persistent challenge. This is particularly so in patients with ARF, many of whom have a coagulopathy and may require surgical intervention. The aim is to anticoagulate the extracorporeal circuit, not the patient, and to protect platelets. Alternatives to standard anticoagulation include regional heparinization with protamine, low-dose heparinization, low molecular weight heparins, heparin-coated and other non-thrombogenic surfaces, prostacyclin, serine protease inhibitors (gabexate mesilate and nafomostat mesilate), regional citrate anticoagulation and saline flush protocols without anticoagulation.

Adequate anticoagulation of the extracorporeal circuit begins with good filter preparation. Meticulous care taken with rinsing and priming the filter with heparinized saline (use 2 litres of saline with 10 000 iu heparin per litre), including if possible a period to allow heparin to soak into the fibres, will prolong filter survival whatever the anticoagulation regimen subsequently employed. The selection of an appropriate regimen then depends on the patient, the type of renal replacement therapy, local experience and preference, the incidence of side effects and, possibly, cost.

Patients with sepsis and ARF may have significant coagulopathy with or without thrombocytopenia. Under these circumstances, clotting of the extracorporeal circuit is unlikely to occur and filter survival without anticoagulation is not significantly different from that achieved with low-dose heparin (500 iu/h of unfractionated high molecular weight heparin delivered pre-filter) or with regional heparinization. In patients without significant coagulopathy regional heparinization was found to be superior to low-dose heparin, particularly in unpumped, low blood flow CAVHD. The incidence of haemorrhagic complications (3.2%) was no greater in patients receiving heparin than in those who were not anticoagulated. Heparin-induced thrombocytopenia was not observed, although patient numbers were small (Bellomo et al 1993b).

Prostacyclin, with or without heparin, can provide adequate anti-coagulation and is particularly useful in those with thrombocytopenia and in patients at high risk of haemorrhage. Prostacyclin may either be infused systemically or via the arterial limb of the extracorporeal circuit. Starting at a low infusion rate and gradually increasing to 5 ng/kg/min avoids the potential complications of hypotension from systemic vasodilatation, and hypoxia from pulmonary shunting. Heparin requirements when used in combination with prostacyclin are seldom greater than 250–500 iu/h. It is reported that prostacyclin infusion leads to improved cardiac index, oxygen delivery and oxygen consumption in patients with sepsis and multiple organ failure (Kishen 1992). Beneficial effects on gastric intra-mucosal pH have also been reported. In our experience initial anti-coagulation of patients with ARF and multiple organ failure using prostacyclin plus or minus low dose heparin, particularly in those with an associated bleeding diathesis, has significantly reduced the complications of anticoagulation.

To date, experience with low molecular weight heparin has been pre-dominantly confined to haemodialysis. Effective and safe anticoagulation was achieved using a low molecular weight heparin and saline filter prime and a bolus of 3000–4000 anti-factor Xa units followed by infusion at 750 u/h (Anastassiades et al 1990). Patients were dialysed for 4–7 h with no complications. A similar regimen has been used in haemofiltration with equal efficacy (Schrader et al 1988). Reports of experience in ARF are awaited.

A recent report advocated the use of 'a totally antithrombogenic continuous ultrafiltration system' (Arakawa et al 1991). The system utilized a polyacrylonitrile-polyethyleneoxide membrane with an ionically heparin-bound catheter and tubing. After preliminary animal experiments, the system was employed in 2 septicaemic patients with ARF using femoral arterial and venous access. Filter survival was good, but no better than that reported in similar patients without anticoagulation (Bellomo et al 1993b). Experience with the serine protease inhibitors has also been encouraging. In their report and review of anticoagulation for patients with ARF at high risk of bleeding, Ward & Mehta (1993) recommend the use of citrate anticoagulation. Although avoiding the potential problems of heparin there is a requirement for a special dialysate, close monitoring and adjustment of ionized calcium levels, and in some cases treatment of alkalosis.

VASCULAR ACCESS FOR CONTINUOUS RENAL REPLACEMENT THERAPY

In a recent United Kingdom survey of the treatment of ARF in intensive care units without on-site renal services, information was sought about vascular access preferences. Double lumen central venous catheters were used in 47% of cases, Scribner shunts in 31% and arteriovenous catheters in 22% (Stevens & Rainford 1992). Each has associated advantages and disadvantages, and local experience and skill are important in choosing which mode to employ (Stevens & Davies 1990).

Percutaneous cannulation of the femoral artery and vein provides excellent blood flow rates for unpumped CAVH or CAVHD but there is a significant complication rate (3–11%) and the catheters should be changed routinely every 5–7 days (Tominga et al 1993). Complications include catheter-related infection, bleeding, thrombosis (venous and arterial), pseudoaneurysm formation and arteriovenous fistulae.

Scribner shunts may also yield blood flow rates sufficient for unpumped CAVH and CAVHD. Their complication rate is, however, highly dependent on the skill, experience and interest of the individual placing the device. Thus, Bellomo et al (1992b) reported a revision rate of 33%. Nevertheless, in our unit, shunts provide the mainstay of access for ARF and revision has proved necessary in only 1% of cases. Properly inserted and well looked after, a shunt will provide vascular access for the duration of the illness. Where recovery of renal function does not occur, wrist shunts may be converted to permanent access. Leg shunts can continue to be used whilst such access is being created. An advantage of the arteriovenous approach is continuous access to arterial blood for gas analysis. Use of a simple 'Y' connector or 3-way tap on the arterial line in an unpumped circuit may also provide arterial blood pressure monitoring when required.

Venovenous access is usually achieved via a double lumen catheter placed in the subclavian, internal jugular or femoral vein. Their obvious advantages are ease of insertion, good flow rates, and preservation of peripheral vessels. Complications are related to insertion (arterial puncture, pneumothorax, haemorrhage), infection and thrombosis. Subsequent venous stenosis may occur and is related both to infection (Hernandez et al 1993) and to racial origin (Barrett et al 1988). This has major implications for future vascular access in patients who survive but fail to recover renal function. We therefore favour the use of the internal jugular route when venovenous access is used.

CLINICAL IMPLICATIONS OF CONTINUOUS RENAL REPLACEMENT THERAPY (CRRT)

The advantages of CRRT compared to conventional haemodialysis in critically ill patients with ARF are simplicity and improved haemodynamic stability. CRRT techniques can be implemented without the requirement for trained haemodialysis staff or machines, by any intensivist capable of obtaining the necessary vascular access. The techniques are well tolerated by critically ill patients with haemodynamic compromise.

Ultrafiltration rates with spontaneous CAVH are, however, not always sufficient to achieve adequate small solute clearance. Modifications designed to yield ultrafiltration rates high enough to control catabolic ARF require vigilant observation of fluid and electrolyte balance. CAVHD has the advantage of adequate solute clearance in catabolic ARF even in its simplest form, although this technique is extremely labour intensive for nursing staff. The high flux membranes used can lead to large ultrafiltration volumes in excess of clinical requirements, and to significant phosphate and bicarbonate loss. The addition of pumps to control blood flow, dialysate flow and ultrafiltration rate has overcome some of these disadvantages but at the expense of increased complexity.

Replacement fluids specifically formulated for use with these techniques have been marketed but there has been some concern over the buffers used, in particular the potential problem of lactate accumulation in patients with combined hepatic and renal dysfunction (Davenport et al 1990). Successful treatment of severe lactic acidosis by haemofiltration using a bicarbonate-based replacement fluid has been reported, but was extremely labour intensive (Barton et al 1991). High ultrafiltration rates require the replacement of significant amounts of calcium and magnesium but association of these electrolytes with bicarbonate in prepackaged sterile solutions risks precipitation, hence the use of acetate and lactate as buffers in these solutions (see Table 11.3). Recently Gonella et al (1993) described a new reinfusate composition for use with haemodiafiltration. Initial studies have been in patients with chronic renal failure. By using a combination of 2 sterile prepackaged fluids administered via a 'Y' connector they obtained a reinfusate with an electrolyte composition of sodium 139, potassium 2, calcium 1.75, magnesium 1, chloride 105.5, acetate 4 and bicarbonate 36 mmol/l. Absence of precipitates in the final solution was ascertained in vitro prior to clinical study. Studies in patients with ARF are awaited.

Conventional haemodialysis has the advantage of higher solute clearance compared with any of the haemofiltration and continuous dialysis techniques and avoids the need for substitution fluids. Dialysis can be tailored to the patient and more than one may be treated using a single machine in a 24-hour period. Disadvantages are that haemodialysis trained staff are required and conventional haemodialysis used in isolation is poorly-tolerated by critically ill patients. Improved cardiovascular stability has been reported with bicarbonate buffered dialysis (Leunissen et al 1986). The use of *isovolaemic* recirculating haemodialysis to control uraemia, combined with slow continuous ultrafiltration to maintain isovolaemia between dialyses confers good cardiovascular stability. In critically ill patients with combined renal and respiratory failure; isovolaemic, recirculating acetate buffered haemodialysis did not cause a reduction in cardiac index, mean arterial pressure, systemic vascular resistance or tissue oxygen delivery (Stevens & Rainford, unpublished observations). Similar findings have been reported in patients undergoing CAVHD, CVVHD and CVVH (Lauer et al 1988, Bellomo et al 1992a, Davenport et al 1993). Intermittent machine haemofiltration on the other hand, has been reported to produce a significant fall in cardiac index and oxygen delivery (MacKenzie et al 1991, Davenport et al 1993).

NUTRITIONAL CONSIDERATIONS

Hypercatabolism (an increase in skeletal muscle breakdown) and hypermetabolism (an increase in basal metabolic rate) are important features of ARF in critically ill patients. They occur as a consequence of alterations in the internal milieu, enhanced proteolytic activity, the influence of dialysis itself and the patient's underlying (and superimposed) illness. Metabolic responses include those related to tissue injury in general, and those specific to ARF (Table 11.6). The physiological consequences of the response to tissue injury include increased acute-phase protein synthesis, skeletal muscle breakdown, glycogenolysis, gluconeogenesis and lipolysis (Cerra 1987, Wilmore 1991). In animal models of ARF peripheral insulin resistance leads to reduced amino acid uptake and insulin-mediated protein synthesis (Clarke & Mitch 1983). Parathormone enhances skeletal muscle breakdown (Garber 1983), and metabolic acidosis can also increase protein

Table 11.6   Metabolic responses in critically ill patients with ARF

Metabolic responses to injury
  ↑ sympathetic activity
  ↑ glucocorticoid levels
  ↑ glucagon levels
  ↑ insulin levels
  Cytokine release (TNF, IL-1, PAF, PGs, LTs)

Additional responses in ARF
  ↓ metabolism of glucagon, insulin and parathormone
  ↑ peripheral insulin resistance
  Metabolic acidosis

IL-1 = interleukin-1; LTs = leukotrienes; PAF = platelet activating factor; PGs = prostaglandins; TNF = tumour necrosis factor.

Protein loss ∴ ITU patients c̄ ARF – up to 200g/day. Usually non-essential AAs (arginine, tyrosine, serine, cysteine) may become essential ∴ ARF – supplemented c̄ a[...] EAA or BCAA is potentially dangerous ∴ ARF.

catabolism (May et al 1987). Culmination of all the factors causing protein breakdown can result in the loss of 150–200 g protein per day in the critically ill patient with ARF (Feinstein et al 1981). In addition, the catabolic consequences of extracorporeal treatment modalities may further accelerate protein breakdown (Gutierrez et al 1992).

Use of biocompatible membranes reduces the contribution of dialysis to catabolism but nevertheless significant amounts of amino acids are dialysed/filtered. At least 10% of the daily administered protein replacement may therefore be lost during CAVHD, leading to low plasma concentrations of a number of essential and non-essential amino acids (Davies et al 1990). Similar protein losses were reported by Bellomo et al (1991), despite 20.5 g intravenous nitrogen per day (equivalent to 127 g of protein) patients remained in a negative nitrogen balance. The difficulty of maintaining nutritional support is illustrated by a study in which 8 critically ill, septic, postoperative patients lost lean body mass despite receiving total parenteral nutrition containing 1.7 g/kg/day of amino acids and 34.1 kcal/kg/day of non-protein energy (Streat et al 1987). Although enteral nutrition is highly desirable in critically ill patients it is apparent that their daily protein requirements may not always be met by enteral nutrition alone, particularly as only 69% of nasogastric feed prescribed to patients with ARF in the intensive care unit was actually administered (Lee & Talbot 1990).

Estimation of protein requirements is difficult. Urea kinetic modelling may be used to calculate the protein catabolic rate from urea nitrogen generation (Murray 1986). However, calculations become complicated in dialysed patients with additional urine urea losses and it is reasonable to assume that requirements will be those of the underlying cause of ARF with an adjustment for therapy-induced nutrient losses. Thus, when catabolism is moderate, for example following elective surgery complicated by infection, protein replacement of 0.8–1.2 g/kg/day plus a further 0.2 g/kg/day to compensate for renal replacement therapy losses is a suitable goal. With severe catabolism, for example with severe injury, multiple organ failure or burns, protein replacement of 1.0–1.5 g/kg/day together with the additional 0.2 g/kg/day should be aimed for (Druml 1994). It is unwise to increase amino acid intake above 2.0 g/kg/day as this simply enhances formation of urea and other nitrogenous waste products.

Although patients who are severely intolerant of standard amino acid solutions and protein formulas may benefit from the short-term use of essential amino acid (EAA) or branch chain amino acid formulas, these should not be used for more than 1 week for fear of limiting a non-essential amino acid (NEAA) in protein metabolism. A number of studies have suggested that in ARF several NEAAs (arginine, tyrosine, serine, cysteine) may become indispensable (Druml 1994). Similarly, although there is some evi-

Energy requard probs. only c. 30 kcal/kg/day (ie 2000kcal for "avege").
Lipolysis may be impaird = ARF, only 20% of energy from lipids ie
glucose (+ insulin) needed. PO_4^{3-} + HCO_3 suppletn ofn needed.

RENAL REPLACEMENT THERAPY   251

dence of an anticatabolic effect from mixtures enriched with branch chain amino acids, which can lead to a dose-related increase in nitrogen balance in hypercatabolic patients (Cerra et al 1983), they may aggravate amino acid imbalance in ARF (Druml 1993). Thus, complete amino acid solutions, or those which include tyrosine-containing dipeptides which are therefore adapted to the metabolic alterations of uraemia (Druml 1993), should be used.

Energy requirements in patients with ARF have tended to be overestimated in the past and excessive intake may lead to respiratory compromise from increased CO_2 generation, elevated body temperature, increased release of stress hormones and fatty liver. Energy requirements should be estimated from the calculation of basal energy expenditure (BEE), through use of either the Harris-Benedict or Schofield equations. A correction must then be made for stress and activity. Generally this results in energy requirements of 25–30 kcal/kg/day in moderately catabolic patients and 30–40 kcal/kg/day in the severely catabolic. Energy substrates include glucose and fat. Glucose is the main energy substrate in ARF and insulin is frequently necessary because of impaired glucose utilization. Advantages of intravenous fat emulsions include a high energy content, low osmolality, provision of essential fatty acids and phospholipids, and reduced CO_2 production. Although lipolysis and fatty acid oxidation may be preserved in the systemic inflammatory response syndrome (SIRS), in ARF lipolysis is impaired and elimination of intravenously infused fat emulsions is retarded due to inhibition of the lipoprotein lipase system. This limits the percentage of energy requirements which may be met by infused lipids to around 20–25%. Utilization of infused lipids may be assessed by measurement of triglyceride levels (aim for <350 mg/dl). Alternatively, if no lipid is visible on visual inspection of a sample of blood drawn 4 hours after cessation of the infusion, it is likely that adequate lipid utilization is occurring.

Modern renal replacement therapy has little impact on lipid balance, but excessive administration may result in more rapid filter clotting. Carbohydrate requirements may be significantly altered by the glucose in dialysate and replacement solutions. Bellomo et al (1991) calculated that using a 1.5% glucose-based dialysate in continuous dialysis 140 and 230 g glucose per day will be delivered to the patient at dialysate flow rates of 1 l/h and 2 l/h respectively.

No additional supplementation of trace elements, or lipid- and water-soluble vitamins other than those given with conventional parenteral feeding regimes is generally necessary, although some loss of water-soluble vitamins does occur. Losses of phosphate, on the other hand, may be substantial and require monitoring and replacement. Bicarbonate supplementation is also frequently required with continuous renal replacement therapies and should be monitored by arterial blood gas analysis.

PHARMACOLOGICAL CONSIDERATIONS

[handwritten margin note: Mark blood labs + response as, especially i differs beda is 'difficult' to predict.]

Drug clearance is difficult to predict in those undergoing continuous renal replacement therapy. Different techniques utilize varying degrees of diffusion and convection and a number of different membranes are available for each technique. Using different treatment modalities necessitates knowledge of their efficiency at extracorporeal drug removal, and their influence on drug pharmacokinetics and the possible dosage adjustments required. Even when such data are available, the use of a different dialyser membrane to that studied may result in very different drug concentrations from those expected. In addition, the values for pharmacokinetic parameters, such as drug volume of distribution in patients with multiorgan failure, may not correspond to those values obtained from the study of other patient groups. Despite these limitations, clinically useful guidelines for drug dosage during continuous renal replacement therapy can still be given (Stevens 1994).

During haemofiltration using highly permeable synthetic membranes, drug protein binding is the major factor determining the appearance of the drug in the ultrafiltrate. The degree to which any drug is filtered by a specific membrane is expressed by its sieving coefficient. This is defined by the equation:

$$S = 2[UF] / [A] + [V]$$

Where [UF] is the ultrafiltrate drug concentration
[A] and [V] are plasma drug concentrations in blood entering and leaving the haemofilter respectively (Colton et al 1975)

For clinical purposes this may be simplified to:

$$S = [UF] / [A] \text{ (Golper et al 1985)}$$

The amount of drug removed during haemofiltration is then expressed by:

$$C = S \times UF$$

Where C is the drug clearance rate in ml/min
UF is the ultrafiltration rate in ml/min

Thus the measurement of a drug concentration in two samples allows the removal of that drug during haemofiltration to be calculated.

For a number of drugs, sieving coefficients for a variety of membranes are known. Where the sieving coefficient is unknown, a reasonable approximation can be regarded as the fraction of drug unbound to plasma protein (Golper 1991).

During continuous haemodialysis, diffusion and ultrafiltration occur so that plasma drug clearance is less easy to predict. It is expressed by the equation:

$$\text{Clearance} = (Q_d + Q_{UF}) \times [\text{drainage fluid}] / [\text{Plasma}]$$

Where [drainage fluid] is drainage fluid (ultrafiltrate plus dialysate) drug
    concentration
    [Plasma] is plasma drug concentration
    Q_d is dialysate flow rate in ml/min
    Q_{UF} is ultrafiltration rate in ml/min

In addition to the dialysate flow and ultrafiltration rates, clearance is also
dependent on the size of the drug, its ionic charge and its degree of protein
binding. Clearance will also be influenced by the pore size, surface area
and ionic charge of the membrane. Drug binding to hydrophobic synthetic
membranes may also occur (Golper 1991).

Molecular weights of the majority of drugs used in clinical practice are
between 200 and 2000 daltons. Small molecules are readily removed by
diffusion whereas larger molecules diffuse far more slowly and are more
effectively removed by the process of convection. Therefore, where the
degree of protein binding is small, clearance of lower molecular weight drugs
should be similar to that of other small solutes. Clearance of higher molecular weight drugs is, however, dictated more by the ultrafiltration rate
and membrane pore size.

Extracorporeal removal of any drug is only one factor which determines
its pharmacokinetics, plasma concentrations and dose regimen in an individual patient. Where there is a large non-renal component to drug elimination the impact of extracorporeal removal made by any form of continuous
renal replacement therapy is likely to be low, irrespective of other factors
such as molecular weight, protein binding, membrane selection and
ultrafiltration and dialysate flow rates. Thus, the clearance of morphine is
little affected by continuous haemofiltration or dialysis. However, because
of reduced drug protein binding and a failure to clear its active metabolite,
patients exhibit increased sensitivity and there is a prolongation of its effect necessitating dose reductions in renal failure. By contrast, the clearance of gentamicin, which is exclusively renally excreted, is heavily
dependent on the extracorporeal clearance achieved.

Advice regarding appropriate dosages is available from drug information
centres. For a review of dosage adjustments suggested for many of the agents
commonly used in intensive care practice, see Reetze-Bonorden et al 1993.
Wherever possible, however, monitoring of blood levels should be performed
to ensure optimal treatment during continuous renal replacement therapy.
Such therapeutic monitoring is mandatory for potentially toxic drugs and
those with a narrow therapeutic index such as aminoglycosides.

DURATION OF OLIGURIA, SURVIVAL AND COST

Episodic hypotension during ARF is thought to lead to fresh lesions of
acute tubular necrosis (Conger et al 1991). The improved cardiovascular
stability conferred by continuous renal replacement therapy might there-

fore be expected to be associated with a more rapid recovery of function. A reduction in the period of oliguria using an isovolaemic technique was first reported by Stevens & Rainford (1990), and a similar trend has since been observed by Bellomo et al (1992c). Neither study demonstrated a significant increase in overall survival, but both showed improvements in patients with multiple organ failure. Stevens & Rainford found the age of survivors treated with the isovolaemic technique was significantly higher, and that there was a reduction in the incidence of cardiovascular mortality. However, no significant difference in mortality was reported in patients with combined renal and respiratory failure treated with conventional haemodialysis (82.8%) versus continuous dialysis (70.8%) (Simpson & Allison 1993). This 6-year prospective, randomized study compared conventional bicarbonate haemodialysis using a cuprophan (non-biocompatible) membrane with continuous dialysis using a polysulfone (biocompatible) membrane. These results contrast with those of Hakim et al (1994) where improved survival and more rapid recovery of function was observed in those patients dialysed with polymethylmethacrylate membranes as against cuprophane membranes. On this issue, the jury is obviously still out.

It was envisaged that continuous renal replacement therapy would allow patients with ARF hitherto denied access to treatment the opportunity for survival. In the United Kingdom in intensive care units without onsite renal services 54.2% of patients were treated with either CAVH/CVVH or CAVHD/CVVHD, 19.7% by conventional haemodialysis and 20.7% by peritoneal dialysis (Stevens & Rainford 1992). Only 20% were transferred to regional renal units. The incidence of combined renal and respiratory failure was 66% and overall survival was 48%, comparable to published series from regional centres. Only 1.9% of patients died because renal replacement therapy was unavailable, suggesting that prior to the advent of CAVH/CVVH and CAVHD/CVVHD this figure would have been much higher.

It is unlikely that the cost of treating ARF is any lower with these newer techniques, although a reduction in the period of oliguria reduces the length of stay in intensive care. The burden of cost will have shifted from regional dialysis units to District General Hospitals. Development of the various techniques has led to machines just as complex, and in certain cases more expensive, than those needed to provide conventional haemodialysis. Furthermore, it is seldom possible to treat more than one patient at a time with one machine. Bellomo et al (1992b) estimated that the cost of CAVHD/CVVHD was roughly twice that of conventional haemodialysis, although these costs represent a fraction of the overall intensive care bill. We would do well to recall the words of Oscar Wilde who observed that 'Nowadays we know the cost of everything and the value of nothing.'

*Outcome not obviously improved - continuous renal replacement v. haemodialysis.
Not obviously cheaper (might more expensive)*

KEY POINTS FOR CLINICAL PRACTICE

- Institute treatment early once a diagnosis of ARF is established. Evidence suggests that use of an isovolaemic technique in critically ill patients confers improved cardiovascular stability and reduces the period of oliguria.
- Choose a technique that is familiar to both medical and nursing staff. If staff are unfamiliar with current techniques training courses are available. Choice of technique will also be dictated by the anticipated workload (the incidence of ARF is approximately 50 per million population per year).
- Use the right membrane for the right technique (e.g. polyamide is good for CAVH/CVVH, but not for CAVHD/CVVHD). Become familiar with the sieving and ultrafiltration characteristics of the membrane(s) chosen. There is experimental evidence to suggest that highly porous biocompatible membranes may confer advantages in patients with sepsis.
- Choice of vascular access will be dictated by the techniques used and by local expertise and skill. Vascular access should be gained by the medical staff responsible for day-to-day management who have the greatest interest in preventing complications.
- Anticoagulation regimes should be dictated by clinical circumstances and local experience. All should be closely monitored. In patients with sepsis there is some evidence to suggest that prostacyclin may confer additional advantages. Good filter preparation will prolong its life as will warming the dialysate if using CAVHD/CVVHD.
- Remember that considerable protein loss may occur with continuous renal replacement therapy and adjust prescriptions accordingly. Phosphate and bicarbonate losses may also be high and require replacement. Fluid and electrolyte balance is easier to control in continuous dialysis as opposed to haemofiltration techniques.
- Drug dosages in ARF should be adjusted according to data sheet recommendations. As a general rule, doses of drugs not cleared by the kidney do not need to be altered but remember active metabolites may accumulate. ARF alters the protein-binding characteristics of several drugs. Different dialysis techniques may have differing effects on clearance. Monitor levels wherever possible.

REFERENCES

Anastassiades E, Ireland H, Flynn A et al 1990 A low-molecular weight heparin (Kabi 2165, 'Fragmin') in repeated use for haemodialysis: Prevention of clotting time and prolongation of the venous compression time in comparison with commercial unfractionated heparin. Nephrol Dial Transplant 5: 135–140

Arakawa M, Nagao M, Geyjo F et al 1991 Development of a new antithrombogenic continuous ultrafiltration system. Artificial Organs 15: 171–179

Barrett N, Spencer S, McIvor J, Brown E A 1988 Subclavian stenosis: a major complication of subclavian dialysis catheters. Nephrol Dial Transplant 4: 423–425

Barton I K, Streather C P, Hilton P J, Bradley R D 1991. Successful treatment of severe lactic acidosis by haemofiltration using a bicarbonate-based replacement fluid. Nephrol Dial Transplant 6: 368–370

Bellomo R, Martin H, Parkin G et al 1991 Continuous arteriovenous haemodiafiltration in the critically ill: influence on major nutrient balances. Intensive Care Med 17: 399–402

Bellomo R, Parkin G, Love J, Boyce N 1992a Management of acute renal failure in the critically ill with continuous venovenous haemodiafiltration. Renal Failure 14: 183–186

Bellomo R, Parkin G, Love J, Boyce N 1992b Use of continuous haemodiafiltration: an approach to management of acute renal failure in the critically ill. Am J Nephrol 12: 240–245

Bellomo R, Mansfield D, Rumble S et al 1992c Acute renal failure in critical illness – Conventional dialysis versus acute continuous haemodiafiltration. ASAIO Journal 38: M654–M657

Bellomo R, Parkin G, Love J, Boyce N 1993a A prospective comparative study of continuous arteriovenous haemodiafiltration and continuous venovenous haemodiafiltration in critically ill patients. Am J Kidney Dis 21: 400–404

Bellomo R, Teede H, Boyce N 1993b Anticoagulant regimens in acute continuous haemodiafiltration: a comparative study. Intensive Care Med 19: 329–332

Bellomo R, Tipping P, Boyce N 1993c Continuous veno-venous haemofiltration with dialysis removes cytokines from the circulation of septic patients. Crit Care Med 21: 522–525

Bergstrom J, Asaba H, Furst P, Oules R 1976 Dialysis, ultrafiltration and blood pressure. Proc Eur Dial Transplant Assoc 13: 293–305

Betz M, Haensch G M, Rauterberg E W et al 1988 Cuprammonium membranes stimulate interleukin 1 release and arachidonic acid metabolism in monocytes in the absence of complement. Kidney Int 34: 67–73

Cerra F 1987 Hypermetabolism, organ failure, and metabolic support. Surgery 101: 1–14

Cerra F, Mazusky J, Teasley K 1983 Nitrogen retention in critically ill patients in proportion to BCAA load. Crit Care Med 11: 775–778

Chenoweth D E 1988 Complement activation produced by biomaterials. Artif Organs 12: 502–504

Clarke A S, Mitch W E 1983 Muscle protein turnover and glucose uptake in rats with acute uraemia. J Clin Invest 72: 836–845

Colton C K, Henderson L W, Ford C A, Lysaght M J 1975 Kinetics of haemodiafiltration. I. In vitro transport characteristics of a hollow-fibre blood ultrafilter. J Lab Clin Med 85: 355–371

Conger J D, Robinette J B, Hammond W S 1991 Difference in vascular reactivity in models of ischaemic acute renal failure. Kidney Int 39: 1087–1097

Davenport A, Will E J, Davidson A M 1990 Paradoxical increase in hydrogen ion concentration in patients with hepatorenal failure given lactate based fluids. Nephrol Dial Transplant 5: 342–346

Davenport A, Will E J, Davidson A M 1993 Improved cardiovascular stability during continuous modes of renal replacement therapy in critically ill patients with acute hepatic and renal failure. Crit Care Med 21: 328–338

Davies S P, Reaveley D A, Kox W et al 1990 Amino acid clearances and nutritional losses in patients with acute renal failure treated with continuous arteriovenous haemodialysis. Nephrol Dial Transplant 5: 312–313

Descamps-Latscha B, Herbelin A, Nguyen A T, Urena P 1991 Respective influence of uraemia and haemodialysis on whole blood phagocyte oxidative metabolism and circulating interleukin-l and tumour necrosis factor. Adv Exp Med Biol 297: 183–192

Dodd N J, Turney J H, Parsons V et al 1982 Continuous haemofiltration maintains fluid balance and reduces haemodialysis requirements in acute renal failure. Proc Eur Dial Transplant Assoc 19:329–333

Druml W 1993 Nutritional management of acute renal failure. In: Mitch W E, Klahr S (eds) Nutrition and the kidney, 2nd edn. Little Brown, Boston, pp 314–345

Druml W 1994 Nutrition in acute renal failure and sepsis. Nephrol Dial Transplant 9 (Suppl 4): 219–223

Feinstein E I, Blumenkrantz M J, Healy M et al 1981 Clinical and metabolic responses to parenteral nutrition in acute renal failure. A controlled double-blind study. Medicine 60: 124–137

Garber A J 1983 Effects of parathyroid hormone on skeletal muscle protein and amino acid metabolism in the rat. J Clin Invest 71: 1806–1821

Geronemus R, Schneider N 1984 Continuous arteriovenous haemodialysis: a new modality for the treatment of acute renal failure. Trans Am Soc Artif Intern Organs 30: 610–612

Ghezzi P M, Gervasio R, Tessore V et al 1992 Haemodiafiltration without replacement fluid – An experimental study. ASAIO Journal 38: 61–65

Golper T A 1991 Drug removal during continuous haemofiltration or haemodialysis. Contrib Nephrol 93: 110–116

Golper T A, Ward R A 1990 Membranes for use in acute renal failure. In: Rainford D J, Sweny P (eds) Acute renal failure 1990 Farrand Press, London, pp 285–298

Golper T A, Wedel S K, Kaplan A A, Saad A M et al 1985 Drug removal during CAVH: Theory and clinical observations. Intern J Artif Organs 8: 307–312

Gomez A, Wang R, Unruh H et al 1990 Haemofiltration reverses left ventricular dysfunction during sepsis in dogs. Anaesthesiology 73: 671–685

Gonella M, Calabrese G, Pratesi G et al 1993 New reinfusate composition in U F haemodiafiltration: electrolyte solution combined with bicarbonate. Nephrol Dial Transplant 8: 54–59

Grootendorst A F, Van Bommel E F H, Van der Hoven B et al 1992 High volume haemofiltration improves right ventricular function in endotoxin-induced shock in the pig. Int Care Med 18: 235–240

Gutierrez A, Alverstrand A, Bergström J 1992 Membrane selection and muscle protein catabolism. Kidney Int 42 (Suppl 38): S86–S90

Hakim R M 1993 Clinical implications of haemodialysis membrane incompatibility. Kidney Int 44: 484–494

Hakim R M, Wingard R L, Parker R A 1994 Effect of the dialysis membrane in the treatment of patients with acute renal failure. N Engl J Med 331: 1338–1342

Henderson L W, Besarab A, Michaels A, Bluemle L W Jr 1967 Blood purification by ultrafiltration and fluid replacement (diafiltration). Trans Am Soc Artif Intern Organs 13: 216–226

Hernandez D, Diaz F, Suria S et al 1993 Subclavian catheter-related infection is a major risk factor for the late development of subclavian stenosis. Nephrol Dial Transplant 8: 227–230

Himmelfarb J, Zaoui P, Holbrook D, Hakim R M 1992 Modulation of granulocyte LAM-1 and MAC-1 during dialysis – A prospective, randomized controlled trial. Kidney Int 41:388–395

Hyghebaert M F, Dhainaut J F, Monsallier J F, Schlemmer B 1985 Bicarbonate haemodialysis in patients with acute renal failure and sepsis. Crit Care Med 12: 840–843

Ilvento M C, Diez R A, Estevez M E et al 1992 Haemodialysis decreases spontaneous migration of polymorphonuclears in chronic renal failure. Dial Transplant 21: 705–708

Kaplan A A 1985 Predilution versus postdilution for continuous arteriovenous haemofiltration. Trans Am Soc Artif Intern Organs 31: 28–32

Kaplan A A, Longnecker R E, Folkert V W 1983 Suction assisted continuous arteriovenous haemofiltration. Trans Am Soc Artif Intern Organs 29: 408–413

Kirkendol P L, Devia C J, Bowler J D, Holbert R D 1977 A comparison of the cardiovascular effects of sodium acetate, sodium bicarbonate and other potential fixed base in haemodialysate solutions. Trans Am Soc Artif Intern Organs 22: 399–404

Kirkendol P L, Robie N W, Gonzales F M, Devia C J 1978 Cardiac and vascular effects of infused sodium acetate in dogs. Trans Am Soc Artif Intern Organs 24: 714–718

Kishen R 1992 The management of multiple organ failure: a clinical approach. Therapy Express No 49

Kitaevich Y, Bissler J, Benzing G et al 1993 Development of a high precision extracorporeal haemodiafiltration system. Biomedical Instrumentation & Technology 27: 150–156

Kramer P, Wigger W, Rieger J et al 1977 Arteriovenous haemofiltration: a new and simple method for treatment of overhydrated patients resistant to diuretics. Klin Wochenschr 55: 1121–1122

Kudoh Y, Iimura O 1988 Slow continuous haemodialysis – New therapy for acute renal failure in critically ill patients. Jpn Circ J 52: 1171–1182

Lauer A, Saccaggi A, Ronco C et al 1983 Continuous arteriovenous haemofiltration in the critically ill patient. Ann Intern Med 99: 455–460

Lauer A, Alvis R, Avram M 1988 Haemodynamic consequences of continuous arteriovenous haemofiltration. Am J Kidney Dis 12: 110–115

Lee H A, Talbot ST 1990 Nutrition in acute renal failure management. In: Rainford D J, Sweny P (eds) Acute renal failure 1990. Farrand Press, London, pp 245–255

Leung A C, Simpson K, Gribben J et al 1983 Arteriovenous haemofiltration. Br Med J 287: 1722

Leunissen K M L, Hoorntje S J, Fiers H A et al 1986 Acetate versus bicarbonate haemodialysis in critically ill patients. Nephron 42: 146–151

Liang C S, Lowenstein J M 1978 Metabolic control of the circulation. Effects of acetate and pyruvate. J Clin Invest 62: 1029–1038

Lysaght M J, Boggs D R, Ritger P et al 1986 Membranes and transport phenomena in CAVH and CAVHD. In: LaGreca G, Fabris A, Ronco C (eds) Proceedings of the International Symposium on Continuous Arteriovenous Haemofiltration. Wichtig Editore, Milan, pp 77–86

MacKenzie S J, Nimmo G R, Armstrong I R, Grant I S 1991 The haemodynamic effects of intermittent haemofiltration in critically ill patients. Int Care Med 17: 346–349

Mason J C, Cowell T K, Hilton P J, Wing A J 1985 Continuous arteriovenous haemofiltration (CAVH) as complete replacement therapy in acute renal failure: management of fluid balance assisted by computer monitoring. In: Sieberth H G, Mann H (eds) Continuous arteriovenous haemofiltration (CAVH). International Conference on CAVH, Aachen 1984. Karger, Basel, pp 37–44

Masterton R G 1990 Infective complications of acute renal failure. In: Rainford D J, Sweny P (eds) Acute renal failure 1990. Farrand Press, London, pp 197–220

May R C, Kelly R A, Mitch W E 1987 Mechanisms for defects in muscle protein metabolism in rats with uraemia: Influence of metabolic acidosis. J Clin Invest 79: 1099–1103

Murray R 1986 Protein and energy requirements. In: Krey S H, Murray R (eds) Dynamics of nutrition support. Norwalk, C T, Appleton-Century-Crofts, pp 185–217

Paganini E P, Nakamoto S 1980 Slow continuous ultrafiltration in oliguric renal failure. Trans Am Soc Artif Intern Organs 26: 201–204

Pattison M E, Stanley M L, Ogden D A 1988 Continuous arteriovenous haemodiafiltration: An aggressive approach to the management of acute renal failure. Am J Kidney Dis 11: 43–47

Peachy T D, Ware R J, Eason J R, Parsons V 1988 Pump control of continuous arteriovenous haemodialysis. Lancet ii: 878

Quinton W E, Dillard D, Scribner B H 1960 Cannulation of blood vessels for prolonged haemodialysis. Trans Am Soc Artif Intern Organs 6: 104–113

Raja R, Kramer M, Goldstein S, Caruana R, Lerner A 1986 Comparison of continuous arteriovenous haemofiltration and continuous arteriovenous dialysis in critically ill patients. Trans Am Soc Artif Intern Organs 32: 435–436

Reetze-Bonorden P, Bohler J, Keller E 1993 Drug dosage in patients during continuous renal replacement therapy. Pharmacokinetic and therapeutic considerations. Clin Pharmacokinet 24(5): 362–379

Ranco C 1994 Continuous renal replacement therapies in the treatment of acute renal failure in intensive care patients — Part 1. Theoretical aspects and techniques. Nephrol Dial Transplant 9 (Suppl 4): 191–200

Rouby J J, Rottembourg J, Durande J P et al 1980 Haemodynamic changes induced by regular dialysis and sequential ultrafiltration haemodialysis: A comparative study. Kidney Int 17: 801–810

Schrader J, Stibbe W, Armstrong V W et al 1988. Comparison of low molecular weight heparin to standard heparin in haemodialysis/haemofiltration. Kidney Int 33: 890–896

Schulman G, Fogo A, Gung A et al 1991 Complement activation retards resolution of acute ischaemic renal failure in the rat. Kidney Int 40: 1069–1074

Sigler M H, Teehan B P 1987 Solute transport in continuous haemodialysis: A new treatment for acute renal failure. Kidney Int 32: 562–571

Silverstein M E, Ford C A, Lysaght M J, Henderson L W 1974 Treatment of severe fluid overload by ultrafiltration. N Engl J Med 291: 747–751

Simpson K, Allison M 1993 Dialysis and acute renal failure: can mortality be improved? Nephrol Dial Transplant 8: 946

Skeggs L T, Leonards J R, Kahn J R 1952 Removal of fluid from normal and oedematous dogs by continuous ultrafiltration of blood. Lab Invest 1: 488–494

Smith L H, Post R S, Teschan P E et al 1955 Post-traumatic renal insufficiency in military casualties. II. Management, use of an artificial kidney, prognosis. Am J Med 18: 187–206

Spertini O, Kansas G S, Munro J M et al 1991 Regulation of leukocyte migration by activation of the leukocyte adhesion molecule-1 (LAM-l) selectin. Nature 349: 305–306

Stein B, Pfenninger E, Grunert A et al 1990 Influence of continuous haemofiltration on haemodynamics and central blood volume in experimental endotoxic shock. Int Care Med 16: 494–499

Stevens P E 1994 Drug clearance – the kidney and the shocked state. Anaesthetic Pharm Rev 2: 92–102

Stevens P E, Davies S P 1990 Artificial kidneys. In: Dobb G J (ed) Intensive care: developments and controversies. Bailliere's clinical anaesthesiology. Bailliere Tindall, London, pp 503–529

Stevens P E, Davies S P, Brown E A et al 1988 Continuous arteriovenous haemodialysis in critically ill patients. Lancet ii: 150–152

Stevens P E, Rainford D J 1990 Isovolaemic haemodialysis combined with haemofiltration in acute renal failure. Renal Failure 12: 205–211

Stevens P E, Rainford D J 1992 Continuous renal replacement therapy: Impact on the management of acute renal failure. Br J Int Care 2: 361–369

Streat S J, Beddoe A H, Hill G L 1987 Aggressive nutritional support does not prevent protein loss despite fat gain in septic intensive care patients. J Trauma 27: 262–266

Tam P Y-W, Huraib S, Mahan B et al 1988 Slow continuous haemodialysis for the management of complicated acute renal failure in an intensive care unit. Clinical Nephrology 30: 79–85

Tominga G T, Ingegno M, Ceraldi C, Waxman K 1993 Vascular complications of continuous arteriovenous haemofiltration in trauma patients. The Journal of Trauma 35: 285–289

Urena P, Herbelin A, Zingraff J et al 1992 Permeability of cellulosic and non-cellulosic membranes to endotoxin subunits and cytokine production during in-vitro haemodialysis. Nephrol Dial Transplant 7: 16–28

Vanholder R, Ringoir S, Dhondt A, Hakim R 1991 Phagocytosis in uremic and haemodialysis patients: A prospective and cross-sectional study. Kidney Int 39: 320–327

Vanholder R, Van Haecke E, Veys N, Ringoir S 1992 Endotoxin transfer through dialysis membranes: small- versus large-pore membranes. Nephrol Dial Transplant 7: 333–339

Vincent J L, Vanherweghem J L, Degaute J P et al 1982 Acetate induced myocardial depression during haemodialysis for acute renal failure. Kidney Int 22: 653–657

Ward D M, Mehta R L 1993 Extracorporeal management of acute renal failure patients at high risk of bleeding. Kidney Int 43 (S41): S237–244

Wehle B, Asaba H, Castenfors J et al 1979 Haemodynamic changes during sequential ultrafiltration and dialysis. Kidney Int 15: 411–418

Wilmore D W 1991 Catabolic illness: Strategies for enhancing recovery. N Engl J Med 325: 695–702

Wizemann V, Soetanto R, Thormann J et al 1993 Effects of acetate on left ventricular function in haemodialysis patients. Nephron 64: 101–105

① Intermittent haemodialysis via Quinton a-v shunt : fluid overload between dialysis
   sessions + haemodynamic instability during dialysis (other authors say ↑
   can be prevented by fluid trends prior to dialysis) (dual HCO_3^- buffer?)

② Continuous haemofiltration : convective solute transport   (cf PD)
                                                                        ↓
           CAVH — limited clearance of small solutes   difficult in acutely ill, persisting
              ↑   uraemia likely
          suction CAVH
          predilution CAVH   ┌─────────────────────────────────┐
          pumped CAVH   │ METABOLIC SUPPORT: ARF   │
              ↓   │ "septic" catabol + amino-acid   │
                                      │ loss thru' filter.   │
      (pumped) CVVH : sufficient e- : severely catabolic ARF with high │
                       ultrafiltrate rates.   See P 249 – 251   │
                                                    └──────────────────┘
              ↓   (add slow dialysis (fluid pole of ultrafiltrate capacity))

      CVVHD (or CAVHD)—small solute→ ISSUES (a) route / vascular access
                          clearance   (b) membranes
      ┌──────────────────────────────────┐   (c) extracorporeal anticoagulation
      │   ┌┄┄┄┄┄┐   │
③ Circuits :   ┊   ┊ (dialysate)
    Blood ——△——[ ]   └─(dialysate pump) ┌─────────────────────────────┐
              bubble trap   │ Solute removal — seiving coefficient
    FILTER   │   — plasma conc^n
   ────── pump   │ ultrafiltrate { — hydraulic conductivity/area
    Blood ▷●◁   │ α ΔP, α   — pressure gradient
                                                  │ blood flow   (π + P)
    Anticoagulant ▷●   │ (90 – 250 ml /min)
                  ●   │
          [▓▓▓] [∿∿∿∿] (dialysate) ultrafiltrate collection
          controller   │ Fluid replacement → ⊖ BALANCE
              ↓   └─────────────────────────────┘
          [∿∿∿] replacement fluid
   ──────△──●
   balanced fluid replacement.

④ Clearance with CAVHD ≡ (ultrafiltrate + dialysate) rates (blood fl 50 – 190 ml/min)
   Pumped CVVHD is equivalent.

⑤ Synthetic membranes preferable for haemofiltration (eg polyacrylonitrile) ; biocompatibility of
   cellulose-based membranes is appreciably less. Synthetic membranes may be ((fresh)
   permeable up to 30 kD ; ?cytokine removal by polyacrylonitrile membranes ?? no proven benefit ?

⑥ Anticoagulation + platelets (what specific coagulopath....) . Prime 2000ml saline/20,000 u. heparin

Index